Breast Cancer Advances in Biology and Therapeutics

John Libbey Eurotext
127, avenue de la République
92120 Montrouge
Tél. : 46 73 06 60

John Libbey and Company Ltd
13, Smiths Yard, Summerley Street
London SW18 4HR, England
Tel. : 1 947 27 77

John Libbey CIC
Via L. Spallanzani, 11
00161, Rome, Italie
Tel. : 06 862 289

©John Libbey Eurotext, 1996
ISBN : 2-7420-0138-7

Il est interdit de reproduire intégralement ou partiellement le présent ouvrage - loi du 11 mars 1957 - sans autorisation de l'éditeur ou du Centre Français du Copyright, 6 *bis*, rue Gabriel-Laumain, 75010 Paris, France.

Breast Cancer Advances in Biology and Therapeutics

21st Meeting of the International Association for Breast Cancer Research

July 3-4-5, 1996
Paris

Edited by
F. Calvo
M. Crépin
H. Magdelenat

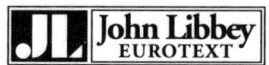

Contents

Foreword IX

**1. Predisposition to breast cancer. Carcinogenesis
   Early breast cancer screening and management** 1

Breast and ovarian cancer susceptibility: implications for presymptomatic testing and screening
M. Skolnick and D. Shattuck-Eidens 3

Psychological aspects of familial breast cancer
H. Lynch and C. Lerman 11

Experimental breast cancer studies: paradigms for human breast cancer
R.C. Moon 19

Human breast cancer risk factors: development of experimental paradigms
L. Holmberg 23

Oncogenes and onco-suppressor genes in the prevention and therapy of breast cancer
D.A. Spandidos, M. Koffa, G. Sourvinos and H. Kiaris 27

Molecular basis of human breast epithelial cell transformation
J. Russo, N. Barnabas, N. Higgy, A.M. Salicioni, Y.L. Wu and I.H. Russo 33

Diet and endogenous hormones as risk factors for cancer of the breast: intervention studies
N.F. Boyd, L. Martin, G. Lockwood, C. Greenberg, D.L. Tritchler 45

Multiple mechanisms of conjugated linoleic acid in mammary cancer prevention
C. Ip 53

n-3 polyunsaturated fatty acids and breast cancer
C. Lhuillery, S. Cognault, E. Germain, V. Chajes and Ph. Bougnoux 59

Breast cancer screening. The scientific basis and the Danish programme
E. Lynge 67

Breast cancer screening. The relations with the hospitals and sanitary organisations in the United Kingdom
J. Patnick 73

The French national breast cancer screening programme
R.A. Ancelle-Park, B. Seradour, P. Schaffer and H. Allemand 77

Breast cancer screening in Canada
A.W. Lees 81

The cost-effectiveness of breast cancer screening in France: from research to policy
S. Wait 87

Minimal breast cancer: diagnosis, strategy and decisional trees
C. Frouge 93

Is there now a consensus on the treatment of minimal breast cancer?
P. Rouanet, C. Charlier and H. Pujol 97

Minimal breast cancer: place of the plastic surgery
J.Y. Petit, M. Rietjens, C. Garusi and P. Veronesi 105

2. Tumor biology. Prognostic factors 109

Molecular and clinical aspects of metalloproteases in breast cancer
P. Basset, A. Okada, R. Kannan, J. Byrne, I. Stoll, A. Noël, V. Dive, M.P. Chenard,
J.P. Bellocq and M.C. Rio 111

Characterization of the PEA3 group of ets-related transcription factors: role in breast cancer
Y. de Launoit, J.L. Baert, A. Chotteau, D. Monte, P.A. Defossez, L. Coutte, H. Pelczar,
M.P. Laget and F.Leenders 115

Steroid metabolism in normal and malignant breast tissue compartments
W.R. Miller and P. Mullen 123

Signal transduction of prolactin and cytokine receptors
V. Goffin, C. Bole-Feysot, F. Ferrag, R. Maaskant, V. Vincent, E. Weimann
and P.A. Kelly 131

Targeting the product of the HER2/neu protooncogene for therapy
P. Carter 139

Targeting of EGF receptors: approaches and clinical results
C. Dean, H. Modjtahedi, S. Eccles, E. Jackson, G. Box, T. Hikish, I. Smith
and M. Gore 147

Pharmacological targeting of signal transduction processes
P.T. Kirschmeier, J.J. Catino, R.J. Doll, F.G. Njoroje, D.M. Carr, L.J.James, K. Grey,
L.M. Perkins, D. Whyte, F. Zhang and W.R. Bishop 159

The role of angiogenesis in tumour progression of breast cancer
M.D. Giampietro Gasparini 167

VEGF and breast cancer
J. Plouet, S. Sordello, B. Malavaud and N. Ortega 175

Why is cathepsin D involved in breast cancer? A 1996 overview
H. Rochefort, V. Laurent, E. Liaudet, N. Platet, D. Derocq, C. Rougeot, J.P. Brouillet
and M. Garcia 183

Clinical significance of the serine protease uPA (urokinase) and its inhibitor PAI-1 as well as the cysteine proteases cathepsin B and L in breast cancer
M. Schmitt, C. Thomssen, F. Jänicke, H. Höfler, K. Ulm, V. Magdolen, U. Reuning,
O. Wilhelm and H. Graeff 191

Urokinase plasminogen activator receptor in breast cancer
N. Brünner, C. Holst-Hansen, A.N. Pedersen, C. Pyke, G. Hoyer-Hansen, J. Foekens
and R.W. Stephens 201

Mutiparameter analysis of prognostic factors in breast cancer
W.L.J. van Putten, J.G.M. Klijn, M.E. Meijer-van Gelder, M.P. Look and J.A. Foekens 209

Interpretation of data in prognostic studies
G.M. Clark 217

3. Therapy 223

Clinical circumvention of antioestrogen resistance
A. Howell and E. Anderson 225

Breast cancer: should we control rather than kill tumor cells?
H. Schipper, M. Baum and E.A. Turley 235

High dose sequential chemotherapy in poor prognosis breast cancer patients
J.M. Extra, C. Cuvier, M. Espie, P. Cottu and M. Marty.. 245

Summary of clinical results of vinorelbine (Navelbine®) in the treatment of breast cancer
G.N. Hortobagyi... 251

Docetaxel in the treatment of breast cancer: current status, ongoing trials and future directions
M.J. Piccart, A. Di Leo, A. Awada and D. de Valeriola 257

In vivo evaluation of docetaxel (Taxotere®) and vinorelbine (Navelbine®) as single agents and in combination in mammary tumor models
M.C. Bissery, P. Vrignaud and F. Lavelle... 265

Clinical data of Navelbine-Taxotere association in breast cancer patients
P. Fumoleau, V. Delecroix, G. Perrocheau, O. Borg-Olivier, C. Maugard, R. Fety, N. Azzli, J.P. Louboutin and A. Riva 273

A short history of drug discovery
P. Potier 279

The expression levels of episialin in human carcinomas are sufficiently high to potentially interfere with adhesion and promote metastasis
J. Hilkens, H.L. Vos, J. Wesseling, J. Peterse, J. Storm, M. Boer, S.W. van der Valk and M.C.E. Maas 281

The detection of micrometastases in the lymph nodes, peripheral blood and bone marrow of patients with breast cancer using immunohistochemistry and the polymerase chain reaction
A. Schoenfeld, K.H. Kruger, J. Gomm, H.D. Sinnett, J.C. Gazet, N. Sacks, H.G. Bender, Y. Luqmani and R.C. Coombes 289

Immunotherapy of breast cancer using a recombinant Vaccinia virus expressing the human *MUC1* and *IL2* genes
N. Bizouarne, J.M. Balloul, C. Schatz, B. Acres and M.P. Kieny 303

The *MUC1* gene as an immunogen: use of naked DNA and role of dendritic cells
J. Burchell, R. Graham, M. Shearer, M. Smith, L. Heukamp, D. Miles and J. Taylor-Papadimitriou 309

Tumour immunotherapy against MUC1 expressing tumours using mannan MUC1
V. Apostolopoulos, G.A. Pietersz, B. Acres, C. Osinski, G. Thynne, P.X. Xing,
V. Karanikas, H.A. Vaughan, L. Hwang, V. Popovski, C. Lees, C.S. Ong
and I.F.C. McKenzie 315

Review of the epidemiologic data on hormone replacement therapy in relation to the risk of breast cancer
L.F. Voigt, N.S. Weiss and J.L. Stanford 321

Influence of percutaneous administration of estradiol and progesterone on the proliferation of human breast epithelial cells
J.M. Foidart, C. Colin, X. Denoo, J. Desreux, S. Fournier and B. de Lignières 329

Clinical and biological prognostic factors in breast cancer diagnosed during postmenopausal hormone replacement therapy
P. Bonnier, S. Romain, P.L. Giacalone, F. Laffargue, P.M. Martin and L. Piana 335

Estrogen replacement therapy in breast cancer survivors
P.J. DiSaia 347

Breast cancer in young women: the University of Pennsylvania experience
L.J. Solin, J. Haas, D.J. Schultz 351

Author index 355

Subject index 357

Foreword

This book is based on the 1996, 3-day « 21st Meeting of the International Association for Breast Cancer Research » in Paris, France.

Contributions from leading authors in the field of clinical and biological breast cancer research constitute these three chapters: predisposition to breast cancer, carcinogenesis, and early breast cancer screening and management; tumor biology and prognostic factors; and therapeutic aspects of breast cancer.

We are indebted to the contributors for their diligence, expertise and kindness, which enabled this book to be published in time for the first day of the meeting, and we are grateful to the staff of AIRMEC and John Libbey Eurotext for their help and patience.

We hope that the content of these chapters will prove to be of value to the readers, and we wish to dedicate this work to all the patients who are faced with this illness.

F. Calvo, MD, PhD
M. Crépin, PhD
H. Magdelenat, PhD

1

Predisposition to breast cancer
Carcinogenesis
Early breast cancer screening and management

Breast and ovarian cancer susceptibility genes: implications for presymptomatic testing and screening

Mark Skolnick and Donna Shattuck-Eidens

Myriad Genetics Inc., 390 Wakara Way, Salt Lake City, Utah 84108, USA

The early detection of women at exceedingly high risk is a promising approach for reducing the unacceptably high incidence and mortality associated with breast and ovarian cancer. These women, once identified, can be targeted for more aggressive prevention programs. Because the strongest known epidemiologic risk factor for breast cancer is a positive family history [1] and because studies of breast cancer patients and their relatives consistently find statistical evidence for involvement of an autosomal dominant gene [2, 3, 4], the identification of specific genetic effects have long been the focus of efforts to identify women at exceedingly high risk. *BRCA1* [5], a gene which confers greatly increased susceptibility to breast and ovarian cancer, was isolated in October 1994 [6], creating great interest among both oncologists and women with a personal or family history of breast cancer. Recently another breast cancer susceptibility gene, *BRCA2*, has been identified and fully sequenced [7, 8]. The focus of this presentation is on scientific issues in diagnostic testing specifically related to *BRCA1* and *BRCA2*.

BRCA1 is a large gene, containing 5,592 nucleotides spread over approximately 70,000 bases of genomic DNA; it is composed of 22 coding exons producing a protein of 1,863 amino acids. Much of *BRCA1* shows no homology to other known genes, with the exception of a 126 nucleotide sequence at the amino terminus which encodes a RING finger motif. This motif is found in other proteins which interact with nucleic acid and/or form protein complexes, suggesting a role for *BRCA1* in DNA transcription. *BRCA2* is an even larger gene, composed of 26 exons encoding 3,418 amino acids. There is no detectable homology between *BRCA2* and *BRCA1* or any other previously identified protein.

The utility of any screening test, genetic or otherwise, depends on three basic factors: the prior probability of having the condition of interest; the sensitivity of the test (the chance that a person with the condition will have a positive test result); and the specificity of the test (the chance that a person without the condition will have a negative test). For *BRCA1* and *BRCA2*, we must consider the probability that a woman diagnosed with breast cancer at a particular age or with a specific family history harbors a mutation in either gene, the probability that a mutation will be detected using a given screening technique, and the probability that a benign sequence variant will be interpreted as a deleterious mutation.

Only 10% of breast cancer is considered to be hereditary. Much of what is currently known about the risks of breast cancer due to susceptibility genes comes from analyses of data collected as part of an international effort to study breast cancer families for linkage to the *BRCA1* region of chromosome 17q [9, 10, 11]. The probabilities of various constellations of personal and family history being attributable to *BRCA1* can be calculated from statistical models of the penetrance of the *BRCA1* locus. These penetrance estimates have been obtained from analyses of large numbers of *BRCA1*-linked kindreds and on analysis of population-based studies of familial breast and ovarian cancer. The probability of a woman with breast or ovarian cancer bearing a *BRCA1* mutation based on such modeling is given in *Table I*. These risks may be overestimated since they depend in part on results obtained from high-risk families suitable for linkage analysis. These studies on *BRCA1* began when the chromosomal location of the gene was announced in 1990.

Table I. Estimated prior probabilities of a particular constellation of cases being due to the *BRCA1* gene [14]. Calculations were made using the model of Easton *et al.* 1993 [9] and estimates of heterogeneity reported in Easton *et al.* 1995 [15].

Criterion	Prior probability case has a *BRCA1* mutation
(a) Families	
Breast only (3+ cases dx <50)	0.40
2+ Breast with 1+ Ovarian case	0.82
2+ Breast with 2+ Ovarian cases	0.91
(b) Sister pairs	
Br <40, Br <40	0.37
Br 40-49 Br 40-49	0.20
Br <50 Ov <50	0.46
Ov <50, Ov <50	0.61
(c) Single affected	
Br <30	0.12
Br <40	0.06
Br 40-49	0.03
Ov <50	0.07

The chromosomal location of the *BRCA2* gene was announced in 1994 and less information has been collected so that similar predictions of the probability of carrying a *BRCA2* mutation are not available. Now that the *BRCA1* and *BRCA2* genes have been isolated, more precise estimates of the proportion of women diagnosed with breast and ovarian cancer at a given age and with a given family history which is attributable to mutations in these genes can be determined. Especially interesting are the recent reports that germ-line *BRCA1* mutations can be present in young women with breast cancer who do not belong to families with multiple affected individuals. In these studies alterations in *BRCA1* were identified in approximately 10% of breast cancer patients diagnosed before age 35 [12, 13].

Data will be presented from the preliminary experiments of many groups of investigators in screening the *BRCA1* and *BRCA2* genes. Investigators have screened samples ascertained from a wide variety of sources and have utilized a variety of techniques to detect *BRCA1* mutations. The samples analyzed for *BRCA1* mutations include families which by linkage analysis have a high probability of segregating *BRCA1* mutations, small families with two or three affected individuals and no linkage data, and samples from early-onset cases unselected for family history. The analysis of these samples has been used to generate a mutation profile and these data can be used to predict the complexity of an eventual diagnostic test. Only data from the initial reports of *BRCA2* mutations is available at this time. Those studies focus on families which by linkage analysis have a high probability of segregating *BRCA2* mutations [7, 8].

The DNA samples which were screened for mutations were extracted from blood or tumor samples from patients with breast or ovarian cancer (or known carriers by haplotype analysis) who were participating in research studies on the genetics of breast cancer. All subjects signed appropriate informed consent. All putative mutations were resequenced to verify the original observation. Where possible, DNA sequence variations were tested for cosegregation with breast or ovarian cancer in the family. Further evidence of a causal role of a sequence variant in cancer was provided by proving the absence of the putative mutation in a set of control individuals. Screening for specific, previously identified mutations in large sets of selected samples was perfomed using allele-specific oligonucleotide hybridization (ASO).

Over 100 different mutations in *BRCA1* have been found in a diverse set of samples by numerous laboratories using a variety of screening methods. Moreover, mutations have been found in many different regions of the gene; phenotypically severe mutations have been found both in the extreme 5' end of *BRCA1* as well as in the extreme 3' portion of the gene. One such mutation found in a family with seven early-onset breast cancer cases produces a protein that is only missing the terminal 10 amino acids, indicating that this region of *BRCA1* plays a role in normal gene function [16]. It is noteworthy that the overwhelming majority of alterations in *BRCA1* have been either frameshift or nonsense mutations. Of the total of 158 independent individuals with mutations identified by complete screening of the coding sequence, 140 (88%) are frameshift, or nonsense, splice, or regulatory mutations which result in a truncated protein product. There is as yet no apparent clustering of mutations in *BRCA1*.

BRCA1, like many other cancer predisposing genes, is characterized by some mutations that have been detected relatively frequently. In *BRCA1*, to date, five mutations appear to be relatively common. A two base pair deletion in exon 2, 185delAG, has been identified in more that 20 Jewish families with familial breast or ovarian cancer. A recent population survey of Ashkenazi Jews, which were chosen without regard to family history of breast cancer, found that about 1 percent carries this mutation [17]. Apparently it is derived by descent from a common ancestor. It is important to note that six of these mutations were found in premenopausal breast cancer cases selected without regard to family history and that three mutations were found in unselected ovarian cancer cases. Thus the mutations which were common in the linked and otherwise high-risk families have also been found repeatedly in probands which are more representative of a general clinic population.

A much smaller set of mutations have been identified in *BRCA2*. To date 15 independent mutations have been identified in 15 families with good evidence for linkage to *BRCA2*. All of the mutations are frameshift mutations which result in premature termination of the protein. There is no apparent clustering of *BRCA2* mutations.

Somatic *BRCA1* mutations in sporadic tumors

The initial report announcing the cloning of *BRCA1* was accompanied by a report by Futreal *et al.* [18] of mutation screening a collection of breast and ovarian tumors which exhibited loss of heterozygosity (LOH) at the *BRCA1* locus but were from women unselected for a family history of breast or ovarian cancer.

Observations from several labs of LOH in sporadic tumors for markers in the *BRCA1* region of 17q suggested that *BRCA1* would be mutated in these tumors. In the Futreal *et al.* study, no *BRCA1* mutations were found in tumor cells which were not also found in the germline DNA of the patient. Since that report several groups have looked extensively for somatic *BRCA1* mutations in breast and ovarian tumors. Two groups have reported somatic mutations in ovarian tumors. Merajver *et al.* [19] analyzed 47 unselected ovarian tumors and found 4 somatic mutations. The tumors with *BRCA1* mutations also demonstrated LOH for a marker in *BRCA1*. In that study one germline mutation was also reported. Hosking *et al.* [20] reported one somatic *BRCA1* mutation in a collection of 17 ovarian tumors selected for LOH at *BRCA1*. The frequency of somatic mutations in ovarian tumors is low, and to date no somatic mutations have been found in breast tumors. However, it is possible that the spectrum of mutations in sporadic tumors is different than in familial tumors, and that the alterations in sporadic tumors occur in the noncoding intronic or promoter regions and therefore have escaped detection. Findings in a report by Thompson *et al.* [21] are consistent with a role for *BRCA1* in sporadic breast tumors in that the level of *BRCA1* mRNA is reduced in invasive breast tumor cells. They also reported that an antisense oligonucleotide mediated down regulation of *BRCA1* expression and stimulated the proliferation of normal and malignant mammary epithelial cells. More recently it has been reported that in normal cells the BRCA1 protein is primarily localized in the nucleus but in 16 of 17 breast and ovarian cell lines and 17 of 17 samples of cells obtained from malignant effusions, BRCA1 protein is mainly in the cytoplasm [22] . Certainly much more research is necessary to define the role of *BRCA1* in sporadic tumors but these findings suggest that *BRCA1* abnormalities may be involved in the pathogenesis of non-familial breast cancer as well.

Factors affecting sensitivity

There are a small number of families reported in which the genetic linkage evidence for involvement of *BRCA1* is very strong but for which mutations have not been identified. For example, Michigan families 28 and 30 which have multiple cases of ovarian cancer and convincing evidence for linkage fall into this category, as do a number of families studied by the Berkeley group [23, 16]. Although these could be due to coding mutations missed by SSCP, similar families have been found among groups using direct sequencing (e.g., family 102 in Simard *et al.* [24] and kindred 1925 in Miki *et al.* [6]). Such families could be analyzed initially for the presence of a single transcript through analysis of the polymorphisms described in the region in cDNA and genomic DNA [6], or by a functional assay when available. It is expected that the frequency of these presumed regulatory mutations lying outside of the regions currently being analyzed (exons and intron/exon junctions) will be low. However, they should be considered in the evaluation of the sensitivity of any sequence-based test for *BRCA1* mutations.

Factors affecting specificity

In the preceding paragraphs we have focused on factors affecting the sensitivity of an assay for *BRCA1* mutations, i.e., the chance that a true, clinically meaningful alteration in the *BRCA1* gene will be detected using a particular screening method. However, we must also consider the specificity of such an assay, or equivalently, the rate of false positives. In practical terms this usually involves the proper interpretation of observed missense mutations. How can one be certain that an observed amino acid substitution found in a patient or relative of a patient is clinically meaningful? Missense mutations which are recurrent in cancer cases but absent or very rare in the general population are likely to be clinically meaningful; cosegregation of the missense mutation with the disease in relatives of the proband provides further support that the missense mutation is indeed causal. Unfortunately, there may still be ambiguity regarding the causal nature of missense mutations. This difficulty is exemplified by a Ser 1040 Asn putative missense mutation, which was described as a polymorphism by Castilla et al. [23] where it was found not to segregate with the disease and was also detected in three out of 232 control chromosomes. In the report of Friedman et al. [16], however, this alteration did segregate with the disease in the family in which it was identified and was absent in 120 control chromosomes. Another example is provided by Utah family K2039 in which a missense mutation changing an arginine to a glycine in amino acid 1347 was detected and was found to be absent in 156 control chromosomes. However, this same variant was found in a patient studied by the Berkeley group who also had a frameshift mutation; thus its functional significance is questionable. This type of variant accounts for less than 15% of the *BRCA1* alterations identified to date. Two of these variants occur to change amino acid residues in conserved positions of the RING finger motif. These are very likely causal missense mutations. Ultimately a functional assay, when available, will be useful for distinguishing causal mutations from neutral polymorphisms in cases where the interpretation of a missense mutation is problematic.

Interpretation of a negative *BRCA1* test result

A negative *BRCA1* test result indicates a risk which combines the probability of non-detection with risks based on empiric data for women with a particular family history such as those provided by Claus et al. [3]. Unless a *BRCA1* mutation has been identified in an affected first degree relative, failure to find a mutation in an at-risk individual only moderately lowers her risk because *BRCA1* accounts for only about half of hereditary breast cancer. When it is determined that an at-risk woman has not inherited the mutant *BRCA1* allele present in her affected relative, her risk of breast and ovarian cancer becomes equal to those in the general population. In all cases, risk calculations should also incorporate non-genetic risk factors, particularly if they are shown to interact with the genetic susceptibility conferred by *BRCA1*.

Conclusion

This presentation has, of necessity, focused on issues involved in testing exclusively for *BRCA1* mutations. Now that *BRCA2* has been identified similar studies are in progress to address these same issues in regard to that gene. In addition, a genetic disorder ataxia-telangiectasia (A-T) may be associated with cancer predisposition, especially breast cancer. This gene, *ATM*, has also now been cloned [25]. In the future a test for breast cancer susceptibility will likely include

BRCA1, *BRCA2*, and perhaps other genes. In each case the issues of risk assessment, as well as the sensitivity and specificity of the tests as outlined here, must be addressed to the determine the utility of these tests in making decisions concerning patient care.

References

1. Kelsey JL, Gammon MD. The epidemiology of breast cancer. *CA A Cancer J Clinic* 1991; 41: 147-65.
2. Newman B, Austin MA, Lee M, King M-C. Inheritance of human breast cancer: Evidence for autosomal dominant transmission in high risk families. *Proc Natl Acad Sci* 1988; 85: 3044-8.
3. Claus EB, Risch N, Thompson WD. Age of onset as an indicator of familial risk of breast cancer. *Am J of Epidemiology* 1990; 131: 961-72.
4. Claus EB, Risch N, Thompson WD. Genetic analysis of breast cancer in the cancer and steroid hormone study. *Am J Hum Genet.* 1991; 48: 232-41.
5. JM, Lee MK, Newman B, *et al*. Linkage of early-onset familial breast cancer to chromosome 17q21. *Science* 1990; 250: 1684-9.
6. Miki Y, Swensen J, Shattuck-Eidens, D *et al*. A Strong candidate for the 17q-linked breast and ovarian cancer susceptibility gene *BRCA1*. *Science* 1994; 266: 66-71.
7. Wooster R, Bignell G, Lancaster J, *et al*. Identification of the breast cancer susceptibility gene *BRCA2*. *Nature* 1995; 378: 789-91.
8. Tavtigian S, Simard J, Rommens J, *et al*. The complete *BRCA2* gene and mutations in chromosome 13q-linked kindreds. *Nature Genetics* 1996. In Press.
9. Easton DF, Bishop T, Ford D, Crockford GP. the Breast Cancer Linkage Consortium. Genetic linkage analysis in familial breast and ovarian cancer: results from 214 families. *Am J Hum Genet* 1993; 52: 678-701.
10. Easton DF, Narod SA, Ford D, Steel CM. The genetic epidemiology of *BRCA1*. *Lancet* 1994, 344; 761 1994.
11. Ford D, Easton DF, Bishop DT, Narod SA, Goldgar DE. Risks of cancer in *BRCA1* mutation carriers. *Lancet* 1994; 343: 692-5.
12. Langston AA, Malone KE, Thompson JD, Daling JR, Ostrander EA. *BRCA1* mutations in a population-based sample of young women with breast cancer. *N Engl J Med* 1996; 3: 137-42.
13. Fitzgerald MG, MacMonald DJ, Krainer M, *et al*. . Germ-line *BRCA1* mutations in Jewish and non-Jewish women with early-onset breast cancer. *N Engl J Med* 1996; 3: 143-9.
14. Shattuck-Eidens D, McClure M, Simard J, *et al*.. A collaborative study survey of 80 mutations in the *BRCA1* breast and ovarian cancer susceptibility gene. *J Am med Assoc* 1995; 273: 535-41.
15. Easton DF, Ford D, Bishop DT. Breast Cancer Linkage Consortium (1995): Breast and ovarian cancer incidence in *BRCA1* mutation carriers. *Am J Hum Genet* 1995; 56: 265-71.
16. Friedman LS, Ostermeyer EA, Szabo CI, Dowd P, Lynch ED, Rowell SE, King M-C. Confirmation of *BRCA1* by analysis of germline mutations linked to breast and ovarian cancer in ten families. *Nature Genetics* 1994; 8: 399-404.
17. Struewing J, Abeliovich D, Peretz T, *et al*.. The carrier frequency of the *BRCA1* 185delAG mutation is approximately 1 percent in Ashkenazi Jewish individuals. *Nature Genetics* 1995; 11: 198-200.
18. Futreal PA, Liu Q. Shattuck-Eidens D *et al*. *BRCA1* mutations in primary breast and ovarian carcinomas. *Science* 1994; 266: 120-2.
19. Merajver SD, Pham TM, Caduff RF, *et al*. Somatic mutations in the *BRCA1* gene in sporadic ovarian tumor. *Nature Genetics* 1995; 9: 439-43.
20. Hosking L, Trowsdale J, Nicolai H, *et al*. A somatic *BRCA1* mutation in an ovarian tumor. *Nature Genetics* 1995; 9: 343-4.
21. Thompson M, Jensen R, Obermiller P, Page D, Holt J. Decreased expression of *BRCA1* accelerates growth and is often present during sporadic breast cancer progression. *Nature Genetics* 1995; 9: 444-50.
22. Chen Y, Chen C-F, Riley D, *et al*. Aberrant subcellular localization of *BRCA1* in breast cancer. *Science* 1995; 270: 789-91.

23. Castilla L, Couch F, Erdos M, *et al*. Mutations in the *BRCA1* gene in families with early-onset breast and ovarian cancer. *Nature Genetics* 1994; 8: 387-91.
24. Simard J, Tonin P, Durocher F, *et al*. Recurrent mutations of the *BRCA1* gene in Canadian breast and ovarian cancer families. *Nature Genetics* 1994; 8: 392-8.
25. Savitsky K. Bar-Shira A, Gilad S, *et al*. A single ataxia telangiectasia gene with a product similar to PI-3 kinase. *Science* 1995; 268: 1749-53.

Breast Cancer. Advances in biology and therapeutics.
F. Calvo, M. Crépin, H. Magdelenat, eds. John Libbey Eurotext © 1996, pp. 11-18.

Psychological aspects of familial breast cancer

Henry Lynch and Caryn Lerman*

Department of Preventive Medicine and Public Health, Creighton University Omaha, NE 68178, USA;
* Bio-behavioral Research, Georgetown University Medical Center, Lombardi Cancer Center, 2233 Wisconsin Avenue, NW, Suite 535, Washington, DC 20007-4104, USA

Quality of life and health behavior

As our knowledge of breast cancer risk factors has increased, so has attention to the impact of risk assignment on women's quality of life. In one of the first empirical studies to examine this systematically, Kash and her colleagues [1] showed that over one-fourth of women with a family history of breast cancer exhibited psychological distress that warranted counseling. Significant distress was also reported in a subsequent population-based study of first-degree relatives of breast cancer patients [2]. In this study, 53% of women reported intrusive thoughts about breast cancer, 33% reported impairments in daily functioning due to breast cancer worries, and 20% reported sleep disturbance. Psychological distress in high risk women parallels that of women diagnosed with invasive breast cancer [3], and is increased significantly compared to women who do not have a family history of this disease [4]. Younger high risk women, such as those aged 35 and younger, appear to be at greatest risk for cancer-related distress [5, 6].

In addition to its effects on quality of life, breast cancer-related distress can also influence health behavior in high risk women. One adaptive aspect of distress is that it may motivate women to seek counseling about their risk and options for prevention and surveillance. In a study of predictors of participation in a breast cancer health promotion trial, high risk women who were more distressed about their risk were significantly more likely to participate than those with low levels of distress [7]. However, while distress may increase motivation for counseling, it may interfere with comprehension of the information provided during the counseling session. In the same trial, Lerman and colleagues [8] found that women who had high levels of breast cancer-related distress prior to the risk counseling session were significantly less likely to improve in terms of their comprehension of personal risk. Moreover, anxieties and fears about breast cancer can lead some high risk women to avoid breast cancer detection practices. Psychological distress has been associated with decreased adherence to guidelines for clinical breast examination, breast self-examination and mammography [1, 2].

Interest in genetic testing for breast cancer susceptibility

In anticipation of the widespread availability of genetic testing for breast cancer susceptibility, several studies have examined interest in testing and anticipated reactions to positive and negative test results. Overall, interest in genetic testing for inherited breast cancer risk has been reported to be very high. In a sample of women with a family history of ovarian cancer, 75% said they would definitely want to be tested for mutations in the *BRCA1* gene and 20% said they probably would want to be tested [9]. Interest in testing was significantly greater among women who perceived themselves to be at higher risk for cancer and those who were more worried about their risk. Similar levels of interest have been observed among women in the general population [10], and female members of hereditary breast-ovarian cancer (HBOC) families [11, 12]. However, with the exception of the study by Lynch and colleagues [12], these studies utilized hypothetical scenarios to assess interest in testing and actual test results were not available.

It is, therefore, possible that the actual demand for genetic testing for breast cancer susceptibility will not be as great as that suggested by these preliminary studies. Prior to the initiation of predictive testing for Huntington's disease (HD), over two-thirds of persons at-risk expressed interest in testing [13]. Since HD predictive testing has become available, fewer than 15% of those who initially expressed interest have come forward [14, 15]. However, one critical difference between HD and breast cancer is that the latter disease can be treated and cured if found early. This potential for early detection and treatment of breast cancer, and the high levels of anxiety about this disease, may generate great demand for genetic testing once it is commercially available.

For those persons who ultimately do decide to receive genetic testing for breast cancer susceptibility, there may be a significant burden associated with the knowledge that one is a carrier of a cancer-predisposing mutation. In the hypothetical studies described above, a substantial proportion of women indicated that they would become very depressed and anxious if they tested positive [9]. Interestingly, many women also anticipated adverse effects of negative results, including guilt (*i.e.*, that other family members had inherited the mutation but they had not) and continued worry. An earlier descriptive report by Lynch and colleagues did not provide evidence for serious adverse emotional effects of disclosure of *BRCA1* mutation status in hereditary breast-ovarian cancer families (HBOC); however, the need for controlled trials of the impact of testing was acknowledged [12].

Prospective study of *BRCA1* testing in HBOC families: work in progress

In collaboration with Dr Henry Lynch and with grant support from the Department of Defense (1994-1998), we are conducting a prospective controlled trial of *BRCA1* testing in a large cohort of HBOC families. The goals are to: (1) examine processes of *BRCA1* test decision-making and (2) evaluate the psychological and behavioral impact of *BRCA1* testing in a large cohort of HBOC families. The schematic for this study is shown in *Figure 1*. Thus far, introductory letters have been mailed to 231 male and female members of HBOC families who are aged 18 and older. Of those, 176 (76%) completed the baseline telephone interview and 55 (24%) refused to participate in the interview portion of the study. Of the 176 interview respondents, fifty-two individuals (29%) declined to receive education or counseling and 125

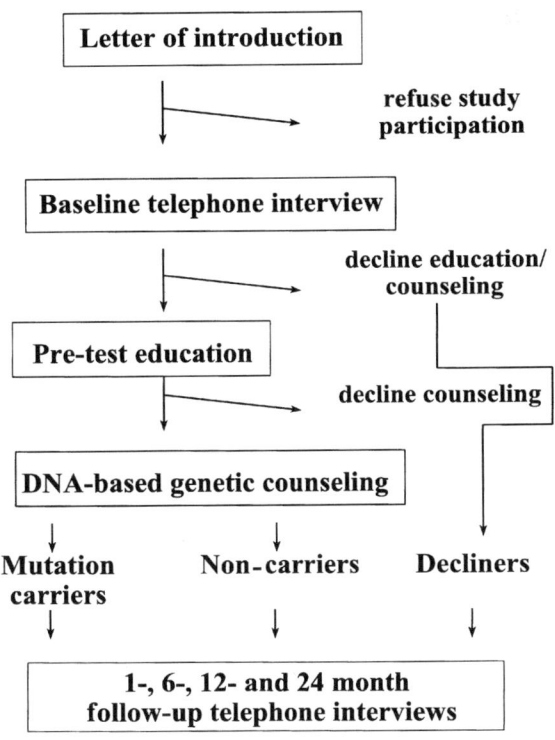

Figure 1. Design of prospective study of BRCA1 testing.

(71%) received pre-test education. All but one of these individuals receiving pre-test education decided to obtain the results of *BRCA1* testing. One-month follow-up interviews have been completed with 110 testing participants.

Factors associated with use of *BRCA1* testing

Figure 2 shows the reasons cited by family members at baseline for wanting *BRCA1* testing and for not wanting testing. The most widely cited reasons for wanting testing were to learn about one's children's risks and to increase use of screening tests. Of interest, almost one-half of individuals surveyed reported childbearing decisions as a « very important » reason for wanting *BRCA1* testing. This is surprising, since reproductive decision making generally is not a focus in genetic counseling for cancer susceptibility. Overall, fewer individuals reported strong reasons for not having testing. This is consistent with the high level of acceptance of testing in this population. However, concerns about the effect of testing on one's family and worries about losing health insurance were cited most frequently as barriers to receiving *BRCA1* test results.

We also examined whether persons who came forward for *BRCA1* testing had different sociodemographic backgrounds than those who declined. This was suppported by our data. Individuals who decided to be tested were predominantly female, under age 50, had at least a high school education, and had health insurance. Thus, *BRCA1* test decliners were mostly males over age 50 who had not completed high school and had no health insurance. In a logistic regression model, the following factors were significant independent predictors of acceptance of testing: gender (OR=3.8, CI=1.8-8.1), age (OR=2.9, CI=1.3-6.2), education (OR=3.4, CI=1.1-11.2), and health insurance status (OR=5.1, CI=1.5-17.0). Thus, females were almost four times more likely than males to request testing; individuals under age 50 were 3,5 times more likely than those over age 50; and individuals with health insurance were about five times more likely than those who did not have insurance.

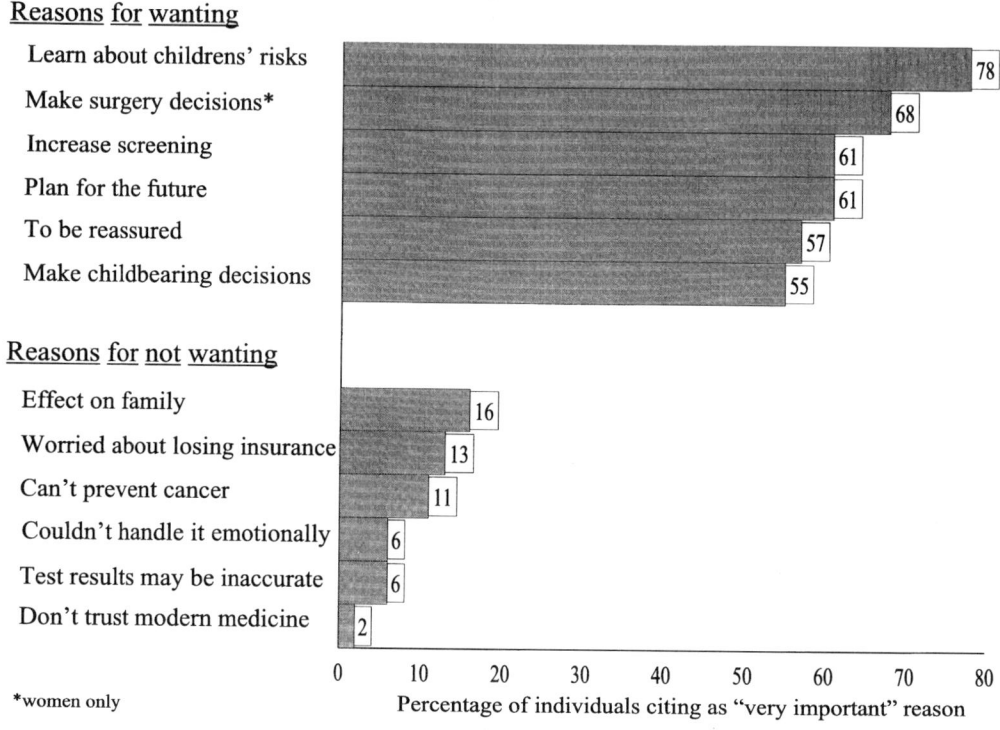

Figure 2. Reasons for wanting and not wanting BRCA1 testing.

Short-term impact of *BRCA1* testing on quality of life

The psychological and behavioral impacts of *BRCA1* testing are being evaluated using validated psychometric tools that are administered during baseline and follow-up telephone interviews. These interviews are conducted with individuals who test positive, negative, and with those who decline testing. Outcomes of interest in this study include perceptions of risk, depression, functional health status, screening behaviors, and medical and reproductive decision-making.

Preliminary data were collected from the initial 110 individuals who received *BRCA1* testing and who completed one-month follow-up interviews. Depression symptoms reported at baseline by individuals in these HBOC families do not differ from general population norms for depression using the Center for Epidemiologic Studies Scale *(Figure 3)* [16]. Reports of impairment in functional health status *(Figure 4)* are in the low to moderate range. This is somewhat surprising in light of previous studies showing elevated distress levels in women at risk for breast cancer [1, 2] . It is possible that members of hereditary breast cancer families develop stronger coping mechanisms as a result of repeated experiences of having relatives diagnosed with cancer. Alternatively, the low levels of distress could reflect the education and counseling received as part of their membership in the hereditary cancer registry.

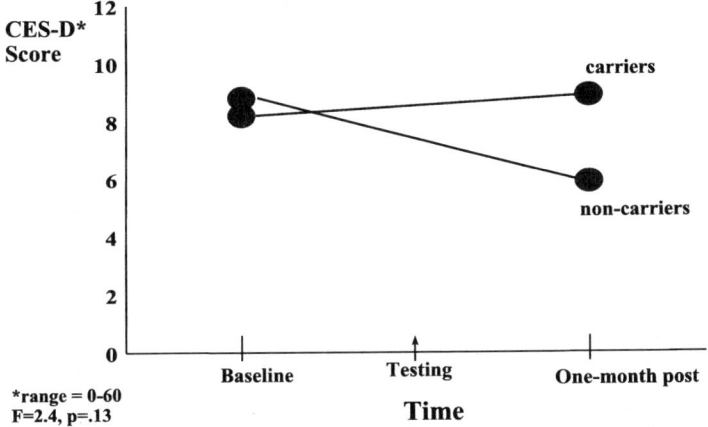

Figure 3. Impact of *BRCA1* testing on depression symptoms.

The effects of disclosure of *BRCA1* status on depression and functional health status are shown in *Figures 3* and *4*, respectively. Carriers show minimal change in depressive symptoms over time (about .10 standard deviations), while noncarriers show a slight decline in depression (about .25 standard deviations). These changes in depression in carriers and noncarriers are not statistically or clinically significant. By contrast, there is evidence for a significant effect of disclosure of *BRCA1* test results on functional health status (role functioning measure from the medical outcomes study; [17]). As shown in *Figure 4*, both carriers and noncarriers show a decrease in functional impairment. The significant time by carrier status interaction effect ($F=5.8$, $p=.02$) indicates that the decrease in impairment is significantly greater in noncarriers vs. carriers.

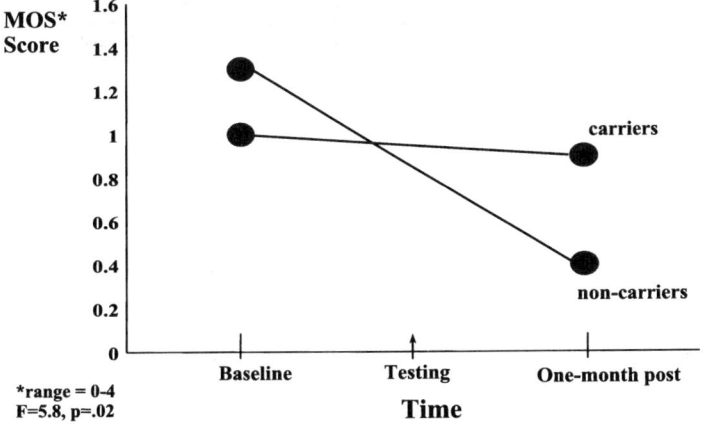

Figure 4. Impact of *BRCA1* testing on role functioning.

15

While these preliminary results are encouraging, caution must be taken in generalizing these findings to all individuals who may participate in *BRCA1* testing. Individuals in this study received extensive education and counseling as part of their involvement in prior linkage studies.

The psychological effects of *BRCA1* testing may differ for individuals who are less aware of their personal risk and who receive test results outside of a controlled research setting. In addition, patients' scores on the depression measure at one-month follow-up show large standard deviations. This suggests that there is substantial variability within the groups of carriers and noncarriers in their responses to testing. This supports the clinical observation that individuals vary widely in how they respond psychologically to genetic information. Once sufficient numbers of individuals have been accrued to this trial, it will be important to identify and characterize the subset of participants who may experience adverse effects following receipt of positive or negative results of *BRCA1* testing.

Impact of *BRCA1* testing on medical decision-making

Other important consequences of *BRCA1* testing involve its effects on decisions about medical care and reproduction. As shown in *Table I*, receipt of a positive *BRCA1* test result may impact the reproductive decisions of many individuals (67%), and some individuals with negative results may be affected as well (19%). Of those who indicated that testing affected their decision-making, most mutation carriers reported that they now are less likely to have children. By contrast, many noncarriers reported that they were now more likely to have children. Among women who were tested, 12% of mutation carriers reported that they decided to have prophylactic mastectomies and 29% decided to have prophylactic oophorectomies. However, many of these women said that they were uncertain, suggesting that supportive counseling may help women make these difficult decisions. Of interest, 4 women who tested negative for the *BRCA1* mutation in their family had already had prophylactic mastectomies and 16 had already had prophylactic oophorectomies. The psychological impact of these decisions will be an important area for future research.

Table I. Impact of *BRCA1* testing on decision-making at 1-month follow-up.

	Test Result	
	Positive	Negative
Impact of childbearing decisions (n=22)*		
% less likely	75	0
% more likely	25	40
% uncertain	0	60
Decided to have prophylactic mastectomy (n=52)*		
% yes	12	0
% no	71	97
% uncertain	17	3
Decided to have prophylactic oophorectomy (n=46)**		
% yes	29	0
% no	59	97
% uncertain	12	3

* Small sample sizes are due to « not applicable » responses from subjects who were beyond childbearing years.
** Small sample sizes are due to exclusion of males and « not applicable » responses from subjects who had already received surgery (either for prevention or treatment).

Insurance issues

The possibility of loss of insurance by persons tested for cancer-predisposing genes is a concern raised in the genetics community [18, 19] and also among persons considering testing [9]. Thus far, in a sample of 88 individuals tested for *BRCA1* mutations, 4 of them indicated problems in obtaining or maintaining insurance; however, in each of these cases the difficulties predated receipt of test results. Four out of 38 individuals who tested positive indicated changes in their insurance since testing; however, these changes were unrelated to genetic testing. While it may be too early to determine the actual rates of insurance discrimination among participants in genetic testing programs, our data indicate that insurance concerns may have an effect on decisions to receive *BRCA1* testing *(Figure 2)* and on medical decision-making. For example, 18% of mutation carriers indicated that insurance concerns affected their decisions about receiving prophylactic surgery. Thus, it is critical that the potential for insurance discrimination be addressed during the pre-test education session. In addition, as genetic testing programs become more widespread, it will be critical to evaluate the extent to which participants are discriminated against in their employment or insurance, and also to urge policy makers to pass legislation that would preclude these detrimental practices.

References

1. Kash KM, Holland JC, Halper MS, Miller DG. Psychological distress and surveillance behaviors of women with a family history of breast cancer. *J Natl Cancer Inst* 1992; 84: 24-30.
2. Lerrnan C, Daly M, Sands C, Balshem A, Lustbader E, Heggan T, Goldstein L, James J, Engstrom P. Mammography adherence and psychological distress among women at risk for breast cancer. *J Natl Cancer Inst* 1993; 85: 1074-80.
3. Lerman C, Schwartz M. Adherence and psychological adjustment among women at high risk for breast cancer. *Breast Cancer Res & Treat* 1993; 28: 145-55.
4. Valdimarsdottir HB, Bovbjerg DH, Kash KM, Holland JC, Osborne MP, Miller DG. Psychological distress in women with a familial risk of breast cancer. *Psycho-Oncology* 1995; 4: 133-41.
5. Schwartz MD, Lerman C, Miller SM, Daly M, Masny A. Coping disposition, perceived risk, and psychological distress among women at increased risk for ovarian cancer. *Health Psychology* 1995; 14: 232-5.
6. Lemman C, Kash K, Stefanek M. Younger women at increased risk for breast cancer: Perceived risk, psychological well-being, and surveillance behavior. *J Natl Cancer Inst Monographs* 1994; 16: 171-6.
7. Lemnan C, Rimer BK, Daly M, Lustbader E, Sands C, Balshem A, Masny A, Engstrom P. Recruiting high risk women into a breast cancer health promotion trial. *Cancer Epidemiol Biomarkers & Preven* 1994; 3: 271-6.
8. Lerman C, Lustbader E, Rimer B, Daly M, Miller S, Sands C, Balshem A. Effects of individualized breast cancer risk counseling: A randomized trial. *J Natl Cancr Inst* 1995; 87: 286-92.
9. Lerman C, Daly M, Masny A, Balshem A. Attitudes about genetic testing for breast-ovarian cancer susceptibility. *J Clin Oncol* 1994; 12: 843-50.
10. Chaliki H, Loader S, Levenkron JC, Logan-Young W, Hall J, Rowley PT. Women's receptivity to testing for a genetic susceptibility to breast cancer. *Am J Public Health* 1995; 85: 1133-5.
11. Struewing JP, Lerman C, Kase RG, Giambarresi TR, Tucker MA. Anticipated uptake and impact of genetic testing in hereditary breast and ovarian cancer families. *Cancer Epidemiol Biomarkers & Preven* 1995; 4: 169-73.
12. Lynch HT, Watson P, Conway TA, Lynch JF, Slominski-Caster SM, Narod SA, Feunteun J, Lenoir G. DNA screening for breast/ovarian cancer susceptibility based on linked markers. *Archives Intern Med* 1993; 153: 1979-87.

13. Evers-Kiebooms G, Swerts A, Van den Berghe H. The motivation of at risk individuals and their partners in deciding for or against predictive testing for Huntington's disease. *Clinical Genet* 1989; 35: 29-40.
14. Craufurd D, Dodge A, Kerzin-Storrar L, Harris R. Uptake of presymptomatic predictive testing for Huntington's disease. *Lancet* 1989; 2: 603-5.
15. Bloch M, Fahy M, Fox S, Hayden, MR. Predictive testing for Huntington disease. II. Demographic characteristics, lifestyle patterns, attitudes, and psychosocial as sessments of the first fifty-one test candidates. *Am J Med Genet* 1989; 32: 217-24.
16. Radloff LS. The CES-D scale: A self-report depression scale for research in the general population. *Applied Psych Measure* 1977; 1: 385-401.
17. Stewart AL, Ware JE (eds.). *Measuring Functioning and Well-being. The Medical Outcomes Study Approach.* Durham, NC: Duke University Press, 1992.
18. Nuffield Council of Bioethics. *Genetic Screening Ethical Issues.* London, England, 1993.
19. Ostrer H, Allen W, Crandall LA, Moseley RE, Dewar MA, Nye D, Van McCrary S. Insurance and genetic testing? Where are we now? *Am J Human Genet* 1993; 52: 565-77.

Breast Cancer. Advances in biology and therapeutics.
F. Calvo, M. Crépin, H. Magdelenat, eds. John Libbey Eurotext © 1996, pp. 19-22.

Experimental breast cancer studies: paradigms for human breast cancer

Richard C. Moon

Department of Surgical Oncology, University of Illinois at Chicago, Chicago, Illinois, USA

Several tumor models for various target organs are available to study modulation of carcinogenesis by both endogenous and exogenous factors. Such tumor models should exhibit several of the following characteristics: 1) cancer development in high numbers should be relatively rapid, preferably 6 to 12 months; 2) initiation should be accomplished with a single carcinogen (chemical, radiation, etc.) dose or, at most, a few doses; 3) cancer should develop only in the organ or tissue of interest, *i.e.*, exhibit target organ specificity; 4) tumors which develop should be histologically comparable to the human counterpart; 5) tumors should be invasive and/or metastatic and 6) the carcinogen should induce little or no systemic toxicity. Several existing tumor models have been used for the modulation of experimental carcinogenesis of the mammary gland in our laboratory; some offer specific advantages over others and are referred to below. Since the emphasis of this report centers on the modulation of mammary cancer, a further description of the model systems most frequently used in such studies appears warranted.

Mammary cancers can be selectively induced in rats by either 7,12-dimethylbenz(a)anthracene (DMBA) or N-methyl-N-nitrosourea (MNU), and both DMBA and MNU induced mammary tumor models have been successfully utilized for both mechanistic and chemoprevention studies. The MNU-induced tumor model as originally described by Gullino *et al*. [1] has subsequently been modified in our laboratory [2]. The DMBA model as described by Huggins *et al*. [3] has been used essentially unchanged. When DMBA is administered in a single intragastric dose at a concentration of 15 mg/ml sesame oil/rat, a 90-100% incidence of mammary tumors is obtained at 180 days post carcinogen whereas a single intravenous injection of 50 mg MNU/kg body weight (pH 5.0) also can induce 100% mammary tumor incidence in rats during a 6-month period. The majority of the cancers induced by these carcinogens are ovarian hormone dependent with a small percentage of tumors remaining as hormone independent. Earlier studies on the modulation of carcinogenesis were conducted with DMBA-induced cancer model, however, the MNU-induced mammary cancer model has remained a model of choice for most studies for several reasons: 1) DMBA-induced tumors are encapsulated and do not invade or metastasize; 2) DMBA must be metabolized to an active form; and 3) DMBA induces a high incidence of adenomas and fibroadenomas. These complications do not arise in the MNU-induced cancer model. Although numerous studies have been reported on the modulation of mammary cancer in mice, the discussion below will be limited to the rat mammary carcinoma model.

There are several reasons to support the use of the DMBA and MNU rat mammary carcinoma models as paradigms for human breast cancer. Firstly, the models are user friendly and highly reproducible, even in the hands of the relatively inexperienced; secondly, the tumors induced by these carcinogens possess many histogenic and biologic similarities to the human counterpart and thirdly, the hormone responsiveness of rat chemically-induced mammary cancer is strikingly similar to that of human breast cancer, particularly as regards the ovarian steroids. Thus, these models have been used extensively to determine the modulatory effect of several classes of compounds on experimental mammary carcinogenesis, some of which have received considerable attention in the clinic.

It is well established that modulation of the hormonal status of the host profoundly affects the development and growth of breast cancer both experimentally and clinically. Although many studies could be cited showing a parallelism between the rat mammary tumor model and the human, the extensive studies of Jordan and his colleagues [4] on the prevention and treatment of breast cancer with the antiestrogen tamoxifen is a prime example for the use of this model as a paradigm for human breast cancer.

Of equal importance relative to the parallelism between the rat model and humans is the effect of parity on the risk for breast cancer. Early epidemiologic studies showed that nulliparous women were at higher risk for breast cancer than multiparous women [5]. Furthermore, the study of MacMahon *et al* [6] showed that the risk for breast cancer increases with an increase in age at first full-term pregnancy and that the protective effect of parity is essentially limited to the first birth. Moon [7] observed a similar effect of parity in the experimental animal. Using the DMBA rat model, it was shown that rats undergoing a single pregnancy or a single pregnancy followed by a subsequent nursing period exhibited a decrease in mammary cancer incidence and an increase in the tumor latent period. Animals subjected to two pregnancies and/or lactations exhibited a significant decrease in mammary cancer incidence and a prolonged tumor latent period when compared with virgin control animals, although tumor incidence did not vary greatly from that of animals undergoing a single pregnancy and lactation. Thus, the effect of previous pregnancies and lactations on mammary cancer incidence in rats appeared to be similar to that found in the human female. These studies were confirmed by Russo and Russo [8] and more recently by Thordarson *et al.* [9] using the MNU rat model.

Although increased parity is associated with a decreased risk for breast cancer in women, the protective effect is limited essentially to the age at which the woman bears her first full-term child. Since DMBA-induced mammary carcinogenesis in the rat is also influenced by parity, additional studies [10] were initiated to determine whether or not the age at which the first litter is borne has an effect upon DMBA-induced mammary carcinogenesis when initiated at a subsequent period in the life of the animal. In this study, virgin and primiperous rats, mated at 50, 145 and 235 days of age, received DMBA at 300 days of age and were observed for an additional 225-265 days for development of mammary cancer. A single pregnancy without a subsequent nursing period afforded protection against DMBA-induced mammary tumorigenesis as evidenced by a reduction in tumor incidence and average number of tumors per animal. Although tumor incidence apparently decreases with an increase in age at which the first litter is borne, the incidence in mammary cancer was not affected by age at which pregnancy ensues, for all groups of parous animals exhibited a similar incidence of cancer. Thus, it appears that parity affords protection against DMBA-induced mammary carcinogenesis, but the age at which pregnancy ensues bears little relationship to the incidence of mammary cancer. However, in an experiment in which animals were mated at 50 days of age, bore the litter, and then received DMBA at 91 days of age, the incidence of mammary cancer was less than that observed in similar animals receiving DMBA at 300 days of age. This would seem to indicate that the degree of protection afforded by an early pregnancy decreases somewhat from the time of first litter until the carcinogenic insult, although the protection afforded by pregnancy is still existent even late in the animal's life.

It is evident from these studies as well as others that mammary carcinoma in the rat behaves much like mammary carcinoma in the human female. However, the two species do not exactly parallel each other. Although parity in both species protects against the development of mammary cancer, the age at which pregnancy ensues does not appear critical in the rat.

Another area of breast cancer research in which the rat mammary tumor model has proved useful is that of cancer chemoprevention. This model has been used extensively in the National Cancer Institute's Chemoprevention Program [11]. The relevance to the human situation is exemplified by studies involving the retinoids.

The efficacy of several retinoids in inhibiting murine mammary carcinogenesis has been investigated in our laboratory over the past 15 years. Past studies [12] have indicated that 4-hydroxyphenyl retinamide (4-HPR) is the most effective retinoid in reducing mammary cancer incidence, multiplicity and increasing the latency of induced mammary cancers, that is, when the ratio of efficacy to toxicity is considered. Furthermore, 4-HPR is concentrated in the mammary epithelium of both rats and women and administration of the compound can be delayed for an extended period after the carcinogenic insult and still retain efficacy.

In an effort to more closely simulate the clinical situation, we conducted an experiment in which retinoid treatment was not initiated until after the surgical removal of the first palpable tumor. Very little quantitative inhibition of mammary tumorigenesis was evident until approximately 50 days following tumor excision, after which a significantly reduced rate of tumor appearance was noted in the retinoid-treated group in comparison to control animals. These studies also suggest that retinoids suppress the progression of early lesions, such as carcinoma in situ and adenomatous hyperplasias. Although retinoids are generally much more effective against the development of early lesions, recent studies have indicated that at least two retinoids temaroten and 4-HPR may exert chemotherapeutic as well a chemopreventive activity, in that established mammary tumors regress in animals treated with these retinoids.

The evidence supporting the chemopreventive activity of retinoids in rat mammary tumor models is substantial, however, only a few studies to determine the clinical efficacy in breast cancer are underway. The longest ongoing clinical trial with retinoids is that which is being conducted in Milan to determine the efficacy of Fenretinide, 4-HPR, in preventing contralateral breast cancer [13]. A recent preliminary report [14] suggest that the « intervention effect of the retinoid is significantly modified by menopausal status and/or age, with a preventive effect being observed in young, premenopausal women. » If such proves to be the case, then the clinical situation would be similar to that found in the experimental rat model since these animals are young, sexually mature, cycling female rats.

Although hormonal modulations of mammary carcinogenesis is well established, the studies cited above indicate that retinoids also effectively alter mammary carcinogenesis. It is likely, therefore, that combination chemoprevention protocols would be more effective in cancer prevention either through additive or synergistic interactions between the two chemopreventive modalities. Such interactions are supported by studies showing that a combination of tamoxifen and 4-HPR is much more effective in preventing MNU-induced mammary cancer in rats than is either agent alone [15].

In addition to the studies cited above, a number of different agents having different mechanisms of action have been evaluated in these mammary tumor models. Such agents have included antihormones, hormone analogs, enzyme inhibitors, antiproliferatives, inducers of apoptosis and immunostimulants, among others. A number of these are currently undergoing phase I/II clinical trials for breast cancer. Although there are many similarities between breast cancer in the two species, the course of the disease is not the same, particularly as related to the postmenopausal status in women. However, with the advent of an increased number of clinical trials, it should be possible to determine whether or not the rat tumor model can truly serve as a paradigm for human breast cancer.

References

1. Gullino PM, Pettigrew HM, Grantham FH. N-nitrosomethylurea as mammary gland carcinogen in rats. *J Natl Cancer Inst* 1975; 54: 401-14.
2. McCormick DL, Adamowski CB, Fiks A, Moon RC. Lifetime dose response relationship for mammary tumor induction by a single administration of N-methyl-N-nitrosourea. *Cancer Res* 1981; 41: 1690-94.
3. Huggins C, Grand LC, Brillantes FP. Mammary cancer induced by a single feeding of polynuclear hydrocarbons and its suppression. *Nature* 1977; 189: 204-7.
4. Jordan VC. Gaddum Memorial Lecture: A current view of tamoxifen for the treatment and prevention of breast cancer. *Br J Pharmacol* 1993; 110: 507-17.
5. Lewison EF. Prophylactic versus therapeutic castration in the total treatment of breast cancer. A collective review. *Obstet Gynecol Surv* 1962; 17: 769-802.
6. MacMahon B, Cole P, Brown J. Etiology of human breast cancer: A review. *J Natl Cancer Inst* 1973; 50: 21-42.
7. Moon RC. Relationship between previous reproductive history and chemically induced mammary cancer in rats. *Int J Cancer* 1969; 4: 312-7.
8. Russo J, Russo I. Susceptibility of the mammary gland to carcinogenesis. *Am J Pathol* 1980; 100: 497-512.
9. Thordarson G, Jin E, Guzman R, Swanson S, Nandi SK, Talamantes F. Refractoriness to mammary tumorigenesis in parous rats: is it caused by persistent changes in the hormonal environment or permanent biochemical alterations in the mammary epithelia? *Carcinogenesis* 1995; 16: 2847-53.
10. Moon RC. Influence of pregnancy and lactation on experimental mammary carcinogenesis. In: MC Pike, PK Siiteri, CW Welsch (eds.). *Banbury Report 8: Hormones and Breast Cancer*, p. 353, Cold Spring Harbor Laboratory, 1981.
11. Steele VE, Moon RC, Lubet RA, Grubbs CJ, Reddy BS, Wargovich M, McCormick DL, Pereira MA, Crowell JA, Bagheri D, Sigman CC, Boone CW, Kelloff GJ. Preclinical efficacy evaluation of potential chemopreventive agents in animal carcinogenesis models: Methods and results from the NCI Chemoprevention Drug Development Program. *J Cell Biochem*, Suppl. 1994; 20: 32-54.
12. Moon RC, Mehta RG, Rao KVN. Retinoids and cancer in experimental animals. In: Sporn MB, Roberts AB, Goodman DS (eds.). *The Retinoids: Biology, Chemistry, and Medicine*, 2nd edition, Raven Press: New York, 1994, pp. 573-95.
13. Veronesi U, DePalo G, Costa A, Formelli F, Marulini E, Del Vecchio M. Chemoprevention of breast cancer with retinoids. *Natl Cancer Inst Monog* 1992; 12: 93-7.
14. Costa A, Decensi A, DePalo G, Veronesi U. Breast cancer chemoprevention with retinoids and tamoxifen. *Proc Amer Assoc Cancer Res* 1996; 37: 655.
15. Ratko TA, Detrisac CJ, Dinger NM, Thomas CF, Kelloff GJ, Moon RC. Chemopreventive efficacy of combined retinoid and tamoxifen treatment following surgical excision of a primary mammary cancer in female rats. *Cancer Res* 1989; 49: 4472-6.

Human breast cancer risk factors: development of experimental paradigms

Lars Holmberg

Department of Surgery University Hospital, S-751 85 Uppsala, Sweden

Definitions

Risk factor

A risk factor is an exposure or an endogenous characteristic that is associated with the occurrence of breast cancer. It would be tempting to narrow the definition down to factors that actually cause breast cancer, but since it is very difficult to, at the final end, establish causality (and we could also argue at length about the definition of causality) - we must take it as sufficient to define risk factors as factors causing or being indicators of causes of a disease [1, 2].

Experiment

An experiment is an attempt to manipulate in this case risk factors to see if the risk for the disease is altered, thus, overthrowing or corroborating our conjecture that a certain exposure is a risk factor. The classical experiment wants to do this in a *controlled way*. Thus, if we measure the outcome after manipulation of the risk factor, we want to be sure that the result is not due to any extraneous factors acting during the manipulation. The classical way to do this is to create a control group where the risk factor is not manipulated. Sometimes we talk about *natural experiments* [3, 4]. E.g. some people start smoking, others don't and we could view the consequences of this as a result of a natural occurring experiment. However, since the habit of smoking also is associated with many other habits that could have consequences for the occurrence of cancer, the experiment is not « clean », *i.e.* we do not have full control over the extraneous factors. However, viewing the fact that some people smoke and some don't as a natural experiment, can help us to approach these problems in a scientific way, trying to get the most out of the observations made on smoking and non-smoking populations.

Paradigm

According to dictionaries, a paradigm is the rule for bending a verb. A paradigm could be seen as a set of theories that are thought to fit together into a pattern explaining facts, patterns and developments. An example of this is the current view of the natural course of breast cancer: Breast cancer is already early on a systemic disease. Local therapy of breast cancer is important, but a main determinant for the long-term outcome is the overall balance between the host and the tumour at the time of primary treatment. At the time of local removal of the tumour, a substantial proportion of the patients will need systemic therapy due to the systemic nature of the disease.

Experiments in humans

A possibility to do experiments in humans would be to follow the risk of breast cancer if a certain risk factor would removed. However, in breast cancer such experiments are difficult to conduct. In the first instance, most of the breast cancer risk factors that we know of are not very strong [3]. They entail small or moderate risks - most of them entail relative risks around 0.5 - 2.5 - and to show that an attempt to remove a certain risk factor would decrease breast cancer risk would require very large numbers of women studied. Another difficulty is that many of the risk factors that we are aware of, cannot for many different reasons be manipulated easily. Age at menarche, age at menopause, age at birth of the first child, number of children, are none of them suitable for large interventions. Some other risk factors could be conceptually thought of as targets for intervention, such as BMI, intake of certain foods, alcohol intake and alike risk factors. However, these factors are not substantiated enough in epidemiological research [5] to today allow for the ethical and logistic difficulties associated with prevention in these areas. An exception would be if any of these risk factors was thought to be important for other diseases, such as coronary heart disease and a large NIH study have used this fact in an attempt to also study breast cancer risk after dietary interventions.

Beside the large obstacles when it comes to the size of these studies, it is also most of the time unclear over what time frames the factors that could be targets for interventions work. For many risk factors, we have reason to believe that time perspectives are long, even dating back to intrauterine life [6]. Thus, we do not only need large studies but also studies that are followed up over very long time and these studies thus become very expensive both in the sense of the large numbers needed, and in terms of time spent.

Experiments in experimental animals or tissue cultures

Manipulating risk factors known from human studies in animal experiments has many difficulties. If we, on the crude level, manipulate, say, hormonal levels and measure the incidence of breast cancer, we are not at all sure that this could be transferred into the human setting and there are many examples of discordance between the animal experiment and what is realised in the human setting. However, it may be more rewarding if we go several levels deeper. *E.g.* if we have a theory saying that alcohol interplays with oncogene X in the premenopausal breast given certain doses of alcohol and duration of exposure, then this may be a theory that could be tested in the animal experiment, and possibly transferred to tissue culture of human cells. Oncogene X could then in the next step be measured in breast cancer cases and related to their exposure to alcohol, say, in a case-control setting. If several rigorous tests of the same type cannot overthrow the theory, this theory might be taken into intervention programmes. The same type of experiments are also of course interesting for risk factors that are not direct targets for clinical interventions. The experiments could anyway make us better understand the mechanisms under which *e.g.* low age at first birth protects against breast cancer. If so, we can perhaps find artificial ways to mimic the protective effect. Such experiments have been proposed [7]. However, for many known or suspected breast cancer risk factors we lack such theories.

What is needed to develop new experimental paradigms?

At large we need good theories, we need an interplay between clinicians, epidemiologists and laboratory researchers, and if a theory survives long enough to be taken into intervention studies, we need concerted action between many people to accrue large numbers of patients and oberve them over a long time.

We need to develop more detailed and rich theories why certain risk factors are risk factors. A theory is an attempt to solve a problem. We have a problem, *e.g.* understanding why and how alcohol intake could be a risk factor for breast cancer: Does alcohol act directly on breast tissue or via hormones? What kind of cellular changes does the direct interference with the cell cause? When are breast tissue cells most susceptible for alcohol exposure and under what circumstances do these changes progress into a cancer? A good theory, thus, in a way takes a known problem further, enriches its different aspects and in this process we simultaneously create new ideas how to test the hypothesis. The development of details of a theory as the one exampled here can lead to several experimental tests. A good theory is also interesting even if it fails. It is just as interesting a finding if we find that alcohol works directly on the cells as if they don't.

To develop these kind of theories, *i.e.* to interpret and directly take epidemiological data down to theories of cellular mechanisms we need interaction between different kinds of specialists. The same is true also if the process goes the other way, *i.e.* from the laboratory out into the clinic. Despite that so many people talk about this type of interaction, it is astonishingly seldom we see it happen in real life. Most institutions still go deeper and deeper into specialisation in the most narrow sense of the word: much knowledge in a small field, but also isolation of perspective to that field. Dangerously enough, it seems like medical training of today rather stimulates this development. Epidemiologists are more and more high-tech biostatisticians, laboratory workers are more and more often high-tech laboratory engineers, clinicians are specialised down to very narrow fields. We need to find ways how they can meet in a stimulating environment.

Experiments with prevention in clinical practice will require large-scale clinical trials. Concerted action is then absolutely mandatory not to make these experiments too time-consuming or in the worst case non-conclusive. To get many large centres to collaborate, an interactive process in scientific thinking and development is needed between the centres and between specialists. This climate is not established rapidly and we have to consider long time strategies to nourish such a process.

Thus, in summary, to develop experimental paradigms for human breast cancer risk factors different types of specialists need to collaborate in developing theories how risk factors work, test these theories in laboratory experiments, critically assess the results and then try to transfer the new knowledge into clinical experiments. The process oscillates back and forth between population studies, clinical work and laboratory efforts and, thus, the process could begin just anywhere in the circle. A perspective on the main present obstacles presently for this process could be: creative interaction between laboratory workers, clinicians and epidemiologists only works in small isolated spots and seldom on a national or international level. Too little care is taken to develop new innovative theories why risk factors are risk factors. In doing clinical or epidemiological research, there is still too little collaboration.

References

1. Rothman KJ. Causes. *Am J Epidemiol* 1995; 141: 587-92.
2. Rothman KJ. *Modern epidemiology*. pp 10-22. Little Brown and Co. Boston 1986.
3. Rothman KJ. *Modern epidemiology*. pp 56-57. Little Brown and Co. Boston 1986.
4. Bradford Hill A. Observation and experiment. *N Engl J Med* 1953; 248: 995-1001.
5. Adami HO, Persson I, Ekbom A, Wolk A, Ponten J, Trichopoulus D. The aetiology and pathogenesis of human breast cancer. *Mutation Res* 1995; 333: 29-35.
6. Trichopoulus D. Hypothesis: does breast cancer originate in utero? *Lancet* 1990; 335: 939-40.
7. Pike MC, Spicer DV, Dahmoush L, Press MF. Estrogens, progesterogens, normal breast cell proliferation and breast cancer risk. *Epidemiol Rev* 1993; 15: 17-35.

Oncogenes and onco-suppressor genes in the prevention and therapy of breast cancer

D.A. Spandidos, M. Koffa, G. Sourvinos and H. Kiaris

Medical School, University of Crete, Heraklion 71 110, Greece

Abstract

The development of breast cancer requires the accumulation of several genetic alterations. Among oncogenes the activation of c-erbB-2 and the ras genes plays an important role in the development of the disease and is associated with particular clinico-pathological parameters. The activation of c-erbB-2 frequently occurs by gene amplification and results in overexpression while the elevated expression of the ras genes is probably associated with transcriptional activation or mutations in the regulatory regions. The deletion or mutational inactivation of onco-suppressor genes located on 8p, 11q, 17p and 17q are also frequent events. Recently, onco-suppressor genes involved in the hereditary form of the disease have been cloned, located on the 13q and 17q arms. Furthermore, an increase in the mutation rate as reflected in the instability of microsatellite sequences has been reported and associated with the genetic destabilization required for the malignant progression. Clarification of the steps involved in this multistep process may have important effects in the clinical practice, such as in the early detection and therapy of breast cancer. In addition, screening tests may be developed to reveal the presence of genetic factors predisposing for the development of the disease. The aim of our study was to summarise the major molecular alterations required for the development of breast cancer and their potential clinical applications.

Introduction

The activation of oncogenes and the inactivation of tumour suppressor genes (TSGs) is required for the development of cancer. Multistage carcinogenesis is reflected in the accumulation of several genetic changes which confer the malignant phenotype [1]. However, each tumour is not a uniform entity with identical genetic information in all the cancer cells but is characterised

by a relatively high degree of heterogeneity [2, 3]. Although each tumour is clonal with respect to the progenitor cell, it is heterogeneous due to the acquisition of additional mutations. This is probably associated with the existence of multiple molecular pathways for the development of the disease and corresponds to selection procedures during the evolution of the tumour.
Recently, genomic instability in simple repeated sequences (microsatellite instability, MI) has been described in many human tumours and associated with an increase in the mutational rate, providing evidence for the molecular mechanism of the acquisition of multiple somatic changes in the cancer cells [4].
The aforementioned observations when applied in breast cancer, reveal complex genetic changes including the activation of oncogenes either by point mutations or by gene amplification, the deletion of onco-suppressor genes and existence of a mutator phenotype as reflected in the instability of microsatellites. In the present study we reviewed the major genetic alterations involved in breast cancer development [5].

Oncogenes

In breast cancer the activation of oncogenes is almost consistently associated with gene amplification. Amplification of *erb*B-2, *myc* and *int*-2 proto-oncogenes occurs in approximately 40 % of breast tumours. Amplification of *erb*B-2 in particular has been reported in 20 % of the cases and associated with poor prognosis [6, 7]. In ductal carcinoma *in situ* the incidence of *erb*B-2 amplification increases to 50 % of the cases, suggesting that this genetic alteration is important for this particular histological subtype. Amplification of *erb*B-2 results in the overproduction of erbB-2 protein which increases the growth rate.
The proto-oncogene c-*myc* is found frequently amplified in breast tumours and associated with overproduction of the *Myc* protein. However, overexpression of c-*myc* occurs more frequently than gene amplification, suggesting that transcriptional activation of c-*myc* may be more important in the development of breast tumours [8]. As regards the incidence of *int*-2 amplification it is found in approx. 15 % of the cases but is not associated with overexpression of the INT-2 protein. Thus, it has been proposed that other oncogene(s), located adjacent to the c-*myc* are the target of the gene amplification and subsequently c-*myc* is co-amplified [5].
Among oncogenes the members of the *ras* family of genes have been involved in a wide range of human tumours [9]. The activation of *ras* genes occurs by point mutations predominantly at codon 12 but also at codons 13 and 61. Mutations in the *ras* family is generally considered as a rare event in the development of breast cancer [10,11]. Koffa et al. [12] found 8 among 65 (12 %) to harbour an activating K-*ras* mutation. All the mutations were restricted to high grade tumours (II+III) indicating that this particular aberration is a late event in the development of the disease. However, although mutational activation of the *ras* family genes is not a very frequent event in the development of the disease, overexpression occurs frequently and has been found both at the level of p21 protein and the level of mRNA encoded by the *ras* family genes [13]. Considering the structure of the *ras* family genes and the absense of inducible regulatory elements, the transcriptional activation may indicate mutations in regulatory regions. Potential target for the aforementioned mutations is the mini-satellite region, downstream of the H-*ras* gene which possesses enhancer activity and its destabilization has been reported in other tumours [14].

Tumour-suppressor genes

The inactivation of TSGs occurs frequently in breast tumours and is associated with the pathogenesis of the disease. Allelotype studies revealed the position of several TSGs involved in the development of breast tumours [5, 15]. Considerable incidence of loss of heterozygosity (LOH) has been found for the chromosomal arms 1p, 1q, 11p, 16q, 17p, 17q, 18q, 22q and Xp. In some cases, the target of the LOH event has been characterised (*i.e.* the p53 in 17p, the DCC, as well as the nm23 gene, considered as a metastasis suppressor gene), however, in the majority of the cases the target of the deletion remains unknown.

Particular attention has been given recently to the identification of genes involved in the familial breast cancers. Experiments based on linkage analysis revealed the position of two loci, on 17q and 13q arms, which harbour the *BRCA1* and *BRCA2* genes. These genes behave as TSGs and inactivating point mutations in the germline of the patients result in a predisposition for the development of breast cancer and account for approx. 90 % of the familial cases [16,17]. However, in sporadic breast cancer, although the LOH incidence in these genes and in *BRCA1* in particular is relatively high, evidence of somatic mutations in sporadic cases remains scarce [18]. These observations suggest that other TSG(s), located in the near vicinity of *BRCA1* may be more important in the development of sporadic breast cancer.

Recent studies revealed the existence of additional breast cancer genes, which apart from the familial cases may be also important for the development of male breast cancer [19, 20].

Replication errors

Microsatellite instability (MI) due to errors in DNA replication reflect an increase in the mutation rate. This corresponds to the destabilization of the genome of the cancer cells which is required for the development of the malignancy [4].

Although the incidence of MI in breast tumours has not been studied in detail, it is considered as a detectable phenomenon in breast tumours, associated with the earlier stages of the disease [21]. However, the association of this phenomenon with mutations in DNA repair genes has not been studied sufficiently as yet. Recent studies on the detection of MI or other alterations in cytological material revealed that it may have important clinical applications in the early diagnosis of human cancer [22, 23]. This methodology in breast cancer uses cytological material from fine needle aspiration (FNA) to detect either MI or other genetic alterations, in the diagnosis for the malignancy.

Conclusions and perspectives

The development of breast cancer requires the acquisition of several genetic and epigenetic events, such as the inactivation of oncogenes, the activation of tumour suppressor genes and the increase of the mutation rate as reflected in the instability of the microsatellite sequences. The elucidation of the fundamental mechanisms of mammary tumorigenesis may have important applications in the clinical practice, involving the early detection of breast cancer and the development of novel therapeutic strategies.

As regards the early diagnosis of breast cancer, MI is detected in cytological material obtained by FNA. MI occurs early in tumorigenesis and it may be present before the clinical symptoms. Apart from MI, activation of oncogenes (such as the c-*erb*B-2) and the inactivation of TSGs, may be detected in cytological material. Furthermore, detection of particular genetic alterations in biopsy specimens associated with a specific clinical phenotype, may provide clues for the appropriate treatment of the cases.

The detection of germline mutations in the familial breast cancer genes may also be applied in order to reveal a predisposition for the development of the disease. Screening test for the population have already been established, based on the BRCA1 gene in particular, following a series of scientific guidelines concerning the regulation of genetic tests. There is a need for education of health professionals and agreed criteria before the test can be established in clinical practice.

Therapeutic strategies based on the molecular alterations of breast tumours, remain a challenging approach, aiming to correct the malignant phenotype with either the inhibition of the mutant gene or its « replacement » with the normal allele. These experiments are in progress, however, future research is required for their application in the clinical practice.

References

1. Spandidos DA. A unified theory for the development of cancer. *Biosci Rep* 1986; 6: 691-708.
2. Heppner GH. Tumor heterogeneity. *Cancer Res* 1984; 44: 2259-62.
3. Kiaris H and Spandidos DA. Quantitation of the allelic imbalance provides evidence on tumour heterogeneity: A hypothesis. *Mutation Res*. in press.
4. Loeb LA. Microsatellite instability: Marker of a mutator phenotype in cancer. *Cancer Res* 1994; 54: 5059-63.
5. Devilee P and Cornelisse CJ. Somatic genetic changes in human breast cancer. *Bioch Bioph Acta* 1994; 1198: 113-30.
6. Slamon DJ, Golphin W, Jones LA, Holt JA, Wong SG, Keith DE, et al. *Science* 1989; 244: 707-12.
7. Lovekin C, Ellis IO, Locker A, Robertson JFR, Bell J, Nicholson R, Gullick WJ, Elston CW and Blamey RW. *Br J Cancer* 1991; 63: 439-43.
8. Spandidos DA, Pintzas A, Kakkanas A, Yiagnisis M, Mahera H, Patra E and Agnantis NJ. Elevated expression of the *myc* gene in human benign and malignant breast lesions compared to normal tissue. *Anticancer Res* 1987; 7: 1299-304.
9. Kiaris H and Spandidos DA. Mutations of *ras* genes in human tumours. *Int J Oncol* 1995; 7: 413-22.
10. Kraus MH, Yasa Y and Aaronson SA. A position 12-activated H-*ras* in all HS578T mammary carcinosarcoma cells but not in normal mammary cells of the same patients. *Proc Natl Acad Sci USA* 1984; 81: 5384-8.
11. Spandidos DA. Oncogene activation in malignant transformation: a study of H-*ras* in human breast cancer. *Anticancer Res* 1987; 7: 991-6.
12. Koffa M, Malamou-Mitsi V, Agnantis NJ and Spandidos DA. Mutational activation of K-*ras* oncogene in human breast tumors. *Int J Oncol* 1994; 4: 573-6.
13. Spandidos DA and Agnantis NJ. Human malignant tumours of the breast, as compared to their respective normal tissue, have elevated expression of the Harvey *ras* oncogene. *Anticancer Res*c 1984; 4: 269-72.
14. Kiaris H, Spandidos DA, Jones AS, Vaughan ED and Field JK. Mutations, expression and genomic instability of the H-*ras* proto-oncogene in squamous cell carcinomas of the head and neck. *Br J Cancer* 1995; 72: 123-8.
15. Bonsing BA, Devilee P, Cleton-Jansen A-M, Kuipers-Dijkshoorn N, Fleuren GJ, Cornelisse CJ.

Evidence for limited molecular genetic heterogeneity as defined by allelotyping and clonal analysis in nine metastatic breast carcinomas. *Cancer Res* 1993; 53: 3804-11.
16. Miki Y, Swensen J, Shattuck-Eidens K, Futreal PA, Harshman K, Tavtigian K, *et al.* A strong candidate for the breast and ovarian cancer susceptibility gene BRCA1. *Science* 1994; 266: 66-71.
17. Wooster R, Bignell G, Lancaster J, Swift S, Seal S, Mangion J, Collins N, Gregory S, Gumbs C, Micklem G, *et al.* Identification of the breast cancer susceptibility gene BRCA2. *Nature* 1995; 378: 789-92.
18. Boyd J. BRCA1: More than a hereditary breast cancer gene? *Nature Genet* 1995; 9: 335-6.
19. Kerangueven F, Essioux L, Dib A, Noguchi T, Allione F, Geneix J, Longy M, *et al.* Loss of heterozygosity and linkage analysis in breast carcinoma: indication for a putative third susceptibility gene on the short arm of chromosome 8. *Oncogene* 1995; 1023: 6.
20. Chuaqui RF, Sanz-Ortega J, Vocke C, Linehan N, Sanz-Esponera J, Zhuang Z, Emmeri-Buck MR and Merino MJ. Loss of heterozygosity on the short arm of chromosome 8 in male breast carcinomas. *Cancer Res* 1995; 55: 4995-8.
21. Yee CJ, Roodi N, Verrier CS and Parl FF. Microsatellite instability and loss of heterozygosity in breast cancer. Cancer Res 1994; 54: 1641-4.
22. Koffa M, Simiakaki H, Ergazaki M, Papaefthymiou M, Karakatsani K, Diakomanolis E and Spandidos DA. HPV detection in stained cytological cervical specimens and correlation with cytology and histology. *Oncol Rep* 1995; 2: 1085-8.
23. Kiaris H, Ergazaki M, Sakkas S, Athanasiadou E and Spandidos DA. Detection of activating mutations in cytological specimens from lung tumours. *Oncol Rep* 1995; 2: 769-72.

Molecular basis of human breast epithelial cell transformation

J. Russo, N. Barnabas, N. Higgy, A.M. Salicioni, Y.L. Wu and I.H. Russo

Breast Cancer Research Laboratory, Fox Chase Cancer Center, Philadelphia, PA 19111, USA

One of the accepted paradigms in human breast cancer is that the normal breast tissue evolves to cancer through several progressive steps; the neoplastic process starts in the terminal structures of the breast, evolving from typical ductal hyperplasia to an atypical form, and from there to carcinoma *in situ* and invasive carcinoma, which ultimately metastasizes [1-4]. The validation that breast cancer is the result of a series of progressive stages requires an experimental model that adequately reproduces the conditions prevailing *in vivo*, and therefore provides an understanding of the biology and molecular basis of the disease. A major drawback towards this goal is the lack of identification of the specific agent (s) or mechanism(s) responsible of the initiation of the neoplastic process. Recent studies indicate that genetic changes, such as DNA amplification and loss of genetic material in at least five possible loci and in 11 chromosomes, respectively, most notably chromosome 17, have been found during the process of transformation of the breast epithelium [5,6]. These genomic alterations have been reported to be present with different frequencies in both, preneoplastic lesions and the invasive forms of the disease. However, it has not been determined whether these changes are responsible of the initiation and /or the progression of the disease, or whether they result from chromosomal destabilization during neoplastic proliferation, but with no functional role or significance in those processes. The analysis of the role of genomic alterations is hindered by the fact that the sequential stages of cancer progression are not always present in a single patient, or do not manifest themselves in a sequential manner, or when they are present, the available material might be insufficient or inadequate for performing genetic manipulation for testing functionality. These studies require an *in vitro* system that mimics the *in vivo* situation, and at the same time provides the flexibility needed for testing the functional role of each genetic change identified.

Human breast epithelial cells *in vitro*

One of major advances in the understanding of the biology of the breast epithelium has been the knowledge gained on the role of calcium in the proliferation and differentiation of human breast epithelial cells (HBEC) in culture [7]. It is well known that calcium (CA^{++}) plays an important role in the activation of the signal transduction pathway, controlling the cascade of events triggering cell proliferation. Primary cultures of HBEC grown under standard culture conditions in medium containing 1.04mM CA^{++} (identified as high CA^{++}), exhibit a limited number of doublings, becoming squamoid, or differentiated, then entering in a quiescent state of senescence. The reduction of CA^{++} concentration in the medium to 0.04mM (also called low CA^{++}), results in an increased growth rate, with a higher yield of cells (almost 100 folds), and an increased number of doublings (up to 50). This phenomenon is reversible, although finite, since quiescent cells start dividing when transferred to the low CA^{++} medium, and their growth is inhibited by the return to the high CA^{++} medium. Eventually all normal cells enter in a senescent state from which they do not recover any more. An exception have been the mortal cells MCF-10M, derived from the breast tissue sample S#130, obtained from a 36 year old woman [8]. MCF-10M cells started growing equally well in both high and low CA^{++} media after 661 days in culture, an indication that they had escaped CA^{++} control, becoming spontaneous immortalized. These cells grew either attached to the bottom of the flask (MCF-10A), or floated in the medium (MCF-10F) [8, 9].

The establishment of the MCF-10 cell lines has relevance in breast cancer research for the following reasons: 1) This cell line is the only one that is diploid and contains only a reciprocal translocation between chromosomes 3 and 9. The fact that these cells became spontaneously immortalized, without viral infection, cellular oncogene transfection or exposure to carcinogens or radiation, a phenomenon reported in few HBECs, makes of MCF-10F the most near to a normal breast epithelial cell line available; 2) this cell line is phenotypically normal; it forms domes at confluence, it does not present loss of contact inhibition and it is not tumorigenic in a heterologous host, and 3) it constitutes an *in vitro* model adequate for addressing specific questions on the mechanisms of cell immortalization and transformation.

Biological and molecular basis of cell immortalization

Immortality in tissue culture is defined as the unlimited division potential of cells, reflecting a change in cell growth properties. It could be postulated that immortality *in vitro* represents the preneoplastic stage of breast cancer progression occurring in the human breast. If this could proven to be the case, then the molecular events identified during *in vitro* cell transformation could be ascribed to the *in vivo* situation [4]. One of the characteristics of the breast epithelium is that its proliferative ability can be regulated by the extracellular concentration of CA^{++}. Of significant interest is the fact that this phenotype is abrogated during the process of cell immortalization [9-11]. It is well known that CA^{++} plays important roles in: i. Activation of the signal transduction pathway, controlling the cascade of events triggering cell proliferation; ii. Production of milk during lactation, and iii. Formation of microcalcifications, an early clinical event observed in ductal hyperplasias and carcinoma *in situ* [4]. Therefore, it is reasonable to postulate that alterations in one or more of these steps may be involved in altering the signals for cell proliferation, and therefore cell immortalization. The identification of the genetic events responsible of cell immortalization is of utmost importance for understanding the biology of the disease. For these purposes we have constructed cDNA libraries from the mortal cells MCF-10M and MCF-10F cells, and a substracted cDNA library using +/- screening [12]. A set of 15 genes which are not present in the mortal MCF10-M cells has been cloned and isolated from the MCF-10F cell cDNA library. Three of these clones have been sequenced. The first clone (S16) is 387bp in size and shows 83% homology to a human calcium binding protein (SSR-alpha); the second clone (S2) is 459bp in size, and shows 100% homology with human apoferritin-H chain, and the third clone (S27) is 1.3 kb in size and has 98% homology to the human elongation factor 1-a. Northern blot analysis has demonstrated that these genes have transcripts of 0.8, 1.6, and 1.8 Kb in size, respectively. These transcripts, which are absent in the mortal cells, are highly expressed in all the passages of MCF-10F cells, in cells transformed with chemical carcinogens, and in the human breast cancer cell lines T-47D and BT20. It is our interpretation that these genes play a functional role in the mobilization of calcium, the control of the cell's entrance into senescence and partly in the signal transduction pathway *(Figure 1)*.

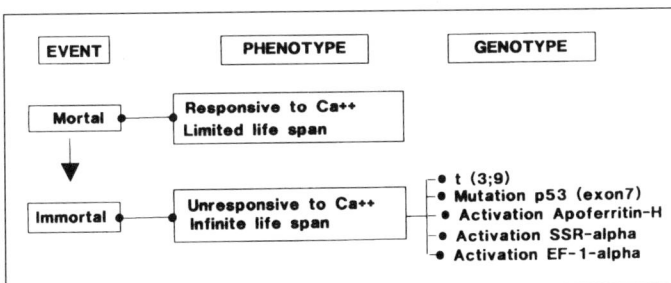

Figure 1. Summary of the phenotypic and genotypic changes taking place during the process of *in vitro* human breast epithelial cell immortalization.

Cell immortalization, such as that induced by either HPV16-E6 or by gamma radiation, has been associated with loss of p53 [13]. The involvement of p53 in cell immortalization has been confirmed by the observation that breast epithelial cells derived from women carrying germline p53 mutations, such as in Li Fraumeni syndrome families, undergo spontaneous immortalization [14]. The p53 gene has been identified as an important tumor suppressor gene in normal cells. Loss of normal p53 function is associated with genomic instability, *in vitro* cell transformation and *in vivo* tumor development [15]. This gene, located in the short arm of the human chromosome 17 at position p13.1, has a product of a 393-aminoacid nuclear phosphoprotein that exhibits antiproliferative activity, regulating the transition from the G_1 to the S phase of the cell cycle, and determining cell death through apoptosis. It functions as a genomic guardian, monitoring the integrity of the genome. By blocking the cell cycle it protects the genome against damaging agents, suppresses cell proliferation and inhibits malignant transformation. In order to determine whether p53 was involved in the immortalization of MCF-10F cells, we compared these cells with the mortal MCF-10M utilizing Northern and Southern blots, polymerase chain reaction (PCR) amplification and sequencing of the p53 gene, and single strand conformation polymorphism (SSCP), which is a rapid and sensitive method for the detection of mutations and/or deletions. Southern and Northern blot analyses did not reveal any changes, whereas SSCP analysis of exons 5-9 of the p53 gene showed a conformational shift in exon 7 in the MCF-10F cell line that was not present in the mortal cells MCF-10M [16]. Sequence analysis using asymmetric PCR-amplified products of exon 7 and an antisense primer revealed an insertional mutation of thymine at codon 254 in MCF-10F, but not in MCF-10M cells. In order to determine whether p53 mutations are the driving force in the immortalization of MCF-10F cells, we transfected these cells with the wild p53 using the pC53-SN3 vector containing neo as selectable marker; this transfection did not restitute the mortal phenotype, indicating that the mutation of p53 is not the only factor responsible of the immortalization. It is possible, however, that the p53 mutation detected in the immortal MCF-10Fcells had resulted in genetic instability that facilitated the emergence of other associated genes leading to immortalization. Although the final answer to the mechanism of cell immortalization is not at hand, our studies have allowed us to conclude that immortality is expressed as the unlimited division potential of human breast epithelial cells cultured *in vitro*, reflecting changes in the responsiveness to Ca^{++}. If immortalization *in vitro* is equivalent to the expression of the preneoplastic phenotype in the human breast, then, further characterization of the molecular events identified during this process might be the starting point for understanding the molecular mechanisms driving the progression of preneoplastic lesions to the full expression of malignancy in the *in vivo* situation *(Figure 1)*.

Molecular changes in the transformation of HBEC

We have developed an *in vitro* system for the transformation of human breast epithelial cells that recapitulates different stages of tumor initiation and progression, culminating in the expression of tumorigenesis in a heterologous host [17, 18]. This paradigm has capitalized in the utilization of the immortalized HBEC MCF-10F, which when treated with the chemical carcinogens 7,12 dimethylbenz(a)anthracene (DMBA) and benz(a)pyrene (BP), express in a progressive fashion, all the phenotypes indicative of neoplastic transformation, from increased survival in agar, formation of colonies in agar methocel, invasiveness in a matrigel *in vitro* system to tumorigenesis in severe combined immunodeficient (SCID) mice [17,18] *(Figure 2)*. The availability of this model, in which isolated clones of cells express different stages of progression from normal-immortalized to preneoplastic to fully transformed, constitutes a useful tool for determining whether the expression of specific phenotypes are the result of specific genotypic alterations.

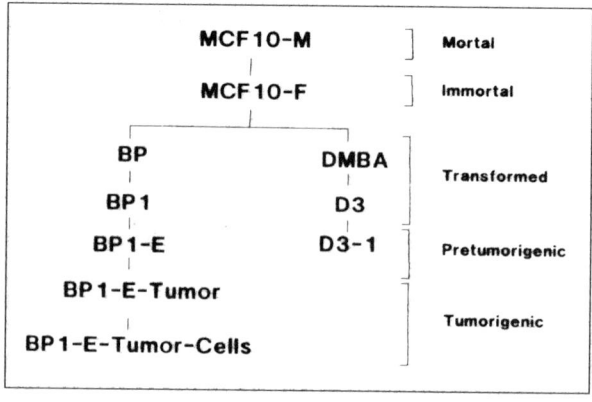

Figure 2. Schematic representation of the evolution of the mortal human breast epithelial cells MCF-10M to the immortal MCF-10F, and the clones derived after treatment with BP and DMBA. The phenotypes expressed by these cells are indicated in the right side column.

The expression of the transformed phenotype in breast cancer is associated with multiple genetic lesions, detected as mutations in tumor biopsy specimens and tumor-derived cell lines. These mutations include the amplification or aberrant expression of protooncogenes such as *c-myc, c-erbB2, int-2/hst-1* and infrequently *Ha-ras*. A type of change frequently observed in both primary and metastatic tumors is the loss of heterozygosity (LOH). Microsatellite instability (MSI) studies have demonstrated that a significant number of primary breast cancers show LOH in chromosomal regions 1p, 1q, 3p, 6q, 7q, 11p, 11q, 13q, 16q, 17p, 17q, and 18q. The diversity of LOH regions observed in breast cancer suggests that some of these events are coincidental noise resulting from errors in DNA metabolism that might have no consequence on the progression of the disease. In our *in vitro* cell transformation system we have found that the immortalization of MCF-10F cells is associated with the presence of a point mutation in exon 7 of the tumor suppressor gene p53 and with the activation of genes regulating calcium mobilization, control of the entrance of cells into senescence and signal transduction pathway [12,16]. Carcinogen-induced transformation was manifested as colony formation in agar methocel and anchorage independence, which were associated with point mutations in codons 12 and 61 of *c-Ha-ras* gene [19]. Other oncogenes involved in this early stage were *c-neu, c-myc and int-2* [20]. The expression of the tumorigenic phenotype was associated with LOH in the telomeric portion of chromosome 17, and overexpression of the *mdm2* gene [21]. The formation of tumors by inoculation of BP1-E cells to SCID mice was associated with MSI in chromosomes 9, 11, 16 and 17 [22, 23] *(Figure 3).*

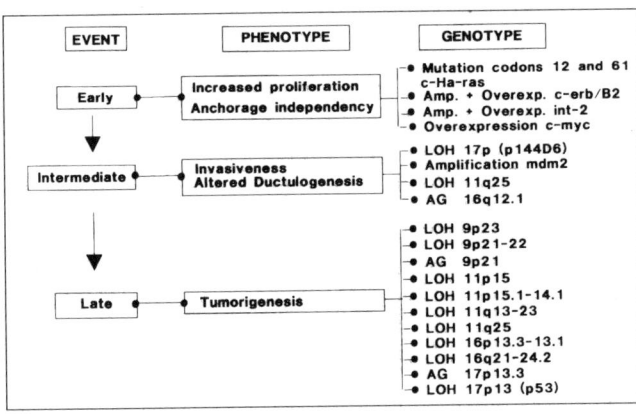

Figure 3. Correlation of the expression of early, intermediate and late events in *in vitro* transformation of human breast epithelial cells with the expression of phenotypical and genotypical changes.

c-Ha-Ras oncogene

There is evidence that the *c-Ha-ras* oncogene plays a role in the development and the progression of human and animal malignancies [24]. Approximately 60-70% of primary human breast carcinomas exhibit overexpression, and 27% LOH of this gene [25,26]. Approximately 10% of all human neoplasms carry a mutated ras gene, although mutations in human breast cancer are rarely found at any stage [19]. The exact mechanism of action of the *c-Ha-ras* gene is not clear; it has been suggested that the mutation may inactivate this locus on chromosome 11, thus leading to cell transformation. Supporting this contention is the finding that clones D1 and D3, derived from DMBA treated MCF-10F cells exhibited mutations in codons 12 and 61 of the *c-Ha-ras* gene. The clones BP1 and BP1-E, derived from BP treated cells exhibited mutations in codon 61, but not in codon 12 . The observations that there was an increase in colony efficiency after a mutation was detected, whereas cells which exhibited a more invasive or the tumorigenic phenotype did not differ in number of mutations from cells exhibiting a less aggressive phenotypes, indicate that mutations of *c-Ha-ras* oncogene are associated with the early events of cell transformation *(Figure 3)*.

LOH in the locus of the *c-Ha-ras* oncogene, on the other hand, has been observed in the BP-1E tumor and tumor derived cell line [23].

c-neu, int-2, and *c-myc* oncogenes

Genetic alterations of the *c-neu, int-2,* and *c-myc* oncogenes have been reported in human breast cancer at different stages of progression of the disease [27]. Amplification of the c-neu oncogene is a frequent event in primary breast cancers, occurring in 18-33% of the cases, and a high percentage of tumors show overexpression of the c-neu protein, indicating that deregulation of the gene might be involved in the neoplastic process. In our *in vitro* system, *c-neu* gene transcript was detected as a 4.5-kb band in the MCF-10F cell line, and the intensity of the signal was increased 8.0-fold in both BP1 and BP1-E cell lines [20]. Southern blot data also showed gene amplification in the same cell lines [20].

The *int-2* gene was first described as a cellular gene activated by insertional mutagenesis using the MMTV provirus in mouse mammary tumors. *int-2* is amplified in 10-20% of human breast cancers. Although the physiological role of this gene has not been clearly established, its homology with the fibroblast growth factor gene family suggests that it might play a role in several biological processes, such as differentiation and development. The *int-2* oncogene produces a 4.6-kb mRNA transcript that was present in the MCF-10F cell line. The intensity of the signal was increased 1.5-, 1.8-, 1.3- and 2.0-fold above the values found in MCF-10F control cells in BP1, BP1-E, D3 and D3-1 cell lines, respectively [20]. Our analysis showed that both, gene amplification and gene rearrangement were associated with increased mRNA levels in BP1, BP1-E and D3-1 cell lines. Genomic DNA changes may affect the level of transcription during the process of cell transformation, which, in turn, may facilitate the evolution of BP1 to BP1-E cells *(Figure 2)*.

The importance of *c-myc* in breast tumorigenesis has been demonstrated in transgenic mice in which overexpression of *c-myc* results in mammary cancer development. Over-expression of the *c-myc* gene as the result of translocation, mutation, or amplification has been implicated in the genesis and progression of a variety of human tumors, including breast cancer [28]. Amplification of the *c-myc* gene is present in 17-33% of primary human breast tumors. Northern blot analysis allowed us the characterization of the *c-myc* gene transcript as a single band of 2.3 kb in MCF-10F cells. The intensity of the signal was increased 1.5-fold only in in D3-1 cells, but none of the other cell lines studied exhibited any changes [20]. Thus, our data show that *c-neu, int-2,* and *c-myc* oncogenes are activated during the process of cell transformation induced by chemical carcinogens *(Figure 3)*.

Analysis of *p53* and *mdm2* genes

Loss of normal *p53* function is associated with cell transformation *in vitro* and tumor development *in vivo* [15]. Mutations in *p53*, mainly within exons 5-9, are observed in primary breast cancer; and are associated with a more aggresive biological behavior of tumors. Breast cancer cell lines have also been found to contain *p53* mutations [29]. During the progression from mortal to immortal, and from immortal to neoplastically transformed, MCF-10F cells and clones derived from carcinogen-treated cells have shown, when subjected to SSCP analysis of exons 5-9 of the *p53* gene, a conformational shift in exon 7 which was not present in MCF10-M mortal cells [16]. LOH of *p53*, on the other hand, was observed only in BP1-E tumor cells and in the cell line derived from BP1-E tumor, but not in any of the pretumorigenic cells (Figure 3). These observations indicate that the conformational shift in exon 7 might be associated with the immortalization, but not the progression of the neoplastic process, whereas LOH of p53 is associated with the emergence of the tumorigenic phenotype. These findings confirm Knudson's two hit hypothesis, according to which for inactivation of a tumor suppressor gene to occur, one allele must contain a point mutation or a small deletion, while the second allele must be lost by either an interstitial deletion, chromosome loss, or an aberrant mitotic recombinant event. Thus, in our case, LOH is manifested at the tumorigenic stage, whereas the mutation in the other allele of *p53* was an early event *(Figure 3)*.

Recent reports suggest that *mdm2* expression may be regulated by wild type *p53* [30]. Since the ability to regulate *mdm2* expression is lost in *p53* mutants, and MCF-10F and transformed cells have a demonstrable *p53* mutation, we hypothesized that *mdm2* expression might be altered in these cells. The Southern blot analysis of the Eco R1 digested genomic DNA of immortal MCF-10F and transformed cells did not reveal any demonstrable amplification of the *mdm2* gene in any of the cell lines studied. Northern analysis of total cellular RNA using *mdm2* specific cDNA, on the other hand, identified a 5.5Kb transcript in all the cell lines. An interesting observation was the 2.5 fold increased expression of the *mdm2* RNA transcript in the BP-1E cell line which was absent in the precursor cell line BP1 [16]. This observation is consistent with the progression of the BP-treated cell lines from BP1 to the tumorigenic and more aggressive clone BP1-E. Since *p53* protein was detectable in all the cell lines, including the parental cell lines, without increased *mdm2* expression, it is reasonable to suggest that upregulation of *mdm2* expression in BP-1E cells may have played a distinct role in the expression of the tumorigenic phenotype by BP-1E cells, apart from its *p53* binding effect *(Figure 3)*. This finding is supported by the reported amplification and overexpression of *mdm2* and *p53* mutation in human soft tissue sarcomas as alternative/exclusive regulatory mechanisms to inactivate the pathway to cell growth suppression.

LOH and fluorescence *in situ* hybridization (FISH) analysis of chromosome 17p

The fact that the highest frequency of allele loss in breast cancer has been reported in chromosome 17p [5, 31] suggests that genes located in that chromosome arm might be likely targets for this event. A gene located in the telomeric portion of chromosome 17p, on 17p13.3, distal to *p53*, has been observed to be lost in primary breast cancer [32]. LOH of this region, studied using the probe p144D6, has been found in 75% of primary breast cancers and in cells that are progesterone receptor negative. LOH of 17p has been associated with high cell proliferation in primry breast tumors, and with a shorter doubling time in the tumorigenic cell line BP1-E. A number of breast tumors have been reported to have lost the tip of 17p without affecting the *p53* gene, suggesting that a second gene, distinct from *p53*, may be involved in breast cancer. With this concept in mind we performed DNA analysis for allelic loss on chromosome 17p 13.3 using probes pYNZ22 and p144D6 for detecting variable number of tandem repeats (VNTR). The Southern blots showed that the cell lines MCF-10M and MCF-10F are heterozygous for probe pYNZ22. Clones D3, D3-1, BP1 and BP1-E, derived from DMBA and BP treated cells, respectively, showed the same heterozygous restriction length polymorphism pattern (RFLP). RFLP analysis with probe p144D6 revealed a heterozygous pattern in MCF-10M, MCF-10F cells and in clones D3, D3-1 and BP1. Only the cell line BP1-E exhibited

LOH when probed with p144D6. This phenomenon was also demonstrated by FISH analysis [33]. Conventional banding analysis did not reveal any alterations of 17p in either MCF-10F or BP1-E cells. FISH analysis showed that both p144D6 and the chromosome 17 centromeric probe hybridized to both copies of chromosome 17 in MCF-10F cells. In these cells, the hybridization signals were in parallel in both chromatids of both homologues. In transformed BP1-E cells, the 17 centromeric probe was positive, but the p144D6 probe did not hybridize both chromatids in the two homologues, but only two chromatids of one homologue were positive, indicating that LOH in the telomeric position of chromosome 17p was observed only in the cell line expressing the pretumorigenic phenotype [33].

Microsatellite instability in chromosomes 9,11, and 16

Five microsatellite markers for chromosome 9, twenty for chromosome 11, and fourteen for chromosome 16 were tested in MCF-10F cells, in clones D3, D3-1, BP1 and BP1-E, in tumors induced in SCID mice by BP1-E cells, and in cell lines derived from these tumors [23].
Microsatellite instability was detected in the loci 9p23 and 9p21-22 (markers D9S199 and D9S157), in BP1-E-induced tumor and in the cell line derived from it. Allelic gain in locus 9p21 was detected with marker D9S169, but no changes were observed with the marker D9S171 for the same locus. No changes were observed using the marker D9S165 that covered the locus 9p13-9q13.
The study of the chromosome 11 revealed LOH in loci 11q23 and 11q25 (markers D11S940 and D11S912, respectively), in the BP1 and BP1-E cells before the tumorigenic phenotype emerged; these changes were maintained in the tumors and in the cell lines derived from these tumors. The observed genetic instability might have contributed to the progression to tumorigenesis *(Figure 3)*. The fact that 17 out of the 20 markers used consistently showed LOH and rearrangement in both arms of chromosome 11 in the BP1-E tumors and in tumor cell lines, indicates that these changes took place during the process of tumorigenesis, a conclusion supported by the reported observations of LOHs in primary breast cancer *(Figure 3)*.
In chromosome 16 the pretumorigenic cell lines D3 and D3-1 showed allelic imbalance in locus 16q12.1, detected with marker D16S285. LOH was observed in BP1-E tumor and tumor-derived cell lines, detected with markers D16S423, D16S404, D16S418, D16S389, D16S398, D16S395, D16S422 and D16S449. LOH in this locus has been reported in 36% of breast cancer.

Summary and conclusions

We have developed an *in vitro* system of induction of neoplastic transformation of human breast epithelial cells with chemical carcinogens that is uniquely fitted for asking specific questions on the mechanisms of cancer initiation and progression. We have demonstrated that immortalization of MCF-10F cells is associated with a mutation in exon 7 of the *p53* tumor suppressor gene and the expression of a new set of genes that control cell proliferation and senescence [12] (Figure 1). One of the earliest genomic changes observed to be associated with the treatment of MCF-10F cells with the chemical carcinogens BP or DMBA was LOH and point mutations in codons 12 and 61 of *c-Ha-ras* gene. We also demonstrated that *int-2*, *c-neu* and *c-myc* oncogenes, known to be involved in breast cancer, are also activated during the process of chemically-induced *in vitro* cell transformation. As an intermediate and late change associated with the pretumorigenic phenotype, we have reported loss of the telomeric portion of chromosome 17p, overexpression of the *mdm2* gene, and MSI in chromosomes 9, 11 and 16 *(Figures 2, 3)*.

From all the models available for *in vitro* study of human breast cancer, the transformation of MCF-10F cells with chemical carcinogens is rather unique, in the sense that it allows researchers to examine the changes from a mortal cell (MCF-10M) from which MCF-10F cells were derived as an immortal cell line to the subsequent transformation with chemical carcinogens, mainly BP, that resulted in a pretumorigenic cell line that evolved to a tumorigenic cell line *(Figure 2)*. This model is a paradigm of the progressive nature of breast cancer. Although a step by step analogy with the pathogenesis of breast cancer, which is currently accepted starts as ductal hyperplasia, progressing to atypical ductal hyperplasia, intraductal carcinoma and invasive carcinoma, still needs to be done, there are several points in common with this *in vitro* model that deserve emphasis, namely: a) The immortalization of MCF-10M to MCF-10F cells may represent the stage of atypical ductal hyperplasia (ADH), since the cells composing these lesions are already clonal and with a higher proliferative activity. It is not known whether they are immortal. Although this phenomenon is difficult to be confirmed, the fact that one out of four ADHs evolve to carcinoma *in situ* may be an indication of immortality; b) Alterations in several oncogenes have been detected in early carcinomas *in situ*, an indication that the phenomenon occurs early in the transformation process; in our *in vitro* model, we observed that amplification and overexpression of several oncogenes emerge as the result of clonal selection; c) The LOH observed in chromosomes 9, 11, 16 and 17 in tumorigenic cells is similar to what is observed in primary invasive breast cancer. These preliminary data indicate that this experimental system will be useful for testing the functional role of these genes in the progression or reversion of the neoplastic phenotype, and for determining whether the expression of the tumorigenic phenotype is the result of a single event, or of a cascade of events, which might need to occur either sequentially or cumulatively.

Acknowledgments

This work was supported by grants R01 CA67238 of the National Institute of Health, PHS, and ESO 7280 from the National Institute of Environmental Health. Reprint requests and correspondence must be addressed to J. Russo, Breast Cancer Research Laboratory, Fox Chase Cancer Center, Philadelphia, PA 19111, USA.

References

1. Russo J, Gusterson BA, Rogers AE, Russo IH, Wellings SR, Van Zwieten MJ. Comparative study of human and rat mammary tumorigenesis. *Lab Invest* 1990; 62: 1-32.
2. Russo J, Rivera R, Russo IH. Influence of age and parity on the development of the human breast. *Breast Cancer Res Treat* 1992; 23: 211-8.
3. Page DL, Dupont WD. Anatomic markers of human premalignancy and risk breast cancer. *Cancer* 1990; 66: 1326-35.
4. Russo J, Calaf G, Sohi N, Tahin Q, Zhang PL, Alvarado ME, Estrada S, Russo IH. Critical steps in breast carcinogenesis. *New York Acad Sciences* 1993; 698: 1-20.
5. Callahan R, Campbell A. Mutations in human breast cancer: an overview. *J Natl Cancer Inst* 1989; 81: 1780-6.
6. Sato T, Tanigami A, Yamakawa K, Akiyama F, Kasumi F, Sakamoto G, Nakamura Y. Allelotype

of breast cancer: Cumulative allele losses promote tumor progression in primary breast cancer. *Cancer Res* 1990; 50: 7184-9.
7. Russo J, Mills MJ, Moussalli MJ, Russo IH. Influence of human breast development on the growth properties of primary cultures. *In Vitro Cell Develop Biol* 1989; 25: 643-9.
8. Soule HD, Maloney TM, Wolman SR, Peterson WD, Brenz R, McGrath CM, Russo J, Pauley RJ, Jones RF, Brooks SC. Isolation and characterization of a spontaneously immortalized human breast epithelial cell line, MCF-10. *Cancer Res* 1990; 50: 6075-86.
9. Tait L, Soule H, Russo J. Ultrastructural and immunocytochemical characterizations of an immortalized human breast epithelial cell line, MCF-10. *Cancer Res* 1990; 50: 6087-99.
10. Ochieng J, Tait L, Russo J. Calcium modulation on microtubule assembly in human breast epithelial cells. *In Vitro* 1990; 26: 318-24.
11. Ochieng J, Tahin QS, Booth CC, Russo J. Buffering of intracellular calcium in response to increased extracellular levels in mortal, immortal and transformed human breast epithelial cells. *J Cell Biochem* 1991; 46: 1-5.
12. Russo J, Zhang PL, Hu YF, Salicioni AM, Higgy NA. Isolation of genes related to the immortalization of breast epithelial cells. *Proc. Am Assoc Cancer* Res. 1996 (In press).
13. Band V, Dalal S, Delmolino L, and Androphy E J. Enhanced degradation of p53 protein in HPV-6 and BPV-1 E6 -immortalized human mammary epithelial cells. *EMBO J* 1993; 12: 1847-52.
14. Shay J W, Tomlinson G, Paityszek M A, Gollohoin L S. Spontaneous in vitro immortalization of breast epithelial cells from a patient with Li Fraumeni syndrome. *Mol Cell Biol* 1995; 15: 425-32.
15. Chang F, Syrjanen S and Syrjanen K. Implications of the p53 tumor-suppressor gene in clinical oncology. *J Clin Oncol* 1995; 13: 1009-22.
16. Barnabas N, Moraes R, Calaf G, Estrada S, Russo J. Role of p53 in MCF-10F cell immortalization and chemically-induced neoplastic transformation. *Int J Oncol* 1995; 7: 1289-96.
17. Russo J, Calaf G, Russo IH. A critical approach to the malignant transformation of human breast epithelial cells. *CRC Critical Rev Oncogen* 1993; 4: 403-17.
18. Calaf G, Russo J. Transformation of human breast epithelial cells by chemical carcinogens. *Carcinogenesis* 1993; 14: 483-92.
19. Zhang PL, Calaf G, Russo J. Allele loss and point mutation in codon 12 and 61 of the c-Ha-ras oncogene in carcinogen-transformed human breast epithelial cells. *Mol Carcinog* 1994; 9: 46-56.
20. Zhang PL, Chai YL, Ho TY, Calaf G, Russo J. Activation of c-myc, c-neu and int-2 oncogenes in the transformation of the human breast epithelial cell line in MCF-10F treated with chemical carcinogens *in vitro*. *Int J Oncol* 1995; 6: 963-8.
21. Russo J, Barnabas N, Zhang PL, Adesina K. Molecular basis of breast cell transformation. *Rad Oncol Invest* 1996 (In Press).
22. Barnabas N, Russo J. Allelic imbalance and loss of heterozygosity in chromosome 16 in human breast epithelial cells transformed by chemical carcinogens. *Proc Am Assoc Cancer Res* 1996 (In Press).
23. Wu YL., Russo J. Chromosome 11 microsatellite instability and loss of heterozygosity in human breast epithelial cells transformed by chemical carcinogens. *Proc Am Assoc Cancer Res* 1996 (In Press).
24. Barbacid M. ras genes. *Annu Rev. Biochem* 1987; 56: 779-827.
25. Rochlitz CF, Scott GK, Dodson JM, Liu E, Dollbaum C, Smith HS, Benz CC. Incidence of activating ras oncogene mutations associated with primary and metastatic human breast cancer. *Cancer Res* 1989; 49: 357-60.
26. Krontiris TG, DiMartino NA, Colb M, Parkinson DR. Unique allelic restriction fragments of the human Ha-ras locus in leukocyte and tumor DNAs of cancer patients. *Nature* 1985; 313: 369-74.
27. Peters G, Brookers S, Smith R, Dickson C. Tumorigenesis by mouse mammary tumor virus: Evidence for common region for provirus integration in mammary tumors. *Cell* 1983; 33: 369-77.
28. Guerin M, Barrois M, Terrier MJ: Overexpression of either c-myc or c-erbB-2 (neu) proto-oncogenes in human breast carcinomas: Correlation with poor prognosis. *Oncogene Res* 1988; 3: 21-31.
29. Bartek J, Iggo R, Gannon J, Lane DP. Genetic and immunochemical analysis of mutant p53 in human breast cancer cell lines. *Oncogene* 1990; 5: 893-9.
30. Juven T, Barak Y, Zauberman A, George DL, Oren M. Wild type p53 can mediate sequence-specific transactivation of an internal promoter within the mdm2 gene. *Oncogene* 1993; 8: 3411-6.

31. Devilee P, Cornelisse CJ. Genetics of human breast cancer. *Cancer Survey* 1990; 9: 605-30.
32. Kirchwerger R, Zellinger R, Schneeberger C, Speiser P, Lovason G, Theillet C. Patterns of allele losses suggest the existence of five distinct regions of LOH on chromosome 17 in breast cancer. *Int J Cancer* 1994; 56: 193.
33. Barnabas N, Bell D, Calaf G, Moraes RCB, Testa J, Russo J. Loss of heterozygosity on chromosome 17p loci in transformed *in vitro* human breast epithelial cells treated with chemical carcinogens. *Proc Am Assoc Cancer Res* 1993; 34: 649a.

Breast Cancer. Advances in biology and therapeutics.
F. Calvo, M. Crépin, H. Magdelenat, eds. John Libbey Eurotext © 1996, pp. 45-51.

Diet and endogenous hormones as risk factors for cancer of the breast: intervention studies

N.F. Boyd, L. Martin, G. Lockwood, C. Greenberg and D.L. Tritchler

Division of Epidemiology and Statistics, Ontario Cancer Institute, Toronto, Ontario, Canada

Problem of breast cancer

Breast cancer remains the commonest cause of death from cancer in women in most of the Western world, and the leading cause of death from all causes among women aged less than 50 [1]. Incidence of the disease has increased by about 1% per year over the past 10 years [2]. Mortality from the disease has not changed appreciably over an extended period of time [3]. There is however evidence that several factors influence the frequency of breast cancer in the population, and if these factors can be modified incidence might be reduced.

Risk factors for breast cancer

Breast cancer risk varies widely around the world and is about 5 times higher in North America, Northern Europe and Australia than in Japan and other Asian [4]. Migrants from lower risk countries to countries with higher risk of breast cancer acquire eventually the risk of the country to which they have moved [5, 6]. These data indicate that some feature of the environment exerts an important influence on risk of the disease. We discuss below the evidence that differences in diet may be responsible for some of the observed international variation in breast cancer rates.
There are also a number of identified factors that are known to affect breast cancer risk, many of them suggesting a role for sex hormone in the etiology of this malignancy which arises in an hormonally responsive tissue. The evidence that endogenous sex hormones influence risk of breast cancer has been reviewed extensively [7-10]. It includes the 100 fold difference in age specific incidence rates between males and females, the absence of the disease before puberty, the increase in risk that is associated with early age at menarche and late age at menopause, and the reduction in risk associated with an early first pregnancy. Risk of breast

cancer is reduced by oophorectomy, protection increasing the earlier in life the procedure is carried out. Several studies have found elevated levels of either total or free oestradiol in association either with breast cancer or in subjects at high risk for breast cancer, relative to controls [see references 9 for a review]. Populations at low risk for breast cancer have also repeatedly been shown to have low levels of oestrogen relative to populations at high risk for the disease. This difference in levels of oestrogens have been found in both pre- and postmenopausal women. For example among women aged 35-44 British women have been found to have oestradiol concentrations study 36% higher on average than those of Chinese women [11]. Comparisons of pre-menopausal Western women with Asian women living in Japan [12-14] or China [12, 15], or recent migrants to Hawaii [16], have also in general found lower oestrogen levels in the group of women at lower risk of breast cancer. In postmenopausal women it has been found that American whites have oestradiol levels 3 times those of recent Asian migrants to Hawaii [16], and similar results have been found in comparisons of British and Chinese women [11], and with rural Japanese women and white women living in Southern California [17]. These observations are consistent with the hypothesis that oestrogens play an important role in the etiology of breast cancer. Further support for the oestrogen hypothesis comes from the observation that obesity is a risk factor for the disease after the menopause, and is associated with elevated levels of oestradiol and reduced levels of sex hormone binding globulin [18, 19]. Parity appears to reduce levels of oestradiol and raise levels of sex hormone binding globulin [19,20], findings which may explain the protective effect of early pregnancy against breast cancer. The time of the menopause also influences risk of breast cancer. The age-incidence curve for breast cancer shows two slopes, with a steeper increase in breast cancer incidence with increasing age before the menopause and a less steep increase after the menopause. An early menopause reduces risk, with a 65-75% reduction in risk of breast cancer after early oopherectomy with no estrogen replacement.

Although controversial [21, 22], there is some recent evidence that exogenous hormones cause a modest increase risk of breast cancer after prolonged use [23-25]. Age at menarche is influenced by nutrition [26, 27] and it has been reported that dietary fat reduction in premenopausal and postmenopausal women reduces plasma levels of oestrogen [28-31]. We provide below further evidence for an effect of diet on ovarian function by describing the effect of dietary intervention on sex hormones and the time of menopause.

Dietary intake and breast cancer risk

Dietary fat intake influences breast cancer risk in animals [see 32-34 for reviews]. Increasing intake of dietary fat increases tumour incidence, increases the number of tumours that develop per animal, and decreases the latent interval before the appearance of tumours. When given with a carcinogen, dietary fat acts as a tumour promoter and appears to have an effect on tumorigenesis that is independent of caloric intake.

Human ecological studies, comparing breast cancer incidence or mortality with dietary fat consumption within countries, show that the more than 5 fold variation in breast cancer rates between countries is strongly correlated ($r = 0.8 - 0.9$) with international variation in estimated dietary fat intake [35]. Countries with the highest estimated fat intake in general also have the highest breast cancer rates, and countries with the lowest fat intake the lowest rates. These associations cannot be explained by differences in intake of total calories, by other dietary constituents, Gross National Product, height, weight, or age at menarche [35]. Further, while international breast cancer incidence rates differ more among postmenopausal than premenopausal women, there is a strong association at all ages between breast cancer incidence and estimates of dietary fat consumption.

Observational cohort and case control studies however have given much less consistent results [see references 36-40 for contradictory reviews]. We have calculated a summary relative risk for all published cohort and case control studies [41]. The summary relative risk for the 23 studies that examined fat as a nutrient was 1.12 (95% CI 1.04-1.21). Cohort studies had a summary relative risk of 1.01 (95% CI 0.90-1.13) and case control studies a relative risk of 1.21 (95% CI 1.10-1.34). Summary estimates of risk for specific types of fat excluded unity for only saturated fat. For the 19 studies that examined food intake, the summary statistically significant increases in relative risk were for meat, milk, and cheese. Regression analysis showed that European studies were more likely than studies done in other countries to show an increased relative risk associated with dietary fat and breast cancer, after taking into account potential modifying factors that included study design and quality. This finding suggests that there is greater variability in dietary fat intake in Europe than North America. A recently published combined analysis of 8 cohort studies found no association between dietary fat intake and risk of breast cancer [42].

The summary relative risks are in keeping with the risk expected based upon international data. The expected risk estimates are small because of homogeneity of fat intake within countries and the measurement error known to be associated with assessment of fat intake. Experimental trials, in which the range of fat intake is increased beyond that seen in most Western populations, are capable of overcoming the constraint imposed on observational epidemiology by the limited range of dietary fat intake seen within most countries, and would provide the strongest evidence available concerning a causal relationship of dietary fat intake to breast cancer risk. Further, such trials are the only means available to determine whether breast cancer risk in high risk subjects can be modified by changing dietary fat intake.

Diet and hormones

Observational evidence suggesting an influence of diet on hormone levels is available from comparisons of vegetarians and non-vegetarians, which have shown significantly higher levels of sex hormone binding globulin and lower urinary oestrogen excretion in vegetarians [43]. Other studies have shown that vegetarians excrete larger amounts of oestrogen in the feces than do omnivores, and significantly lower levels in the urine [44]. Vegetarians have also been found to have lower levels of plasma oestradiol than omnivores [44].

Experimental evidence showing the relationship between change in diet and change in hormone levels is available from several studies. These studies have generally involved small numbers of subjects, and without exception have been of short duration. They show however that the adoption of a low fat/high fiber diet is associated with a significant reduction of plasma oestrogen concentrations in a number of settings.

Previous work

We have adopted an experimental approach to examing the role of diet in the etiology of breast cancer to allow us to examine the effects of a wider range of fat intake on the breast. We are carrying out a multi-centre randomized controlled trial designed to determine whether, given optimal circumstances, the incidence of breast cancer in a high risk population can be reduced by an intervention involving a reduction in dietary fat intake and an increase in intake of complex carbohydrate. The general method used is to recruit subjects with extensive mammographic densities and enrol them in randomized trial of dietary intervention. The dietary intervention involves intensive individual counselling aimed at reducing total dietary fat to a target of 15% of calories. Controls receive general advice about diet but are not counselled to change their intake of fat. The results presented here are concerned only with the early effects of the dietary intervention on serum levels of sex hormones and the time of the menoapsue. Descriptions of other aspects of the trial can be found elsewhere [45-47].

Effect of dietary intervention on sex hormone levels

We have examined the early effects of intervention with a low fat-high carbohydrate diet on serum sex hormone levels in women taking part in this trial. Sex hormones were measured in 234 premenopausal and 91 postmenopausal subjects who have completed at least 2 years in the trial in bloods collected at entry, 12 and 24 months after randomization.

The results *(Table I)* showed that in premenopausal women in the intervention group (n = 123) estradiol fell 13% (51 pmol/L) over 2 years compared to a 0.3% decrease (0.9 pmol/L) in the control group (n = 111). FSH rose over 2 years by 73% (14.3 IU/L) in the intervention group compared to an increase of 36% (6 IU/L) in the controls. Samples taken 2 years after randomization and analyzed according to the time of the menstrual cycle in which blood was taken showed that estradiol was 30% lower in the intervention group in the latter half of the cycle (p = 0.04).

In postmenopausal subjects at 1 year, estradiol fell 30% (65.9 pmol/L) in the intervention group compared to a 20% (28.4 pmol/L) increase in controls (p = 0.04). At 2 years estradiol was 18% lower than baseline in the intervention group and 17% higher than baseline in controls (p = 0,09). At 1 year FSH increased by 12% (10.3 IU) in the intervention group and fell by 9% (7.4 IU) in controls (p = 0.08).

Because of the strong evidence linking ovarian hormonal activity to breast cancer risk these results suggest that a low-fat high-carbohydrate diet may reduce risk of breast cancer by reducing exposure to estradiol, a stimulus to cell division in the breast.

Effect of dietary intervention on time to menopause

We have examined the early effects of the dietary intervention on ovarian function in 695 premenopausal women taking part in this trial, who have completed at least 2 years in the trial, by noting the time after randomization of the menopause, defined as the cessation of menstrual activity for at least 6 months. The results show that membership in the intervention group was associated with an earlier time of menopause (log rank p = 0.05). By 48 months post randomization 20% of the intervention group had entered menopause while the control group didn't achieve 20% until 60 months. The group effect remains after taking into account the influence

Table I. Changes in sex hormones.

Hormone	Premenopausal			Postmenopausal		
	Intervention (n=123)	Control (n=111)	P value	Intervention (n=44)	Control (n=47)	P value
Progesterone (nmol/L)						
- baseline	12.3	16.3	0.21^2 $(0.13)^1$	7.0	4.9	0.51 (0.39)
- Δ at 1 year	-0.42	0.15	0.93^1	-4.5	-2.3	0.53
- Δ at 2 years	-4.3	-2.3	0.55^1	-4.8	-1.6	0.82
Time x Group			0.18^3			0.72
Estrogen (pmol/L)						
- baseline	384	359	0.79 (0.91)	220	143	0.05 (0.07)
- Δ at 1 year	-19.3	-14.3	0.90	65.9	28.4	0.04
- Δ at 2 years	-50.7	-0.9	0.30	-40.6	23.8	0.09
Time x Group			0.14			0.13
FSH (IU)						
- baseline	19.6	16.8	0.17 (0.07)	85.7	86.9	0.69 (0.73)
- Δ at 1 year	4.1	-0.8	0.17	10.3	-7.4	0.08
- Δ at 2 years	14.3	6.0	0.62	7.2	0.4	0.92
Time x Group			0.69			0.28
FSH/E_2						
- baseline	0.17	0.14	0.54 (0.31)	1.97	2.73	0.14 (0.14)
- Δ at 1 year	0.12	-0.01	0.30	0.54	-0.24	0.11
- Δ at 2 years	0.37	-0.02	0.15	0.91	-0.12	0.10
Time x Group			0.26			0.15

[1] Wilcox on 2-sample test.
[2] T test on logs.
[3] Repeated measures on logs.

of age and weight (risk ratio = 0.63; Cox regression p = 0.03). The effect of dietary intervention on time to menoapsue suggests that on emechanism by whci a low fat high carbohydrate diet may influence risk of breast cancer is by advancing the time of the menopause.

References

1. Boring CC, Squires TS, Tong T. Cancer Statisics, 1993. *Cancer J Clin* 1993; 43: 7-26.
2. Statistics Canada. Canadian Cancer Statistics 1992. Health and Welfare Canada 1994.
3. Bailar JC, Smith EM. Progress against cancer? *N Engl J Med* 1986; 314: 1226-32.
4. International Agency for Research on Cancer. Cancer in Five Continents. Vol. 6. Lyon, France: International Agency for Cancer Research, 1992.
5. Haenszel W, Kurihara M. Studies of Japanese migrants; mortality from cancer and other diseases among Japanese in the United States. *JNCI* 1968; 40: 43-68.

6. King H, Locke FB. Cancer mortality among Chinese in the United States. *J Natl Cancer Inst* 1980; 65: 1141-48.
7. Key TJA, Pike MC. The role of oestrogens and progestagens in the epidemiology and prevention of breast cancer. *Eur J Clin Oncol* 1988; 24: 29-43.
8. Pike MC, Spicer DV, Dahmoush L, Press MF. Estrogens, progestins, normal breast cell proliferation, and breast cancer risk. *Eur J Cancer* 1993; 15: 17-35.
9. Bernstein L, Ross RK. Endogenous hormones and breast cancer risk. *Epidemiol Rev* 1993; 15: 48-65.
10. Hulka BS, Margolin BH. Methodological Issues in Epidemiologic Studies Using Biologic Markers. *Am J Epidemiol* 1992; 135: 200-9.
11. Key TJA, Chen J, Wang DY, Pike MC, Borcham J. Sex hormones in women in rural China and in Britain. *Br J Cancer* 1990; 62: 631-6.
12. MacMahon B, Cole P, Brown JB, *et al*. Urine oestrogen profiles of Asian and North American women. *Int J Cancer* 1974; 14: 161-7.
13. Hayward JL, Greenwood FC, Glober G, *et al*. Endocrine status in normal British, Japanese and Hawaiian-Japanese women. *Eur J Cancer* 1978; 14: 1221-8.
14. Gray GE, Pike MC, Hirayama T, *et al*. Diet and hormone profiles in teenage girls in four countries at different risk for breast cancer. *Prev Med* 1982; 11: 108-13.
15. Bernstein L, Yuan JM, Ross RK, *et al*. Serum hormone levels in pre-menopausal Chinese women in Shanghai and white women in Los Angeles: results from two breast cancer case-control studies. *Cancer Causes and Control* 1990; 1: 51-8.
16. Goldin BR, Adlercreutz H, Gorbach SL, *et al*. The relationship between estrogen levels and diets of caucasian American and Oriental immigrant women. *Am J Clin Nutr* 1986; 44: 945-53.
17. Shimizu H, Ross RK, Bernstein L, Pike MC, Henderson BE. Serum oestrogen levels in postmenopausal women: comparison of American whites and Japanese in Japan. *Br J Cancer* 1990; 62: 451-3.
18. Anderson DC. Sex-hormone-binding globulin. *Clin Endocrinol* 1974; 3: 69-96.
19. Moore JW, Key TJA, Bulbrook RD, *et al*. Sex hormone binding globulin and risk factors for breast cancer in a population of normal women who had never used exogenous sex hormones. *Br J Cancer* 1987; 56: 661-6.
20. Bernstein L, Pike MC, Ross RK, Judd HL, Brown JB, Henderson BE. Estrogen and sex hormone-binding globulin levels in nulliparous and parous women. *J Natl Cancer Inst* 1985; 74: 741-5.
21. Prentice RL, Thomas DB. On the epidemiology of oral contraceptives and disease. *Adv Cancer Res* 1987; 49: 285-401.
22. Vessey MP. Exogenous hormones. In: Vessey MP, Gray M, eds. *Cancer Risks and Prevention*. Oxford: Oxford University Press, 1985.
23. UK National Case-Control Study Group. Oral contraceptive use in and breast cancer in young women. *Lancet* 1989; 1: 973-82.
24. Vessey MP, McPherson D, Villard-Mackintosh L, Yeates D. Oral contraceptives and breast cancer: latest findings in a large cohort study. *Br J Cancer* 1989; 59: 613-7.
25. Bergkvist L, Adami HO, Persson I, Hoover R, Schairer C. The risk of cancer after estrogen and estrogen-progestin replacement. *N Engl J Med* 1989; 321: 293-7.
26. Maclure M, Travis LB, Willett W, MacMahon B. A prospective cohort study of nutrient intake and age at menarche. *Am J Clin Nutr* 1991; 54: 649-56.
27. Merzenick H, Boeing G, Wahrendorf J. Dietary fat and sports activity as determinants for age at menarche. *Int J Epidemiol* 1993; 138: 217-24.
28. Rose DP, Boyar AP, Cohen C, Strong LE. Effect of a low-fat diet on hormone levels in women with cystic breast disease. I. Serum steriods and gonadotropins. *J Natl Cancer Inst* 1987; 78: 623-6.
29. Woods MN, Gorbach SL, Longcope C, Goldin BR, Dwyer J, Morrill-LaBrode A. Low-fat, high-fibre diet and serum estrone sulphate in premenopausal women. *Am J Clin Nutr* 1989; 49: 1179-83.
30. Ingram DM, Bennett FC, Willcox D, de Klerk N. Effect of low-fat diet on female sex hormone levels. *J Natl Cancer Inst* 1987; 79: 1225-9.
31. Goldin BR, Woods MN, Spiegelman DL, *et al*. The effect of dietary fat and fiber on serum estrogen concentrations in premenopausal women under controlled dietary conditions. *Cancer* 1994; 74: 25-31.
32. Rogers AE, Lee SY. Chemically induced mammary gland tumors in rats: modulation by dietary fat. In: Ip C, Birt DF, Rogers AE, Mettlin C, eds. Dietary Fat and Cancer. Progress in Clinical and Biological Research. Vol. 222, 1986: 255-82.

33. Freedman LS, Clifford C, Messina M. Analysis of dietary fat, calories, body weight and the development of mammary tumours in rats and mice: a review. *Cancer Res* 1990; 50: 5710-9.
34. Welsch CW. Relationship between dietary fat and experimental mammary tumorigenesis - A review and critique. *Cancer Res* 1992; 52: S2040-8.
35. Prentice RL, Kakar F, Hursting S, Sheppard L, Klein R, Kushi LH. Aspects of the rationale for the women's health trial. *J Natl Cancer Inst* 1988; 80: 802-14.
36. Goodwin P, Boyd NF. Critical appraisal of the evidence that dietary fat intake is related to breast cancer risk in humans. *J Nat Cancer Inst* 1987; 79: 473-85.
37. Willett WC, Stampfer MJ. Dietary fat and cancer: another view. *Cancer Causes and Control* 1990; 1: 103-9.
38. Prentice RL, Sheppard L. Dietary fat and cancer: consistency of the epidemiologic data, and disease prevention that may follow from a practical reduction in fat consumption. *Cancer Causes and Control* 1990; 1: 81-97.
39. Hunter DJ, Willett WC. Diet, body size, and breast cancer. *Epidemiol Rev* 1993; 15: 110-32.
40. Howe GR. Dietary fat and cancer. *Cancer Causes and Control* 1990; 1: 99-100.
41. Boyd NF, Martin LJ, Noffel M, Lockwood GA, Tritchler DL. A meta-analysis of studies of dietary fat and breast cancer risk. *Br J Cancer* 1993; 68: 627-36.
42. Hunter DJ, Spiegelman D, Adami HO, et al. Cohort studies of fat intake and the risk of breast cancer - a pooled analysis. *N Engl J Med* 1996; 334: 356-61.
43. Armstrong BK, Brown JB, Clarke HT, *et al.* Diet and reproductive hormones: a study of vegetarian and nonvegetarian postmenopausal women. *J Natl Cancer Inst* 1981; 67: 761-7.
44. Goldin BR, Adlercreutz H, Gorbach SL, *et al.* Estrogen excretion patterns and plasma levels in vegetarian and ominvorous women. *N Engl J Med* 1982; 307: 1542-7.
45. Lee-Han H, Cousins M, Beaton M, *et al.* Compliance in a randomized clinical trial of dietary fat reduction in patients with breast dysplasia. *Am J Clin Nutr* 1988; 48: 575-86.
46. Boyd NF, Cousins M, Beaton M, Kruikov V, Lockwood G, Tritchler D. Quantitative changes in dietary fat intake and serum cholesterol in women: results from a randomized, controlled trial. *Am J Clin Nutr* 1990; 52: 470-6.
47. Boyd NF, Cousins M, Lockwood G, Tritchler D. Dietary fat and breast cancer risk: the feasibility of a clinical trial of breast cancer prevention. *Lipids* 1992; 27: 821-6.

Breast Cancer. Advances in biology and therapeutics.
F. Calvo, M. Crépin, H. Magdelenat, eds. John Libbey Eurotext © 1996, pp. 53-59.

Multiple mechanisms of conjugated linoleic acid in mammary cancer prevention

Clement Ip

Department of Surgical Oncology, Roswell Park Cancer Institute, Buffalo, NY 14263, USA

Introduction

Conjugated linoleic acid (abbreviated henceforth to CLA) is a collective term that refers to a mixture of positional and geometric isomers of linoleic acid [1]. The two double bonds in CLA are in positions 9 and 11, or 10 and 12, along the carbon chain, thus giving rise to the designation of a conjugated diene. Each of the double bonds can be in the *cis* or *trans* configuration; the combination of *cis/trans* double bonds in the molecule accounts for the geometric isomers. CLA is normally found as a minor constituent in the lipid fraction of many different kinds of food [2]. Meat from ruminants generally contains more CLA than meat from non-ruminants. Milk, cheese and other dairy products are also good sources of CLA, while seafoods and vegetable oils are not. Although the biochemistry of CLA has been documented for decades in the literature, little is known about its nutritional activity or requirement [3]. More than 30 years ago, Bartlett and Chapman first reported that CLA was an intermediate in the microbial biohydrogenation of linoleic acid in butter fat [4]. Kepler *et al.* subsequently discovered that a rumen bacterium, *Butyrivibrio fibrisolvens*, was able to convert linoleic acid to stearic acid *via* CLA [5]. Microorganisms are not necessarily the major producer of CLA. There are additional factors which may facilitate the formation of CLA in cooked and processed foods. For example, grilling ground beef has been shown to increase the CLA content in beef fat by about 4-fold [1].

In contrast to linoleic acid which has been observed consistently to enhance mammary tumorigenesis in rodents over a wide concentration range [6-8], CLA expresses an inhibitory effect at levels of 1% or less in the diet [9, 10]. The studies demonstrating a cancer promoting effect of dietary linoleic acid were often conducted using vegetables oils (*e.g.* corn oil or safflower oil) which are rich in linoleate esterified to glycerol. CLA is likewise present naturally as a component of triglyceride in food. However, it should be noted that CLA was given as a free fatty acid in the previous animal mammary cancer prevention experiments [9, 10]. The reason that triglyceride-CLA is not routinely used *in vivo* is because of the prohibitive cost. In spite of that, the question has remained open as to whether the free fatty acid-CLA effect could be artifactual. We have recently shown that the cancer inhibitory effects of free fatty acid-CLA and triglyceride-CLA are very similar to each other [11]. This is an important observation because it rules out a nonspecific free fatty acid effect. In terms of practical implication, we can continue the *in vivo* research with the less expensive free fatty acid-CLA without compromising the physiological relevance of the data.

Effect of timing and duration of CLA supplementation on mammary cancer prevention

The rat mammary gland undergoes marked morphological changes during the first few weeks after weaning. We were interested in finding out whether exposure to CLA within this critical window of gland development was able to confer a protective effect against mammary carcinogenesis in the absence of sustained treatment. An experiment was undertaken in which rats were injected with methylnitrosourea (MNU) at either 42 or 56 days of age, and a 1% CLA diet was fed from weaning (21 days of age) up to the time of MNU administration. Thus the length of CLA feeding was limited to either 3 or 5 weeks, respectively, prior to MNU in the two supplemented groups. MNU is a direct alkylating agent and does not require metabolic activation. Because the design involved CLA feeding immediately before carcinogen treatment, the MNU model is ideal for this purpose, inasmuch as it obviates any potential confounding influence of CLA on carcinogen metabolism. The results, as reported in a recent paper [11], clearly indicated that exposure to CLA during the early post-weaning and adolescent period of the rat was sufficient in reducing the susceptibility of the mammary gland to subsequent carcinogen-induced neoplastic transformation. Total tumor yield was reduced by 47% or 42%, respectively, in rats which received the MNU dose at 42 or 56 days of age.

A second experiment with the MNU model was aimed at determining the effect of CLA feeding on the post-initiation phase of mammary carcinogenesis. CLA was given to rats immediately after MNU administration (dosed at 56 days of age) and was maintained for either 1, 2 or 5 months. All rats were sacrificed at 5 months post-MNU. The time course of tumor development in the different groups is shown in *Figure 1*. It is evident that short-term exposure to CLA for 1 or 2 months post-MNU was relatively ineffective in cancer protection. Significant inhibition ($P < 0.05$) was observed only in the group that received an uninterrupted supply of CLA in the diet.

Inhibitory effect of CLA in rats fed different levels or types of fat

The above cited studies on CLA chemoprevention [9-11] were carried out in rats fed a 5% (w/w) fat diet formulated with corn oil. Currently, there is no information as to whether an increase in the level of fat or a substitution in the type of fat in the diet might affect the cancer inhibitory efficacy of CLA. The following experiments were designed to address this question [12]. Because the anticancer agent of interest is a fatty acid, it is anticipated that the approach will provide some insight into its mechanism of action. For the fat level experiment, a custom-formulated fat blend was used that simulates the fatty acid composition of the US diet. This fat was present at 10%, 13.3%, 16.7% or 20% by weight in the rat diet. For the fat type experiment, a 20% (w/w) fat diet containing either corn oil (exclusively) or lard (predominan-

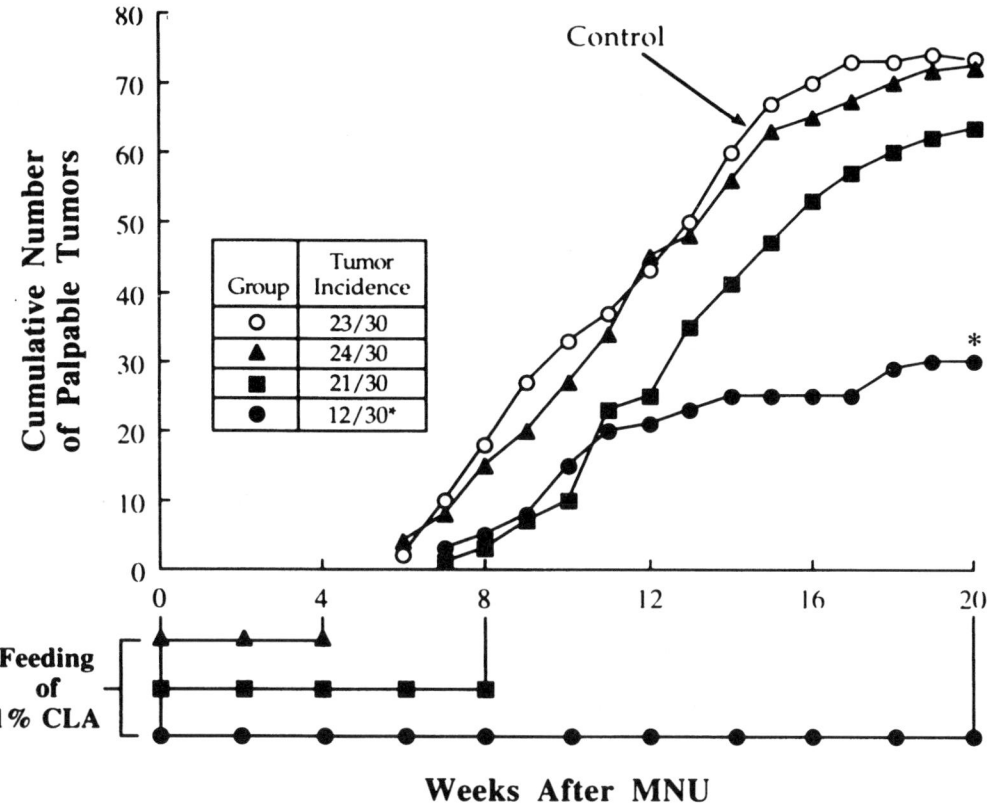

Figure 1. Effect of interrupted versus continuous CLA feeding after MNU administration on mammary carcinogenesis. The duration of CLA feeding in the 3 supplemented groups is indicated along the X-axis time line by the connected symbols (▲, ■ or ●). These symbols also match the time course of mammary tumor development shown on the main body of the diagram. Control group without CLA supplementation is represented by the open circle symbol. The asterisk denotes statistically significant difference ($P < 0.05$) from the control data. Reproduced from [11].

tly) was used. Corn oil and lard differ significantly in their content of linoleate. Therefore, changes in the inhibitory activity of CLA in the presence of these two fat types may point to a possible interaction between CLA and linoleic acid in modulating tumor development. Mammary cancer prevention by CLA under these various dietary conditions was evaluated using the rat dimethylbenz[a]anthracene (DMBA) model.

The results of these experiments indicated that the magnitude of tumor inhibition by 1% CLA was not influenced by the level of fat *(Figure 2)* or the type of fat in diet (data not shown but can be found in [12]). Fatty acid analysis in the mammary tissue showed that CLA was incorporated predominantly in neutral lipids, while the increase of CLA in phospholipids was minimal. Furthermore, there was no evidence that CLA supplementation perturbed the distribution of linoleate or other fatty acids in these two fractions. Collectively, the carcinogenesis and biochemical data suggest that the cancer preventive activity of CLA is unlikely to be mediated by interfering with the disposition or metabolism of linoleic acid.

Additionally, it should be pointed out that in the cancer prevention studies, a similar dose response to CLA at 1% and below was observed in rats fed either a 5% or 20% corn oil diet [9,12]. No further protection, however, was evident with the supplementation of CLA above 1% in both cases (unpublished data). The fact that the effect of CLA maximizes at 1% may indicate a limiting step in the capacity to convert CLA to some active product(s) which is essential for inhibition of carcinogenesis. Suffice it to note that the absorption of CLA is probably not a confounding factor here because tissue accumulation of CLA continues to rise with dietary levels above 1%.

The storage of CLA in mammary gland neutral lipids could portend the importance of this pool in providing a continuous supply of CLA for the generation of some active metabolite(s) in the target tissue. As illustrated by the data in *Figure 1* (similar results were also obtained in the DMBA model), the rate of tumor appearance rose after a short delay upon withdrawal of CLA feeding. We have unpublished data showing that the CLA concentration in mammary tissue neutral lipids decreased very rapidly if CLA was removed from the diet. By 4 weeks after withdrawal, the CLA content in the gland had essentially returned to basal level. Thus the time-dependent disappearance of CLA in mammary tissue neutral lipids seemed to correlate with the short delay in the gradual appearance of mammary tumors in the animals after CLA feeding was discontinued.

Discussion

CLA is not the only fatty acid known to inhibit carcinogenesis. Eicosapentaenoic acid and docosahexaenoic acid, which are representative of the n-3 polyunsaturated fatty acids in fish oil, also fit this category [13]. However, CLA differs from the fish oil fatty acids in two distinct aspects as far as their efficacies are concerned. Whereas fish oil is usually required at levels of about 10%, CLA at levels of 1% or less is sufficient to produce a significant cancer protective effect [10]. Additionally, there are a number of papers which have indicated that an optimal ratio of fish oil to linoleate in the diet is critical in achieving maximal tumor inhibition [14-16]. As can be seen from the present study, the potency of CLA in cancer prevention is largely dissociated from the quantity and type of dietary fats consumed by the host.

We have described the bi-modal activities of CLA in mammary cancer prevention. First, exposure to CLA during the early post-weaning and peri-pubertal period only (from 21 to 42 days of age) is sufficient to block subsequent tumorigenesis induced by a single dose of carcinogen given at 56 days of age. This observation suggests that CLA is able to effect certain changes in the immature mammary gland and render it less susceptible to neoplastic transformation at a later time. Second, CLA is also active in suppressing tumor promotion/progression. However, the mechanism of action is different from the first in that once the mammary cells have been initiated by a carcinogen, a continuous intake of CLA is necessary to achieve maximal inhibition.

According to the previous work of Russo and Russo [17], the rat mammary gland undergoes extensive morphological remodeling during the postnatal, prepubertal and pubertal period. At birth and in the first week of postnatal life, the mammary gland is made up of a single primary duct which branches into several secondary ducts. These ducts end in dilated club-shaped structures called terminal end buds. During the second and third week, additional sprouting of the ducts occurs, leading to a sharp increase in the number of terminal end buds. After reaching a peak at weaning (21 days of age), the terminal end buds begin to reduce markedly in size and number due to their differentiation to alveolar buds and lobules. By about 40 days of age, these latter structures are far more prevalent than the terminal end buds and their population density is approaching a morphological state seen in the mature gland. We reported previously that CLA suppressed the level of bromodeoxyuridine labeling in the lobulo-alveolar fraction [10]. The determination was made at about 55-60 days of age after 5 weeks of CLA feeding, *i.e.* at a time when there were few terminal end buds left. Chemical induced mammary carcinomas in the rat are believed to originate from terminal end bud cells and not from lobulo-alveolar cells [17]. Although it is reasonable to assume that the proliferative activity of the lobulo-alveolar cells may be indicative of that of the progenitor terminal end bud cells, further work is clearly necessary in order to delineate the role of CLA in modulating the kinetics of mammary gland development. In view of our present observation that the feeding of CLA from weaning to 42 days of age (a duration of only 3 weeks) is capable of protecting the mammary gland against tumorigenesis, it is critical to find out whether this protective effect is due to (a) a general decrease in proliferative activity during gland morphogenesis, (b) a change in the time course of gland maturation leading to a quantitative shift in gland composition, or (c) a specific response of target epithelial cells and/or the stromal component which surrounds the epithelial structures.

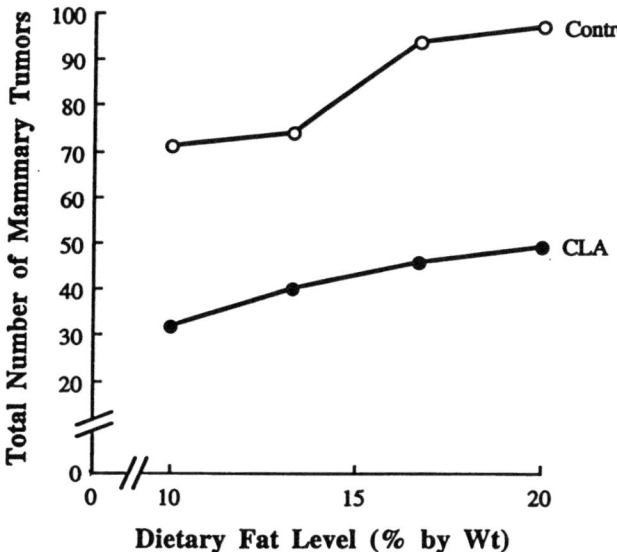

Figure 2. Mammary cancer prevention by CLA in rats fed different levels of fat. The composition of the blended fat used in this experiment was described in [12]. There were 32 rats in each group; all rats were treated with DMBA for the induction of mammary tumors.

For a rationale elucidation of how CLA might interfere with carcinogenesis after the mammary cells have been initiated, it might be profitable to consider the metabolic disposition of CLA in vivo. Being a fatty acid, CLA could potentially be (a) metabolized for energy, (b) incorporated as a component of membrane phospholipids and neutral lipids, or (c) converted to some other biologically active substances. The first route is unlikely to be of interest in the context of cancer prevention, while little is known about the significance of the last two alternatives. The presence of CLA in membrane phospholipids could conceivably be linked to the signal transduction pathway. This mechanism may modify the responsiveness to peptide stimulatory and/or inhibitory factors which are known to play an important role in regulating the proliferation, morphogenesis, differentiation and transformation of mammary epithelial cells. With respect to the neutral lipid CLA, it is possible that this pool may serve as the precursor to some as yet unidentified oxidized metabolites in the target tissue. Oxidation products of linoleic acid including hydroperoxy-, hydroxy- and oxooctadecadienoic acid, have been shown to express potent biological activity in a number of different systems [18,19]. It is possible that similar oxidation metabolites are produced from CLA. The intracellular effects of CLA might be multi-focal. Our objective at this point is to suggest certain potentially fruitful areas of research that could contribute to the understanding of the mechanism of action of CLA in cancer prevention.

References

1. Ha Y, Grimm NK, Pariza MW. Newly recognized anticarcinogenic fatty acids: Identification and quantification in natural and processed cheeses. *J Agricul Food Chem* 1989; 37: 75-81.
2. Chin SF, Liu W, Storkson JM, Ha YL, Pariza MW. Dietary sources of conjugated dienoic isomers of linoleic acid, a newly recognized class of anticarcinogens. *J Food Comp Anal* 1992; 5: 185-97.
3. Chin SF, Storkson JM, Albright KJ, Cook ME, Pariza MW. Conjugated linoleic acid is a growth factor for rats as shown by enhanced weight gain and improved feed efficiency. *J Nutr* 1994; 124: 2344-9.
4. Bartlet JC, Chapman DG. Detection of hydrogenated fats in butter fat by measurement of cis-trans conjugated unsaturation. *J Agric Food Chem* 1961; 9: 50-3.
5. Kepler CR, Hirons KP, McNeill JJ, Tove SB. Intermediates and products of the biohydrogenation of linoleic acid by *Butyrivibrio fibrisolvens*. *J Biol Chem* 1966; 241: 1350-4.
6. Ip C, Carter CA, Ip MM. Requirement of essential fatty acid for mammary tumorigenesis in the rat. *Cancer Res* 1985; 45: 1997-2001.
7. Fischer SM, Conti CJ, Locniskar M, Belury MA, Maldve RE, Lee ML, Leyton J, Slaga TJ, Bechtel DH. The effect of dietary fat on the rapid development of mammary tumors induced by 7,12-dimethylbenz(a)anthracene in SENCAR mice. *Cancer Res* 1992; 52: 662-6.
8. Welsch CW. Relationship between dietary fat and experimental mammary tumorigenesis. A review and critique. *Cancer Res* 1992; 52: 2040s-8s.
9. Ip C, Chin SF, Scimeca JA, Pariza MW. Mammary cancer prevention by conjugated dienoic derivative of linoleic acid. *Cancer Res* 1991; 51: 6118-24.
10. Ip C, Singh M, Thompson HJ, Scimeca J. Conjugated linoleic acid suppresses mammary carcinogenesis and proliferative activity of the mammary gland in the rat. *Cancer Res* 1994; 54: 1212-5.
11. Ip C, Scimeca JA, Thompson H. Effect of timing and duration of dietary conjugated linoleic acid on mammary cancer prevention. *Nutr Cancer* 1995; 24: 241-7.
12. Ip C, Briggs SP, Haegele, AD, Thompson HJ, Storkson J, Scimeca JA. The efficacy of conjugated linoleic acid in mammary gland prevention is independent of the level or type of fat in the diet. *Carcinogenesis* 1996; 17: 101-6.
13. Cave WT Jr. Dietary n-3 polyunsaturated fatty acid effects on animal tumorigenesis. *FASEB J* 1991; 5: 2160-6.
14. Ip C, Ip MM, Sylvester P. Relevance of trans fatty acids and fish oil in animal tumorigenesis studies. *Prog Clin Biol Res* 1986; 222: 283-94.
15. Cohen LA, Chen-Backlund JY, Sepkovic DW, Sugie S. Effect of varying proportions of dietary menhaden and corn oil on experimental rat mammary tumor promotion. *Lipids* 1993; 28: 449-56.
16. Rose DP, Rayburn J, Hatala MA, Connolly JM. Effects of dietary fish oil on fatty acids and eicosanoids in metastasizing human breast cancer cells. *Nutr Cancer* 1994; 22: 131-41.
17. Russo J, Tay LK, Russo IH. Differentiation of the mammary gland and susceptibility to carcinogenesis. *Breast Cancer Res Treat* 1982; 2: 5-73.
18. Buchanan MR, Haas TA, Lagarde M, Guichardant M. 13-Hydroxyoctadecadienoic acid is the vessel wall chemorepellant factor, LOX. *J Biol Chem* 1985; 260: 16056-9.
19. Bull AW, Nigro ND, Marnett LJ. Structural requirements for stimulation of colonic cell proliferation by oxidized fatty acids. *Cancer Res* 1988; 48: 1771-6.

n-3 polyunsaturated fatty acids and breast cancer

Claude Lhuillery*, Sophie Cognault*, Emmanuelle Germain*, Véronique Chajes** and Philippe Bougnoux**

* Laboratoire de Nutrition et Sécurité Alimentaire, INRA, 78352 Jouy-en-Josas, France
** Laboratoire de Biologie des Tumeurs, JE 313, Université de Tours, 37044 Tours, France

Abstract

In a prospective study with breast cancer patients, we have used the adipose tissue fatty acid composition as a biochemical marker of past fatty acid intake and have individualized α-linolenic acid (18:3n-3) to be potentially involved in breast cancer development. We have shown (in experimental carcinogenesis) that n-3 polyunsaturated fatty acid (PUFA) profile in mammary adipose tissue was not modified by mammary tumor growth and that PUFA modifications in breast cancer patients more likely depend on their dietary intake. Our recent results show that dietary n-3 PUFA effect on tumor growth largely depends on the presence in the diet of pro- and anti-oxidant micronutrients and suggest that the tumor-inhibitory effect of n-3 PUFA is linked to the generation of lipoperoxides. These data emphasize the need, in epidemiological and experimental studies, to consider the effects of PUFA in relation with micronutrients involved in oxidative status.

The influence of dietary fat on breast cancer risk and outcome is still highly controversial. Whereas more recent cohort studies [1] indicate that there is no association between total *amount* of dietary fat intake and breast cancer risk, there is, at the time, no clearcut conclusion on the influence of the *type* of ingested fat on breast cancer.
The n-6 and n-3 polyunsaturated fatty acids (PUFA) families are derived from precursor fatty acids: respectively, linoleic acid (18:2n-6) and α-linolenic acid (18:3n-3), which cannot be synthesized by humans and must be obtained from diet. They are therefore considered essential for humans. In experimental carcinogenesis studies, various models have shown that high levels of dietary n-6 PUFA stimulate tumor development whereas long chain n-3 PUFA (as in fish oil) do not [reviewed in 2-3]. Potential mechanisms have been reviewed [4].

The need for an approach based on biochemical indicators of past fatty acid intake

Difficulties in assessing the influence of the type of dietary fat in human studies partly arise from (I) the large variety of fatty acyl composition of ingested oils and fats and (II) the low quantities of some potentially active fatty acids (such as n-3 PUFA, for example). Dietary questionnaires are not precise and sensitive enough to evaluate dietary intake of such minor components and epidemiological studies based on these questionnaires cannot discriminate the potential influence of individualized fatty acids.

In humans, the adipose fatty acid composition is a good reflect of the type of ingested fat in the previous 2-3 years. For that reason, this composition has been used as a qualitative marker of dietary fat. Two recent north-american case-control studies, using adipose tissue composition as a marker, could not provide evidence for an association between specific fatty acids and breast cancer risk [5-6]. We performed a case-control study in breast cancer patients from the central part of France and, in line with the US studies, could not find clear differences between fatty acid profiles of breast adipose tissue from case and controls [7]. Presently, there is no data from prospective (cohort) studies using adipose tissue composition as a marker of past fat intake.

Breast adipose tissue and breast cancer outcome: a prospective study

Instead of using occurrence of breast primary tumor as the indicator of breast cancer in a prospective study with unselected women (incidence rate: 50 to 100 cases/year out of 100 000) we have performed a prospective study in a population of patients treated for breast cancer. We used the occurrence of metastasis (1 out of 3 patients) as the endpoint of the study [8]. A fragment of breast adipose tissue close to the tumor was obtained at the time of initial surgery and its fatty acid content was analyzed. We examined for each patient the relationship between each individual fatty acid in adipose tissue and the risk of subsequent metastasis and found that the likelihood for a patient to develop metastasis was increased (R.R. = 4,3) when α-linolenic acid (18:3n-3) in breast adipose tissue was low *(Figure 1)*.

Thus, human data obtained in this study individualized one essential polyunsaturated fatty acid (18:3n-3) to be potentially involved in tumor invasion and metastatic spread of breast cancer.

Low 18:3n-3 in adipose tissue and breast cancer growth: consequence or cause?

In the above study, it was not established whether low 18:3n-3 in patients with poor prognosis resulted from lower dietary intake of this essential fatty acid or from its increased metabolism due to tumor burden. At this point, it was thus critical to examine the *in vivo* influence of growing mammary tumors on the profile of fatty acids stored in contiguous adipose tissue. To address this question, we used a rat model of chemically-induced mammary carcinogenesis. Female Sprague-Dawley rats were fed a diet containing 10% fat as rapeseed oil (in which 9%

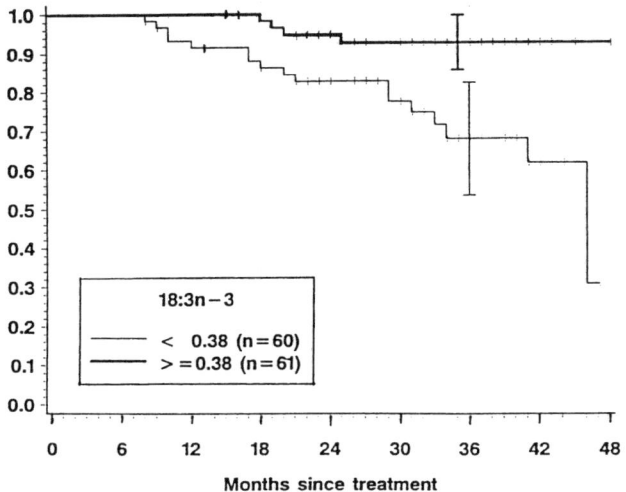

Figure 1. Metastasis-free survival according to breast adipose tissue level of 18:3n-3. The threshold for 18:3n-3 is the median (log-rank value 10.29, p < 0.001). Reprinted from [8].

of total fatty acids is 18:3n-3). Half of rats received an injection of nitroso-methylurea (NMU) to initiate mammary tumors. In control and NMU-treated groups, 3 to 5 animals were sacrificed every 3 weeks during the 5-month experimental time. Tumor growth was followed by weekly palpation of the animals and by the measure of total tumor mass and number in sacrificed rats. Mammary tumoral and adipose tissues were sampled in sacrificed rats. Fatty acid composition of adipose tissue was analyzed and confronted to tumor growth [9].

We found that although mammary adipose tissue fatty acid profile changed throughout the experiment, there was no difference in fatty acid profile between control and NMU-treated rats of the same age. In the NMU-treated group, 18:3n-3 level remained identical throughout the experimental period, irrespective of tumor burden as shown in *Figure 2*.

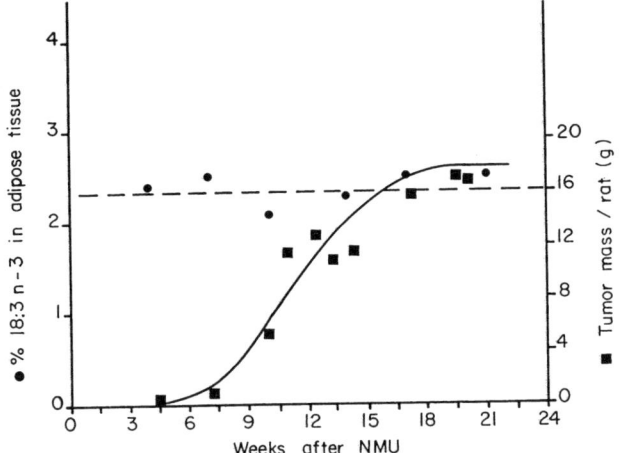

Figure 2. 18:3n-3 in mammary adipose tissue is not modified by the growth of mammary tumor in NMU-treated rats.

These data provide evidence that, in rats with controlled dietary fat intake, tumor growth and tumor burden do not significantly alter the fatty acid composition of mammary fat pad, even at early stages of tumor development. No selective removal of individual fatty acids by growing tumors could be detected. This holds true even for highly mobilizable fatty acids such as a-linolenic acid. These findings indicate that tumor growth does not interfere with host stored lipid composition and validate the use of adipose tissue composition as a marker of past fat intake and host lipid metabolism.

Finally, these data suggest that the low level of α-linolenic acid observed in adipose tissue of breast cancer patients with poor prognosis is not consequent to tumor growth but should be explained by other factors such as differences in lipid metabolism, and/or decreased α-linolenic acid storage in adipose tissue due to decreased supply.

Can dietary 18:3n-3 inhibit mammary tumor growth?

Very few experimental studies have specifically examined the role of this fatty acid on mammary tumor growth. The available data suggest that 18:3n-3 could attenuate tumor growth [10-12]. More information is available for long chain n-3 PUFA (C20 and C22) and it has been shown in various models that n-3 PUFA-enriched diets (such as fish oil diets) may have growth suppressive effects [2]. Various mechanisms have been proposed to explain this modulatory activity, such as interference with eicosanoid metabolism [4]. It has been proposed by different research groups that growth suppressive effects would be mediated -at least in part- through lipoperoxide generation [13]. Moreover, studies with breast cancer cell lines have shown that n-3 and n-6 PUFAs could inhibit cell proliferation, that cell growth could be restored by the addition of antioxidant molecules (vitamin E) or further decreased by the addition of oxidant molecules [14-15]. In the above animal and cell lines studies, growth modulatory effects of PUFA have been inversely correlated to lipid peroxidation products [15-16].

These observations indicating that some PUFA effects on tumor growth rely on lipid oxidation processes imply that the availability of anti- and pro-oxidant molecules to tumor cells may be a determinant factor in these effects.

Using the NMU-rat model of mammary carcinogenesis, we have recently shown that the promoting effect of high levels of dietary n-6 PUFA was considerably reduced when the amount of antioxidant molecules (*i.e.* vitamin E) was decreased in diet. At the end of the experiment, tumor incidence was 100% in the group fed normal amounts of antioxidant and only 40% in the group with a low level of antioxidants. Tumor number and mass were also higher in rats fed diet containing vitamin E than in the vitamin-deficient group *(Figures 3 and 4)*.

Tumor growth results from an inbalance between tumor cell proliferation (which increases tumor mass) and tumor cell loss (which decreases it). Therefore, in the above experiment, we have measured the percentage of tumor cells in S phase (as an index of proliferation) and apoptosis (as an index of cell loss) in tumors from both dietary groups. Preliminary results showed that the proportions of proliferating tumor cells (*i.e.* in S phase) were similar in both groups whereas tumor cell loss by apoptosis was decreased in tumors from high antioxidant group. Therefore, in the presence of high levels of PUFA in diet, antioxidants such as vitamin E may stimulate tumor growth by decreasing cell loss.

Our observations suggest that, although antioxidants such as vitamin E may have protecting effects at the earliest stages of carcinogenesis, they could, in the presence of a concomitant high intake of PUFA have deleterious effects on established tumors at later stages of carcinogenesis.

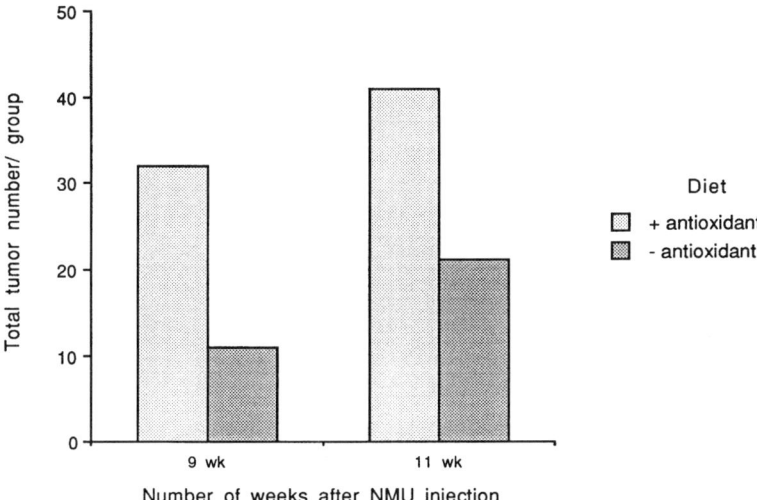

Figure 3. Tumor number is decreased in rats fed a high PUFA diet with a low amount of antioxidants.

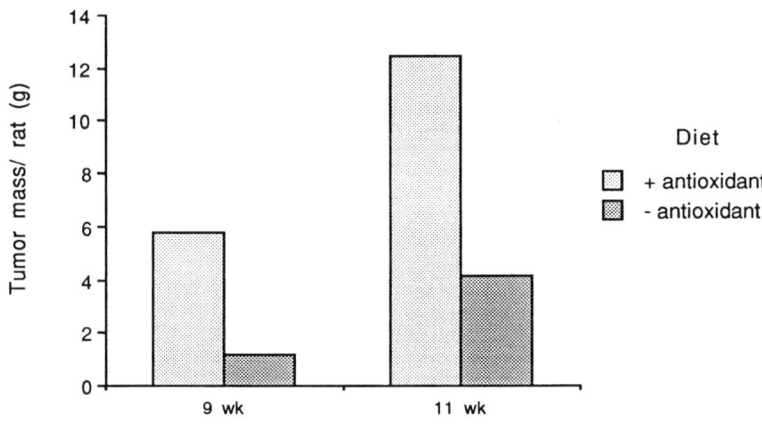

Figure 4. Tumor mass is decreased in rats fed a high PUFA diet with a low amount of antioxidants.

Conclusions

1. The potentiel involvement of n-3 PUFA in human breast cancer *risk* is still unresolved, although populations consuming high levels of n-3 PUFA in their diet (such as Eskimos or Japanese) have lower incidence of cancer. Recent results suggesting that n-3 PUFA could interfere with the *outcome* of breast cancer indicate there is a need for more research in this area.

2. From experimental data, a growing body of evidence shows that PUFA may have different modulatory effects according to their dietary « environment » (ratios n-6/n-3 for eicosanoid metabolism and oxidative status for PUFA in general).

May be it is necessary to remind the simple fact that diet is highly complex and that its overall effects on health are probably different from the effects of its elementary components. This is particularly true for PUFA. As a consequence, it seems important in epidemiological and experimental studies to take into account the effects of PUFA *in association* with other dietary components such as micronutrients involved in oxidative status. The emerging importance of lipid peroxidation (consequent to interactions between PUFA and oxidant or antioxidant molecules) in tumor growth emphasize the need for further research in this field.

Acknowledgements

This work was supported by grants from the INSERM (CRE 930301 and 930309) and from the Ligue Nationale contre le Cancer (Comités Départementaux du Loir-et-Cher et de la Charente).

References

1. Hunter DJ, Spiegelman D, Adami HO, Beeson L, van den Brandt PA, Folsom AR, Fraser GE, Goldbohm A, Graham S, Howe GR, Kushi LH, Marshall JR, McDermott A, Miller AB, Speizer FE, Wolk A, Yaun SS, Willett W. Cohort studies of fat intake and the risk of breast cancer - a pooled analysis. *N Engl J Med* 1996; 334: 356-61.
2. Cave WT. Dietary fat effects on animal models of breast cancer. *Adv Exp Biol Med* 1994; 364: 47-58.
3. Welsch CW. Relationship between dietary fat and experimental mammary tumorigenesis: a review and critique. *Cancer Res* 1992; 52: 2040s-8s (Suppl).
4. Welsch CW. Enhancement of mammary tumorigenesis by dietary fat: review of potential mechanisms. *Am J Clin Nutr* 1987; 45: 192-202.
5. London SJ, Sacks FM, Stampfer M, Henderson IC, Maclure M, Tomita A, Wood WC, Remine S, Robert NJ, Dmochowski JR, Willett W. Fatty acid composition of the subcutaneous adipose tissue and risk of proliferative benign breast disease and breast cancer. *J Natl Cancer Inst* 1993; 85: 785-93.
6. Petrek JA, Hudgins LC, Levine B, Ho MN, Hirsch J. Breast cancer risk and fatty acids in the breast and abdominal adipose tissues. *J Natl Cancer Inst* 1994; 86: 53-6.
7. Klein V. Acides gras alimentaires et risque de cancer du sein: étude cas-témoins basée sur la composition en acides gras du tissu adipeux mammaire de 209 patientes de la région de Tours. Thèse de Médecine. 1994. Université de Tours, France.
8. Bougnoux P, Koscielny S, Chajès V, Descamps P, Couet C, Calais G. α-linolenic acid content of adipose breast tissue: a host determinant of the risk of early metastasis in breast cancer. *Br J Cancer* 1994; 70: 330-4.
9. Lhuillery C, Bougnoux P, Groscolas R, Durand G. Time-course study of adipose tissue fatty acid

composition during mammary tumor growth in rats with controlled fat intake. *Nutr Cancer* 1995; 24: 299-309.
10. Kamano K, Okuyama H, Konishi R, Nagasawa H. Effects of a high-linoleate and high a-linolenate diet on spontaneous mammary tumorigenesis in mice. *Anticancer Res* 1989; 9: 1903-8.
11. Fritsche KL, Johnston PV. Effect of dietary α-linolenic acid on growth, metastasis, fatty acid profile and prostaglandin production of two murine mammary adenocarcinomas. *J Nutr* 1990; 120: 1601-9.
12. Hirose M, Masuda A, Ito N, Kamano K, Okuyama H. Effects of dietary perilla oil, soybeam oil and safflower oil on 7,12-dimethylbenz-(a)-anthracene (DMBA) and 1,2-dimethylhydrazine (DMH)-induced mammary gland and colon carcinogenesis in female SD rats. *Carcinogenesis* 1990; 11: 731-5.
13. Gonzalez MJ. Fish oil, lipid peroxidation and mammary tumor growth. *J Am Coll Nutr* 1995; 14: 325-35.
14. Bégin ME, Ells G, Das UN, Horrobin DF. Differential killing of human carcinoma cells supplemented with n-3 and n-6 polyunsaturated fatty acids. *J Natl Cancer Inst* 1986; 77: 1053-62.
15. Chajès V, Sattler W, Stranztl A, Kostner GM. Influence of n-3 fatty acids on the growth of human breast cancer cells *in vitro*: relationship to peroxides and vitamin E. *Breast Cancer Res Treat* 1995; 34: 199-212.
16. Gonzalez MJ, Schemmel RA, Dugan L, Gray JI, Welsch C. Dietary fish oil inhibits human breast carcinoma growth: a function of increased lipid peroxidation. *Lipids* 1993; 28: 827-32.

Breast cancer screening.
The scientific basis and the Danish programme

Elsebeth Lynge

Danish Cancer Society, Strandboulevarden 49, DK-2100 København Ø, Denmark

Introduction

Breast cancer is the most frequent cancer in women in developed countries. In Denmark 8% of women, who survive to the age of 75 years, will develop breast cancer. Apart from genetic susceptibility known to account for a small proportion of breast cancers, the best documented risk factor is late age at first birth. Based on the available knowledge of the etiology primary prevention of breast cancer is thus difficult.

Although breast cancer is not one of the most lethal cancers; the age-adjusted 5-year relative survival for all breast cancer patients in Denmark is 65%. But the survival has improved only slightly over the past twenty years.

The survival is very sensitive to extend of disease at time of diagnosis, and breast cancer is therefore a disease for which early detection is expected to improve the patients' prognosis.

Evidence for the effect of mammographic screening

Mammography is a method for detection of non-palpable lesions in the breast. The aim of mammography screening is thus early detection of already developed invasive lesions.

This means that the parameter of interest for the successful outcome of a mammographic screening programme is reduction in the breast cancer mortality

Mammography screening has been evaluated in several randomised trials. These studies are listed in *Table I*. In total, 260,000 women have been enrolled in the study arms of these trials, and 226,000 women in the control arms. The latest data on reduction in the mortality from breast cancer from these trials are shown in *Table II*. The first pooled analysis of data from the five Swedish trials included all deaths before 1 January 1990 [4]. For the age-group 50-69 years this analysis showed a 29% reduction in breast cancer mortality among the scree

Table I. Randomised trials for assessment of the effect of breast cancer screening with mammography.

Place	Year of initiation	Age at entry	Design I: Study group II: Control group	Screening method	Screening interval	Participation in round	References
HIP, New York, USA	1963	40-64	HIB-members, individually randomised I: 31,000 II: 31,000	I: Physical examination + 2-view mammography II: Standard service	12 months (4 rounds)	65%	1,2
Malmö, Sweden	1976	45-70	Individually randomised I: 21,000 II: 21,000	I: 2-view mammography 1- or 2-view in subsequent rounds II: Standard service	18-24 months	74%	3,4
Kopperberg and Östergotland, (WE), Sweden	1977-78	40-74	Municipality randomisation I: 78,000 II: 57,000	I: 1-view mammography II: Standard service	40-49: 24 and later 22 months 50-74: 33 and later 24 months	89%	4,5
Edinburgh	1979	45-64	Practices I: 23,000 II: 22,000	I: Physical examination + mammography II: Standard service	24 months for mammography	61%	6,7
Canada	1980	40-49	Volunteers, individually randomised I: 25,000 II: 25,000	I: Physical examination + mammography + BSE II: Physical examination at entry + BSE	12 months	88% (2 rounds)	8
	1980	50-59	Volunteers, individually randomised I: 20,000 II: 20,000	I: Physical examination + mammography + BSE II: Physical examination annually + BSE	12 months	89% (2 rounds)	9
Stockholm	1981	40-65	Individually randomised I: 40,000 II: 20,000	I: 1-view mammography II: Standard service, later mammography	28 months	82%	4,10
Göteborg	1982	40-59	Individually randomised I: 22,000 II: 30,000	I: Mammography II: Standard service	18 months	84%	4

ned women compared with the non-screened. The evidence for a reduction in breast cancer mortality in this age group is somewhat weaker for the three non-Swedish studies [2, 7, 9], but they point in the same direction. It thus seems prudent to conclude that it is possible to reduce the breast cancer mortality in 50-69 year old women by 25-30% by regular mammography screening.

Table II. Relative risks for breast cancer mortality in screening groups compared to control groups in randomised trials for assessment of the effect of breast cancer screening with mammography.

	40-49 years			50-ca. 70 years		
	Follow-up in years	RR 95% CI	Reference	Follow-up in years	95% CI	Reference
Sweden						
Malmø	15y	0.67 (0.35-1.27)	12	11.4y	NR	
Kopperberg (W)	14y	0.67 (0.37-1.22)	12	9.9y	NR	
Östergötland (E)	13y	1.02 (0.59-1.77)	12	8.8y	NR	
Stockholm	11y	1.08 (0.54-2.17)	12	6.7y	NR	
Göteborg	10y	0.59 (0.33-1.06)	12	5.8y	NR	
Sweden total	-	0.77 (0.59-1.01)	12	-	0.71 (0.57-0.90)	4
Other trials						
HIP, New York	18y	0.77 (0.53-1.11)	12	18y	0.79 (0.65-0.97)	2
Edinburgh	min 10y	0.73 (0.43-1.25)	12	10y	0.85 (0.62-1.15)	7
Canada	9y	1.36 (0.84-2.21)	8	9y	0.97 (0.62-1.52)	9
All trials		0.83 (0.69-1.00)	12	-	NR	

For women who started screening at age 40-49, the first pooled analysis of the Swedish trials showed a 13% statistically non-significant reduction in breast cancer mortality. This picture had, however, changed when the results of updated analysis including all deaths before 1 January 1995 were released recently [11]. This update showed a 23% reduction in breast cancer mortality at the borderline of statistical significance. This result is in line with the data from the HIP [11] and Edinburgh [11] trials. The only outlier is the Canadian study which showed a 35% increase in breast cancer mortality in the screened group compared with the controls [8]. The data therefore relatively consistently indicate that a 20-25% reduction in breast cancer mortality is possible among women who start screening at age 40-49 years.

The Danish programme

In Denmark, mammography screening was latest reviewed by the National Board of Health in 1994 [12]. Data were at that time available only from the first pooled analysis of the Swedish trials [4]. The recommendation from the National Board of Health were as follows:
1. all countries should establish an efficient and thoroughly integrated diagnostic system,

2. countries running or planning mammography screening should initiate studies on the psychological consequences,
3. experiences should be collected systematically and the running or planning activities should be evaluated in countries not offering mammographic screening,
4. a national counselling and evaluation group should be established to assist with this evaluation,
5. in setting priorities for the future prevention and treatment, the individual counties should consider the report and recommendations from the National Board of Health, and
6. mammographic screening should be reevaluated by the National Board of Health in 3-5 years time depending on the development.

The Minister of Health approved these recommendations on 26 May 1994.

Three mammography screening programmes are at present running in Denmark, all covering women aged 50-69 years with biannual screening. These programmes in total cover 18% of Danish women aged 50-69 years. The participating rate in the first screening round was 70.6% in Copenhagen [13] and 88.1% in Fyn [personnal communication, Walter Schwartz, 1996]. For comparison 5.3% of women aged 50-69 years were estimated to have a mammogram taken outside the organised screening programmes in the two-year period 1990-91 [14].

Table III. Organised mammography screening and other mammography examinations of women aged 50-69 years in Denmark.

Region	Start of screening programme	Number of women aged 50-69	Participation rate in first screening round	Reference
Copenhagen municipality	1 April 1991	40,000	70.6%	13
Fyn county	2 Nov 1993	50,000	88,1%	personal communication W. Schwartz, 1996
Frederiksberg municipality	Mid June 1994	10,000	NR	NR
Rest of Denmark	None	450,000	5.3%[1]	14

1. Estimated percent of 50-69 year old women with at least one mammogram outside an organised programme during the two-year period 1990-91.

The possible introduction of organised mammography screening has been considered in all the 16 Danish countries; only one additional county has up until now decided in principle to start screening, but the date for starting has not been decided upon yet.

References

1. Shapiro S, Venet W, Strax P, Venet L, Roeser R. Ten- to fourteen-year effect of screening on breast cancer mortality. *JNCI* 1982; 69: 349-55.
2. Chu KC, Smart CR, Tarone RE. Analysis of breast cancer mortality and stage distribution by age for the Health Insurance Plan Clinical Trial. *JNCI* 1988; 80: 1125-32.

3. Andersson I, Aspegren K, Janzon L, Landberg T, Lindholm K, Linell F, Ljungberg O, Ranstam J, Sigfússon B. Mammographic screening and mortality from breast cancer: the Malmo mammographic screening trial. *BMJ* 1988; 297: 943-8.
4. Nyström L, Rutqvist LE, Wall S, Lindgren A, Lindqvist M, Rydén S, Andersson I, Bjurstam N, Fagerberg G, Frisell J, Tabár L, Larsson L-G. Breast cancer screening with mammography: overview of Swedish randomised trials. *Lancet* 1993; 341: 973-8.
5. Tabár L, Fagerberg G, Gad A, Baldetorp L, Holmberg LH, Gröntoft O, Ljungquist U, Lundström B, Manson JC, Ekelund G, Day NE, Pettersson F. Reduction in mortality from breast cancer after mass screening with mammography. *Lancet* 1985; i: 829-32.
6. Roberts MM, Alexander FE, Anderson TJ, Chetty U, Donnan PT, Forrest P, Hepburn W, Huggins A, Kirkpatrick AE, Lamb J, Muir BB, Prescott RJ. Edinburgh trial of screening for breast cancer: mortality at seven years. *Lancet* 1990; 335: 241-6.
7. Alexander FE, Anderson TJ, Brown HK, Forrest APM, Hepburn W, Kirkpatrick AE, McDonald C, Muir BB, Prescott RJ, Shepherd SM, Smith A, Warner J. The Edinburgh randomised trial of breast cancer screening: results after 10 years of follow-up. *Br J Cancer* 1994; 70: 542-8.
8. Miller AB, Baines CJ, To T, Wall C. Canadian National Breast Screening Study: 1. Breast cancer detection and death rates among women aged 40 to 49 years. *Can Med Assoc J* 1992; 147: 1459-76.
9. Miller AB, Baines CJ, To T, Wall C. Canadian National Breast Screening Study: 2. Breast cancer detection and death rates among women aged 50 to 59 years. *Can Med Assoc J* 1992; 147: 1477-88.
10. Frisell J, Eklund G, Hellström L, Glas U, Somell A. The Stockholm breast cancer screening trial - 5-year results and stage at discovery. *Breast Cancer Res Treat* 1989; 13: 79-87.
11. The Swedish Cancer Society and the Swedish National Board of Health and Welfare. The impact of breast cancer screening with mammography in women aged 40-49 years. An International Conference under the auspices of the Swedish Cancer Society and the Swedish National Board of Health and Welfare. Falun: The Swedish Cancer Society and the Swedish National Board of Health and Welfare, 1996.
12. The National Board of Health. Breast cancer - Early detection and examination. A review. Copenhagen: National Board of Health, 1994.
13. Jorgensen T, Jensen LB, Duun S, Hirsch FR, Mouridsen HT, Blichert-Toft M, Rank FE, Christensen LH, Hansen AG, Nissen FH, Pedersen KLD, Nielsen AL, Francis D, Bertelsen S, Schiodt T, Olesen KP. Mammography screening in Copenhagen. *Ugeskr Læger* 1996; 158: 1212-7.
14. Andreasen AH, Andersen KW, Madsen M, Mouridsen HT, Olesen KP, Lynge E. Mammographic examinations in Denmark, 1990-1991. *Ugeskr Læger* 1994; 156: 6517-20.

Breast cancer screening. The relations with the hospitals and sanitary organisations in the United Kingdom

Julietta Patnick

NHS Breast Screening Programme, The Manor House, 260 Ecclesall Road South, Sheffield S11 9PS, England

The United Kingdom, since 1948, has had a National Health Service (NHS), paid for from public taxation and free at the point of delivery. However, each locality has responsibility for its healthcare vested in a local District Health Authority (DHA). Hospitals are run by National Health Service Trusts which sell services to the DHAs. Thus the NHS in the UK operates on an internal market basis, with DHAs being purchasers of health care on behalf of their population, and Trusts being providers.

The operation of the NHS is overseen by the NHS Executive. This is a branch of the civil service and within the Department of Health. It is accountable to elected Government ministers and Parliament. There are 8 regional offices. Scotland, Wales and Northern Ireland each have their own health service.

The NHS Breast Screening Programme was established in 1988 following Sir Patrick Forrest's report to the Health Ministers of England, Scotland, Northern Ireland and Wales. From the beginning it was recognised that, to be effective, a national screening programme should have national standards set and a clear national policy structure established. We could learn from the mistakes of the cervical screening programme which, at that time, was not well organised or coherent. In 1988 the NHS operated under a different structure. Responsibility for implementing breast screening was given to the 14 regional health authorities which existed then. Hospitals were run by district health authorities and the internal market was not yet on the scene. This system was much more top heavy than the one we have today and the screening programme was introduced in a fairly centrist manner.

The NHS Breast Screening Programme is nationally coordinated and locally delivered. The only people it directly employs are the twelve people in the national office. All other staff who work in the programme are employed by the NHS hospital Trusts. The service is funded by purchasers who buy from the Trusts.

The primary health care team is where the screening programme has its roots. Each family doctor's list is held by the local Health Authority. These lists are searched to draw up a batch of women aged 50 to 64 who are due for screening. Once the family doctor has checked the list, the women are invited for screening by the local screening programme based in a Trust. The family doctor is kept informed at all stages of the screening process and is consulted when referral for treatment is required. Quite often there is a standing arrangement between a family doctor and the local screening programme for referral.

So how does it work? In the beginning, health authorities were told how much to spend and where to buy from. But since the advent of the internal market in 1992, this is no longer the way we do things. Nationally we put a great deal of effort into producing guidelines and specifications. They are developed and agreed by professionals in tandem with the Royal Colleges. These guidelines are circulated to Trusts and DHAs who must comply with them. Monitoring of performance is a vital part of making sure the system works. We have in place a quality assurance structure which monitors each individual screening programme. This is funded by purchasers, but is accountable to the local regional office of the NHS Executive. In this way, impartiality is maintained and both providers and purchasers can have their performance monitored. In addition, the national office takes an energetic role and can hold purchasers to account.

Our quality assurance structure *(Figure 1)* brings together groups of professionals who both define our standards and guidelines and monitor performance against them. The system depends upon peer review and professional competence. Formal accreditation does not exist in the UK. We are reliant upon the structure of the NHS to create and maintain good standards of care.

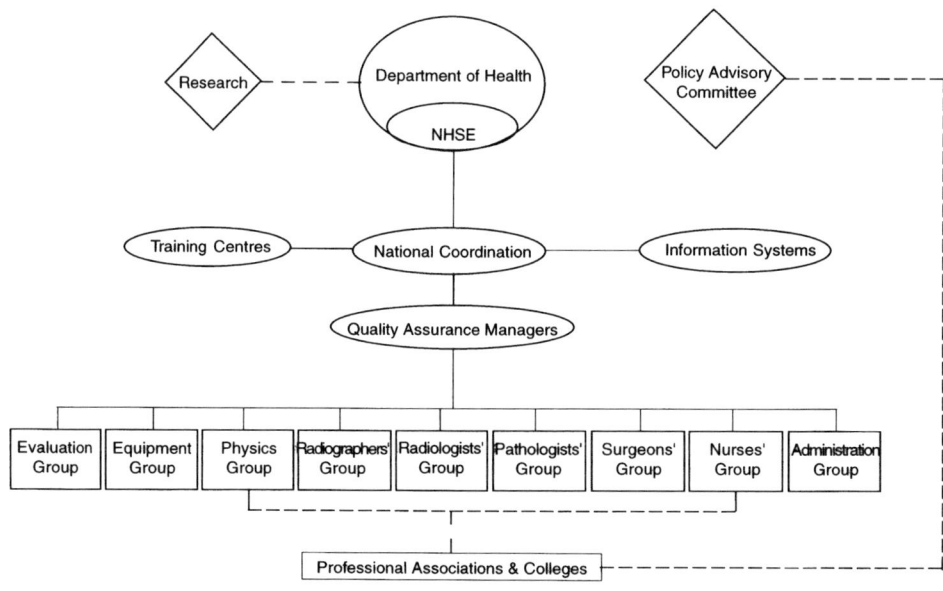

Figure 1. UK quality assurance structure.

The private sector is subject to radiation protection and cancer legislation, but since there is no formal accreditation, standards can vary from the very high to the quite poor. We endeavour to build links with the private screening services. However, since we have a « free » health service, they are not major providers on a national basis although they are prominent in some localities.

The charities in the United Kingdom play a vital role in encouraging women to come forward for breast screening. Almost 2/3 of women aged 50-64 have been screened in the last 3 years.

Uptake amongst invited women is rising and this is, in part, due to our partnership with the voluntary sector.

We work closely with the cancer registries in the UK. This is essential since we wish to identify our interval cancers, monitor incidence and mortality rates and undertake other evaluation exercises. Cancer Registries are organised on a regional basis by the NHS and do not have a national office similar to my own. There are 11 in England alone. This can make coordination difficult at times.

Since the NHS Breast Screening Programme was established in 1988, the NHS has been reorganised into the structure described here. If we have a change of Government, the structure may change again. Our emphasis on quality assurance and national guidelines has proved our strength and allowed us the flexibility to bend and change with the direction of Government policy.

The French national breast cancer screening programme

R.A. Ancelle-Park[1], B. Seradour[2], P. Schaffer[3] and H. Allemand[4]

[1] DGS, Paris ; [2] ARCADES, Marseille ; [3] ADEMAS, Strasbourg ; [4] CNAMTS, Paris, France

Breast cancer is the most frequent cancer in women. In developed countries breast cancer accounts for approximately 30% of cancer deaths in this population. Many studies have been conducted world wide to assess the impact of screening on the reduction of cancer mortality. Many district or regional programmes have been set up in various areas of the world; however, few countries have adopted a national breast cancer screening programme.

In France a pilot programme was set up in 1989 by the prevention department of the national health service fund (CNAMTS) to test the applicability of an organized breast cancer screening programme within a decentralized private radiology sector. This pilot programme comprised 10 districts, six included in 1989 and four in 1991.

In 1994 the French ministry of health decided to establish a national programme to provide, in the frame of a strict organisation, a free mammography test to all french women aged 50 to 69. A national pilot committee together with a programme management group and a coordinating team were set up at the level of the department of health. This paper presents the French breast cancer model and the basic results.

Methods

The programme is organized at a district level and is based on the existing private and public radiologic facilities. Each district programme is run independently. According to the national protocol, the screening programmes invite women aged 50 to 69. Women of the target population are invited every three years to refer to the radiologist of their choice, to perform a free mammography test. Participating radiologists sign an agreement form which commits them to, attend specific training, perform a single-view mammogram, submit their views to double reading (colleague or expert committee), and perform regular control of the quality of their equipment. Pathologists established in the district also sign an agreement form regarding quality control and biopsy data collection.

Evaluation of the programme is undertaken at a national level. Districts are requested to return data to the national coordinating unit on a yearly base according to a standard format.

The aim of the national programme is to progressively extend screening programmes to the whole of the French territory (100 districts). Districts who wish to set up a programme have to present to the national programme management group the organisation they have chosen. The programme management group analyses the proposed programme and assesses whether it is in agreement and fits the national protocol. Nine additional district programmes have been set up since the implementation of the national programme. To date the national programme comprises 19 districts out of 100: six pilot programmes started in 1989, Ardennes, Alpes-Maritimes, Bas-Rhin, Bouches-du-Rhône, Rhône, Sarthe, and four started end 1990 beginning 1991, Isère, Marne, Somme, Val-d'Oise. Three programmes started in 1994, Ille-et-Vilaine, Mayenne, Allier, three programmes started end 1995 beginning 1996 Loire, Puy-de-Dôme, Var and 3 started in june 1996, Haute-Vienne, Loire-Atlantique, Calvados.

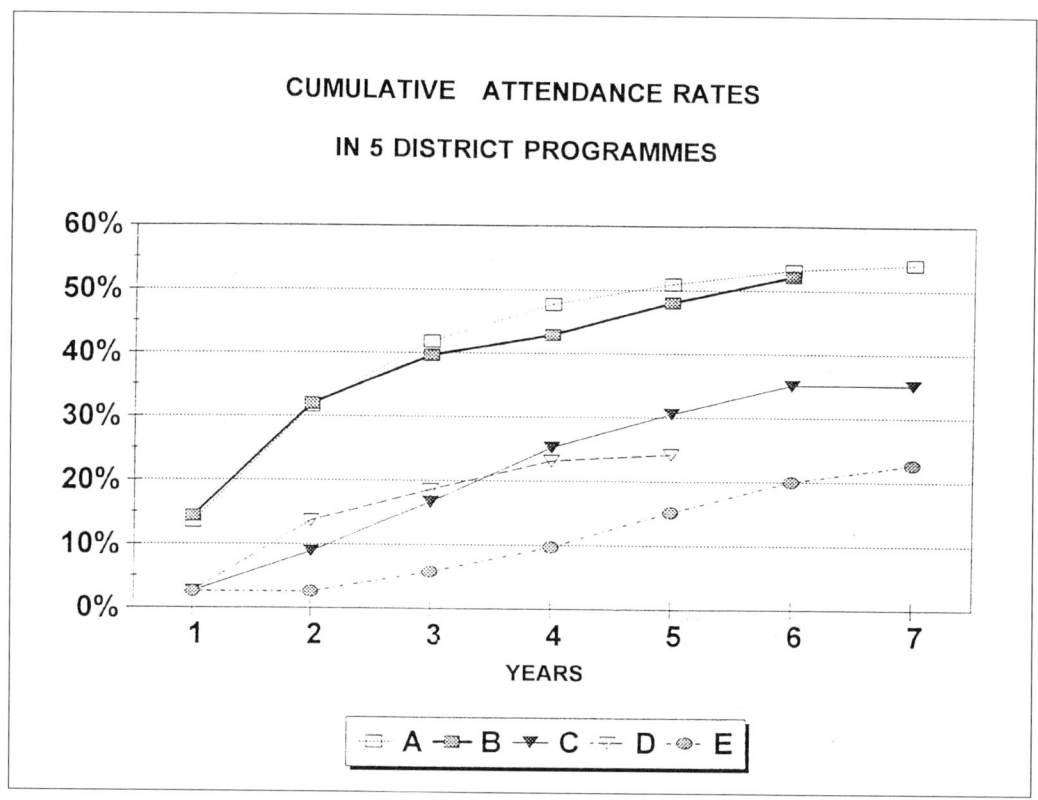

The results presented in this paper account for the first round of the 5 districts in the pilot study who provided comprehensive data at a meeting which was held in Marseille, january 1996.

Results

The target population according to the 1990 census reaches 552,194 women. Screening attendance rates vary widely from one district to an other. After five years participation rates for women attending the first round ranged from 15.2% to 50.9%. Only two programmes presented rates higher than 50%.
The average recall rate reached 7.8% and ranged from 12% to 4.4%. Only one district had a recall rate higher than that of the european reference.
Cancers detected during the first year of activity ranged from 4.7 per thousand to 8.1 per thousand. After 5 years activity these rates decreased and ranged from 4 per thousand to 5.2 per thousand.

Discussion

The existing french health system is based on private practice. Availability of mammographic facilities has progressed rapidly in the late eighties. Any women of any age may request a mammography test whether she is asymptomatic or not.
The programme attendance rates presented in this paper are low. Various surveys have been implemented to assess the level of screening outside the programme either at a local level or at a national level. The results of the 1995 « Baromètre santé » of the french committee for health education (CFES) using a representative sample of women shows that 78% of women aged 50 to 70 years have had at least one mammography in the last three years, which implies that the majority of the tests are performed outside the programme. With 19 districts the national screening programmes addresses 1,600,000 women of the age group, nearly one third of the target population. There is a necessity to improve participation in the programme and reduce the level of screening outside the programme. This is being presently addressed by the national pilot committee.

Breast cancer screening in Canada

Alan W. Lees

Cross Cancer Institute, Department of Radiation Oncology, 11560 University Avenue, Edmonton, Alberta T6G 1Z2, Canada

Introduction

The National Breast Screening Study (NBSS) [1], which recruited participants in fifteen urban centres across the country from 1980-1988, together with results from screening studies in other countries [2-6] focused attention on the potential for reducing breast cancer mortality in Canada by early diagnosis. A National Workshop of experts was convened in Ottawa in 1988 for the purpose of writing a Canadian position paper which would guide the development of screening programs in the provinces and territories. The participants included representatives from key voluntary and professional organizations as well as government. Proposals for screening programs were presented by three provinces (British Columbia, Alberta and Ontario).

Health care in Canada is by provincial health insurance rather than federal, but the provinces are subject to the Canada Health Act which ensures equal access to health care for all Canadians. The federal government also has some fiscal control through transfer payments to the provinces. The National Cancer Institute of Canada (NCIC), the Canadian Cancer Society (CCS), Health Canada and Stats Canada are organizations involved when a program the size of breast cancer screening is conceived. The deputy ministers of health (the civil servants responsible for running the health services) for the provinces and territories meet regularly and were the instigators of the Workshop following a request made Septembre 27 1987 by Dr. Maureen Law, deputy minister of the Department of Health and Welfare (later Health Canada). The Workshop was sponsored by the CCS, the Department of Health and Welfare and the NCIC on behalf of the conference of Federal-Provincial Deputy Ministers of Health.

The Workshop Group wrote a report [7] giving recommendations according to a woman's age. Screening under the age of 40 was not recommended. There was considered to be no definite proof of screening efficacy for women 40-49 and consequently it was left to the provinces to decide whether or not to target this age group. The effectiveness of screening in this age group was tested as part of the NBSS[1].

The main recommendation was to target women aged 50-69 for screening with two view mammograms and physical examination every two years. Breast Self Examination (BSE) would also be taught to participants and reinforced at the screening visits. Women aged over 70 years were not specifically mentioned in the report.

It was recommended that screening be done in dedicated centres as part of a province wide program. Recommendations for the identification and recruitment of target groups were made. Self-contained screening centres would be placed in urban settings (e.g. shopping malls) and linked to diagnostic facilities and mobile vans would be used for the rural communities. Program components were film-screen mammography with two views (cranio-caudal and medio-lateral oblique), protocols for physical examination and BSE. The assessment of suspected abnormal findings required arrangements for special radiological techniques to assure prompt referral for biopsy if indicated.

Recommendations were made about staffing levels, quality control of mammography, physical examination and BSE and evaluation and monitoring of the programs by linking with the provincial cancer registry.

Further to the workshop, Health Canada in 1990, with collaboration from CCS and NCIC, organized a meeting which recommended that a group composed of representatives from Health Canada, Statistics Canada, CCS and interested provincial jurisdictions be established to promote and facilitate collaborative planning and work in the development of ongoing breast cancer screening programs in Canada. Issues to be addressed included the development of a national data-base and the establishment of quality assurance programs. This group has met twice yearly since November 1990.

In 1992, in response to the Fourth Report of the Standing Committee on Health and Welfare, Social Affairs, Seniors and the Status of Women entitled Breast Cancer: Unanswered Questions, the Federal Government launched the Canadian Breast Cancer Initiative with funding of C$25 million over 5 years. One of its five components was the Breast Cancer Screening Initiative. In this, the federal government recommitted to enable a federal/territorial working group on breast cancer screening to implement and evaluate breast cancer screening programs in Canada. Furthermore, Health Canada was given the mandate to support the initiatives of jurisdictions that have established organized screening programs to standardize their data and promote quality assurance of breast cancer screening programs.

Another component of the Canadian Breast Cancer Initiative was the National Forum on Breast Cancer held in Montreal in November 1993. The report of this Forum [8] discussed issues and from this discussion made recommendations about screening.

Subjects for study were identified as:
- Developing and using a national data base derived from the provincial screening programs to assess the costs and outcomes of screening and to look at the differences in outcome resulting from varying policies for screening women under fifty and varying arrangements for physical examination of the breast.
- The teaching of breast examination in medical schools would be assessed with a view to standardizing and improving technique if found necessary.
- Imaging techniques other than mammography should be assessed as to their potential for use in screening.

Subjects for action were identified as:
- Adequate resources should be made available to reach at least 70% of women 50-69 years of age by means of organized provincial programs with the components outlined before.
- Communicating information to the target group by public education, professional, and voluntary groups. There would be special emphasis on hard to reach groups due to language or distance barriers.

- The development of an information package for use in the primary care setting for women under age 50 and over 70 to help them make an informed decision about mammography screening. This information package would also address the issue of screening premenopausal women with a family history of breast cancer in a firstdegree relative.
- The development of a consensus about the teaching and technique of breast self examination throughout Canada.
- The development of a policy with respect to genetic screening.

Following the Forum the national committee became known as the National Committee for the Canadian Breast Cancer Screening Initiative and the current chair is Doctor Heather Bryant of Calgary, Alberta. There are two subcommittees: Public Education, Health Promotion and Program-focused Awareness Issues, and Program Development, Evaluation and Information Sharing Issues. The former has a working group on BSE and a working group on Dissemination and Communication of the Benefits of Organized Screening Programs. The latter has a sub-committee on data base management, a technical sub-committee examining quality elements of organized screening programs, and a planning group for another national workshop to be held in 1997.

Current situation. Description of programs

British Columbia (started 1988) [9, 10], Alberta (1990) [11], Saskatchewan (1990), Ontario (1990) and Nova Scotia (1991) [12] provide the information for this paper. Yukon Territory has a small scattered population and has had a screening facility in Whitehorse operating since 1991. Manitoba and New Brunswick have just started their programs and Newfoundland will start this year.

Target ages are shown in *Table I*, together with the size of the target population and the total population of the province. British Columbia has recently changed its target age to 50-70 though women aged 40-49 will be accepted. The old figures are shown in brackets.

Table I. Population targets.

	Total population (millions)	Target age	Target population size (000's)
B.C.	3.712	50-70 (40+)	324 (800)
Alberta	2.750	50-69	187
Saskatchewan	1.003	50-69	85
Ontario	11.12	50-69	1000
Nova Scotia	0.932	50-69	78

Table II shows the chosen screening interval and the consequent target number of mammograms per year, the percentage of the target population, the capacity of the program and whether screening is available outside the provincial program.

Table III gives figures for prevalence screens and abnormality rates.

Table II. Canadian breast screening programs capacities.

	Screening interval years	Annual target screens (000's)	Total% target population	Capacity of program	Outside screening?
B.C.	1	227 (560)	70%	250	Yes
Alberta	2	75	80%	21	Yes
Saskatchewan	2	34	80%	34	Not 50-69
Ontario	2	350	70%	60	Yes
Nova Scotia	2	27	70%	12	Yes

Table III. Canadian breast screening programs.

Results	
Cancer detection rates, first visit	4.7 - 9.9/1000
Abnormality rates	4.5 - 14%

Comments

The data given above reinforce the points for study and action outlined above in the report of the Breast Cancer Forum.

The age of the target group has a large influence on the numbers of women to be screened because of the demographics of Canada's population. This is demonstrated in *Table I* by the size of British Columbia's target population in comparison with Alberta's. It is therefore very important to plan for giving advice about screening to women under the age of 50. Those 70 years of age and older who are at high risk by age but for whom the potential years of life saved by intervention is less than in the target group also need advice.

The capacity of the programs to achieve their purpose with the exception of Saskatchewan is deficient meaning that more funds are required to support more screening centres or increase the capacity of each centre. The 1988 Workshop suggested that centres be capable of processing at least 10,000 participants each year.

In the Canadian health care system, where all women are insured by the province, there are numerous private facilities offering mammography which compete with high volume low cost mass screening programs The nature of the interface between the systems led to a great deal of debate before screening was able to start. Programs with two year intervals find that some patients are having mammograms in the interval years at diagnostic facilities arranged by family doctors. The frequency is difficult to measure accurately. The attitude of physicians and the public to screening is very important and education about its benefits essential.

If an abnormality is found by screening diagnostic procedures are usually done in the private sector by family doctors following a letter to the patient and her doctor. However, there are diagnostic centres associated with a screening centre e.g. in Nova Scotia where needle core biopsies are available as part of the work-up of screening abnormalities. The increasing use of this facility was attributed to the ease and simplicity of the process offered to primary care physicians compared with them making their own arrangements for work-up [12]. The place of integrated diagnostic centres will be studied by the National Committee.

Physical examination of the breast is commonly delegated to the family doctor but in Ontario nurses examine breasts and teach self examination whereas in Nova Scotia the examination and teaching are done by the radiology technicians. These differences will allow the evaluation of the different techniques.

The prevalence screen has given cancer detection rates and abnormality rates in keeping with the findings of the NBSS.

Conclusions

Despite the size of Canada it has been possible to set up a system with the objective of population screening as most provinces have a program. The establishment of a national database will enable the common factors to be analyzed as well as the differences which will give insight into the diagnostic approach and the technique of physical examination for example. More resources are required to complete the objective.

Full implementation of the programs will also depend on the education of physicians and the public about the potential benefits of systematic screening.

References

1. Miller AB, Baines CJ, To T, Wall C. Canadian National Breast Screening Study. *Can Med Assoc J* 1992; 147: 1459-88.
2. Shapiro S, Venet W, Strax P. Current results of the breast cancer screening trial: the Health Insurance Plan (HIP) of Greater New York study. In Day NE, Miller AB (eds); *Screening for Breast Cancer*, Hans Huber, Toronto, 1988: 3-15.
3. Tabar L, Fagerberg CJG, Gad A, Baldetorp L, Holmberg LH, Grontoft O, Ljungquist H, Lundstrom B, Manson JC, Eklund G, Day NE. Reduction in mortality from breast cancer after mass screening with mammography. *Lancet* 1985; 1: 829-32.
4. Collette HJA, Day NE, Rombach JJ, Waard F de. Evaluating of screening for breast cancer in a non-randomized study (the DOM project) by means of a case-control study. *Lancet* 1984; 1: 1224-6.
5. Verbeek ALM, Hendriks JHCL, Holland R, Mravunac M, Sturmans F, Day NE. Mammographic screening and breast cancer mortality: age specific effects in the Nijmegen project, 1975-82. *Lancet* 1985; 1: 865-86.
6. Palli D, Del Turco MR, Buiatti E, Carli S, Ciatto S, Toscani L, Maltoni G. A case-control study of the efficacy of a non-randomized breast cancer screening programme in Florence (Italy). *Int J Cancer* 1986; 38: 501-4.
7. The Workshop Group. Reducing deaths from breast cancer in Canada. *Can Med Assoc J* 1989; 141199-201.
8. Health Canada. Report on the National Forum on Breast Cancer. *Health Canada Publications* 1994.
9. Warren Burhenne LJ, Burhenne HJ, Hislop TG. The British Columbia Mammography Screening Program: evaluation of the first 15 months. *AJR* 1992; 158: 45-9.
10. Warren Burhenne LJ, Burhenne HJ, Kan L. Quality-orientated mass mammography screening. *Radiology* 1995;194: 185-8.
11. Bryant HE, Desautels JEL, Castor W, Horeczko N, Jackson F, Mah Z. Quality assurance and cancer detection rates in a provincial screening mammography program. *Radiology* 1993; 188: 811-6.
12. Caines JS, Chanziantoniou K, Wright BA, Konok GP, Iles SE, Bodurtha A, Zayid I, Daniels C. Nova Scotia Breast Screening Program Experience: use of needle core biopsy in the diagnosis of screening-detected abnormalities. *Radiology* 1996; 198: 125-30.

The cost-effectiveness of breast cancer screening in France: from research to policy

Suzanne Wait

8, rue Fondary, 75015 Paris, France

Abstract

One of the difficulties of health policymakers is to extrapolate from research findings in order to make health policy decisions. The current debate surrounding the extension of breast cancer screening initiatives to a national level in France and in other countries is illustrative of this situation. From an economic perspective, the literature clearly suggests that breast cancer screening is cost-effective. Nonetheless, existing programmes do not necessarily meet the optimal quality conditions achieved in reference studies. In France, the decentralized model of screening poses particular difficulties which are not addressed by existing economic studies. A strong presence of spontaneous screening threatens to reduce the potential gain in public health terms expected from the programmes. Country-specific economic and epidemiological data will be necessary to best determine the future of breast cancer screening in France.

Introduction

One of the difficulties for health policy makers is to extrapolate from research findings in order to decide on the implementation of health programmes. The current debate surrounding breast cancer screening by mammography is a clear illustration of this dilemma. Although the results of clinical trials, conducted over a period of 30 years, have demonstrated that periodic screening by mammography can reduce breast cancer mortality by up to 15% in women aged 50 to 69 years of age [1,2], very few countries have adopted a nationwide screening policy and programmes remain essentially regionally-based or experimental in purpose. Economists have demonstrated that the cost-effectiveness of high quality breast cancer screening compares favourably with that of other health interventions. Yet the United Kingdom [3] and the Netherlands [4] are the only European countries to have commissioned a specific cost-effectiveness anlysis before deciding to launch a nationwide screening programme. Other study results, although published and widely discussed, have remained essentially in the domain of research and have yet to transgress into the policy arena.

In France, pilot screening programmes have been running since 1989. The decision to extend screening to a national level has been toyed with, however policy-makers and researchers alike remain hesitant. Indeed, the true effect of organized screening on mortality rates in France and the relative cost-effectiveness of screening within the programmes still need to be verified before a national policy on breast cancer screening can be determined.

The purpose of this paper is to address the French breast cancer screening situation from an economic and a health policy perspective. First, this paper will provide a brief overview of the French breast cancer screening situation and present economic data related to existing programmes. Second, it will describe some of the difficulties in applying existing cost-effectiveness study results to the French situation. Finally, the need for a better articulation between economic research and health policy in the field of breast cancer screening will be discussed.

The French breast cancer screening programme

In France, the first screening programmes were begun in 1989 under the auspices of the Prevention Department of the main national Sickness Insurance Fund *(Caisse Nationale d'Assurance Maladie des Travailleurs Salariés, CNAMTS)*. Today, 15 administrative districts *(départements)* run screening programmes. In early 1994, a decision was made by the French Ministry of Health to extend screening gradually to cover all remaining French districts over a 2-5 year period. However, the extension of screening remains uncertain, mainly due to difficulties in reconciling the need for optimal quality with the difficulties inherent in a decentralized screening system. Attendance for screening has been low (mean, 37% in the first screening round) [5] and important competition exists from spontaneous screening within the target population. There is a huge overcapacity of mammographic units, numbered at 2.100 across the country when studies have suggested that as little as 250 full-time machines would be needed to cover the entire target population [6]. Moreover, the programmes address a target population of women used to receiving mammograms as part of premenopausal surveillance in a country lacking a strong prevention tradition.

The cost of breast cancer screening in France

The cost of screening in France was first addressed by Lancry, Fagnani *et al.* in 1988 [7]. Using mostly theoretical data, the authors estimated the direct cost of a screening mammogram at 250 Francs within the context of a programme, as compared to a cost of 285 Francs for a mammogram done on an individual basis. A further cost analysis, which was entirely resource-based, was conducted by Lancry and Wait [8] in 1993 at the request of the Prevention Department of the CNAMTS. This study concerned only the first round of screening for 5 of the oldest screening programmes. The average cost of the first round of screening was found to be 374 Francs (US$63) per woman screened, with important discrepancies between programmes ($56-73) *(Table I)*. A minimum investment of $15 per attender (24% of total costs) was needed in physical and personnel resources to maintain the programme. Organizational aspects of the programme accounted for an average of $25 per woman screened or 40.5% of total costs. The remaining 59.5% accounted for technical aspects of screening, namely the cost of mammograms, their interpretation and quality control of radiologic equipment. Using a predictive model based on current programme costs, it was estimated that the first round of screening in a nation-wide programme in France would cost $135 millions for attendance rates of 30% and $217 millions for attendance rates of 60%. This would represent a cost ranging from $62 to $77 per woman screened.

Table I. Average cost per woman screened and cost distribution (in US dollars per woman screened).

Cost item	Mean cost in US $ (range)	% total cost (range)
Start up and ongoing costs	8.3 (5.7-12.6)	13.0 (9.2-19.2)
Personnel	13.6 (9.5-25.6)	21.5 (16.9-35.9)
Advertising	3.7 (0.1-10.2)	6.0 (0.1-4.2)
Mammogram	37.4 (36.7-40.2)	59.5 (52.8-67.2)
Total cost per woman screened	63.0 (55.8-72.8)	100.0
Total capital costs	15.2 (9.8-21.7)	24 (17.6-29.8)

The cost-effectiveness of breast cancer screening

Cost analyses are helpful in determining the amount of resources required to run a screening programe, however they give no indication of the health effects which can be expected for any given expenditure. Cost-effectiveness studies aim to provide policy-makers with a ratio of spent resources to health gains, expressed, in the case of screening, as a cost per life-year gained. There exist a number of cost-effectiveness studies on breast cancer screening. These studies, based in different medical and epidemiological contexts and testing different screening modalities, reveal cost-effectiveness ratios ranging from $3.400 to $84.000 per life year gained. Meta-analyses have allowed to account for and reduce some of these differences but the range remains large [9,10]. Moreover, these studies offer no solution to the problem of applying results to other national and epidemiological contexts.

The extrapolation of cost-effectiveness results to the French context is particularly complex. *Table II* lists some conditions which must be fulfilled if organized screening is to have a favourable cost-effectiveness ratio. First, most of the studies base their screening scenario on a centralized system using dedicated screening units, whereas France has opted for a decentralized system based in existing radiology clinics. Secondly, the population entering screening is assumed to have had no previous exposure to screening mammography as access to screening is expected to be restricted to the programme. In other words, the reference population of non-attenders is assumed to be « screen-free ». Furthermore, the estimates of the reduction in breast cancer mortality used in cost-effectiveness studies are most often based on Swedish [2] study results, where optimal quality and high attendance exceeding 90% were achieved. In France, the target population has been exposed to screening since before the onset of the programme. A study conducted in 1988 showed that two-thirds of the 1.9 million mammograms performed annually in France were done on a spontaneous rather than on a diagnostic basis [11]. Recent surveys indicate that levels of spontaneous screening are very high, especially among women under the age of 55 [12]. The attending population is thus not entirely screen-free upon entering the programme. Furthermore, the baseline stage distribution of cancers in the reference population is likely to be more favourable than in other countries since spontaneous mammography, even if of lesser quality, will have detected some preclinical cancers. Therefore the marginal gain in life expectancy achieved by introducing organized screening is likely to be reduced. Moreover, the share of breast cancer cases detected by the screening programme may be limited by suboptimal screening quality and low attendance rates. In an estimate of the reduction in breast cancer mortality projected from a nationalized screening programme in Germany, De Koning *et al.* estimated that, if screening only accounted for 16% of cancers detected, the mortality reduction could not be expected to exceed 11% [13].

Table II. Conditions for a favourable cost-effectiveness for organized breast cancer screening.

1. Breast cancer incidence and mortality rates are high.
2. A large proportion of breast cancer cases is detected by the screening program (at least 25%).
3. Attendance rates are high for the programme (> 70%)
4. The direct cost of a mammogram within the screening programme is less expensive than that of a mammogram done on a spontaneous basis (higher quality, fewer views)
5. The population entering the screening programme has had no previous exposure to screening mammography.
6. The size distribution of tumours among attenders is more favourable than that among non-attenders.
7. Specificity and sensitivity of the screening test are high.
8. The main cost savings are incurred by the reduction in treatment costs of advanced stage disease.

These important discrepancies between cost-effectiveness study conditions and the actual French situation render the transposition any of these study results to the French programmes extremely difficult. The need for a country-specific cost-effectiveness study is evident and two such studies are currently being carried out in the districts of the Bouches du Rhône and the Bas-Rhin. The purpose of these studies is to compare the cost-effectiveness of existing screening programmes projected over a 20-year period with a situation in which no organized screening exists, yet access to screening on an individual basis is prevalent at observed levels. The results of these studies are expected in late 1997.

Conclusion

Cost-effectiveness studies in health care have grown tremendously in number over the past 20 years. The purpose of a cost-effectiveness study is to allow policy makers to choose between competing health care strategies by privileging the alternative which provides the best ratio of resources spent to effectiveness gained [14]. The difficulty with breast cancer screening studies is that the cost-effectiveness ratio is contingent on the screening modalities, epidemiological context and methodological choices of the authors. Without in depth knowledge of the reference study conditions, estimating the cost-effectiveness of breast cancer screening in a different national context can be very misleading.

The French programme is illustrative of a non-specialized model of screening, confronted by a highly competitive radiological market where supply greatly outstrips demand. This situation is likely to be applicable to other countries at arms with growing demand for screening mammography. Policy makers face a difficult task in attempting to adapt health policy to the particular medical and cultural context of their country. Economic studies can be helpful in developing appropriate prevention policies although a thorough understanding of published results is necessary to avoid misinterpreting figures. The future of breast cancer screening policy, in France and elsewhere, will undoubtedly rest in part on finding the appropriate articulation between public health and health economics research and health policy agendas.

References

1. Rutqvist LE, Miller AB, Andersson I, *et al*. Reduced breast cancer mortality with mammography screening - an assessment of currently available data. *Int J Cancer 1990*; Suppl 5: 76-84.
2. Nystrom L, Rutqvist LE, Wall S, *et al*. Breast cancer screening with mammography: an overview of the Swedish randomised trials. *Lancet* 1993; 341, 973-8.
3. Forrest, P. Breast cancer screening: Report to the health ministers of England, Wales, Scotland and Northern Ireland by a working group chaired by professor Sir Patrick Forrest. London: Her Majesty's Stationery Office, 1987.
4. De Koning HJ. The effects and costs of breast cancer screening (Dissertation). Rotterdam: Erasmus University, 1993.
5. Wait S, Allemand H. The French breast cancer screening programme: epidemiological and economic results of the first round of screening. *European J Public Health 1996*, 6 (1): 43-8.
6. Montaville B, Lefaure C. Le dépistage du cancer du sein en France: programmes et projets. Paris: INSERM U.240, 1988.
7. Lancry PJ, Fagnani F. Evaluation économique du dépistage systématique des cancers du sein et du col de l'utérus. Paris: COMAC-HSR, Paris.
8. Lancry PJ, Wait S. Evaluation économique des dépistages de masse du cancer du sein. A propos de cinq programs expérimentaux français. Paris: CREDES Rapport N° 997, 1993.
9. Elixhauser A. Costs of breast cancer and the cost-effectiveness of breast cancer screening. *Int J Tech Assess Hlth Care* 1991; 7: 604-15.
10. Brown ML, Fintor L. Cost-effectiveness of breast cancer screening: preliminary results of a systematic review of the literature. *Breast Cancer Res Treat* 1993; 25: 113-8.
11. Fagnani F, Le Galès C, Lefaure C. Analyse économique du dépistage du cance du sein par mammographie: comparaison des différentes organisations. *J d'Econ Méd* 1989; 7 (5): 319-31.
12. Mamelle N *et al*. Réseau Inserm de Santé Publique. *Rapport final: méthodologie d'évaluation comparative des programmes de dépistage du cancer du sein*. Lyon: INSERM U.265, 1994.
13. Beermsterboer PMM, de Koning HJ, Warmerdam PG, *et al*. Prediction of the effects and costs of breast cancer screening in Germany. *Int J Cancer* 1994; 58: 623-8.
14. Williams C, Coyle D, Gray A, *et al*. European School of Oncology Advisory Report to the Comission of the European Communities for the Europe Against Cancer Programme: Cost-effectiveness in Cancer Care. *Eur J Cancer* 1995; 31A (9): 1410-27.

Minimal breast cancer: diagnosis, strategy and decisional trees

C. Frouge

Service de Radiologie, Hôpital de Bicêtre, 78, rue du Général-Leclerc, 94275 Kremlin-Bicêtre Cedex

The first step of the early detection of minimal breast cancer (MBC) is mammography. This examination may be perfomed in a mass screening or after an individual prescription. In both situation, three main signs will be suggestive of malignancy: a fibrous reaction, a cluster of microcalcification and a localized increase of density. In each situation a simple decisional tree may be proposed in an attempt to avoid unnecessary biopsies.

There is a wide range of mammographic and sonographic appearance of MBC depending of the histologic type of breast cancer *(Figure 1)*. A fibrous reaction detected in only one incidence, may be the only sign of breast cancer. The first point is to exclude a superposition of

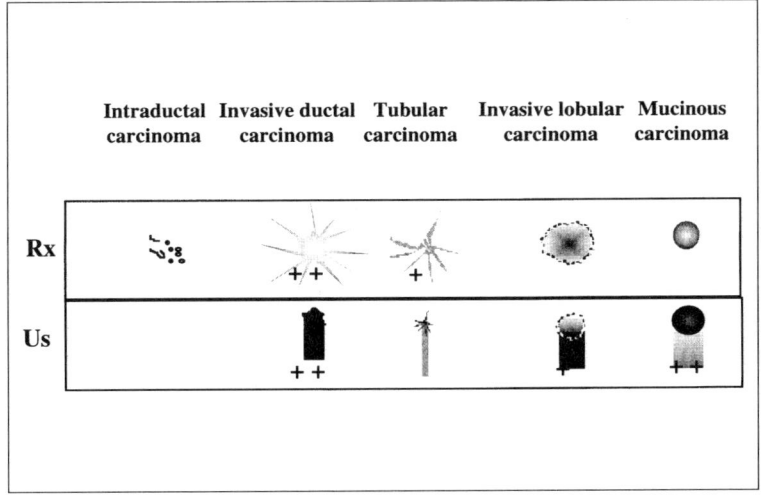

Figure 1. Minimal breast cancers.

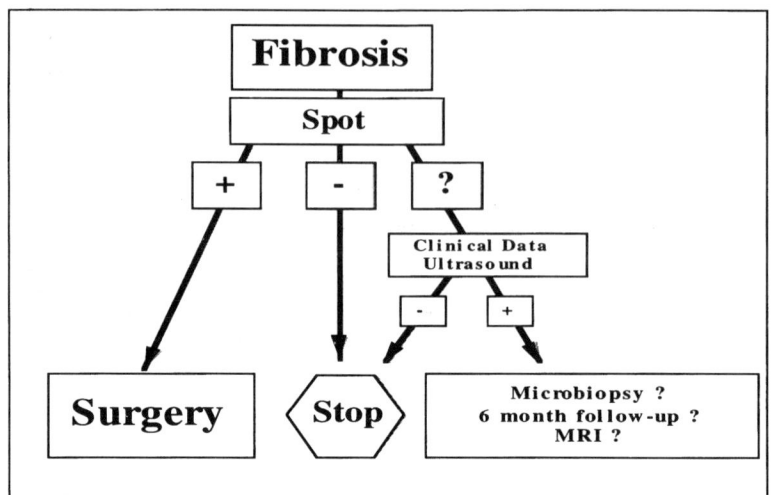

Figure 2

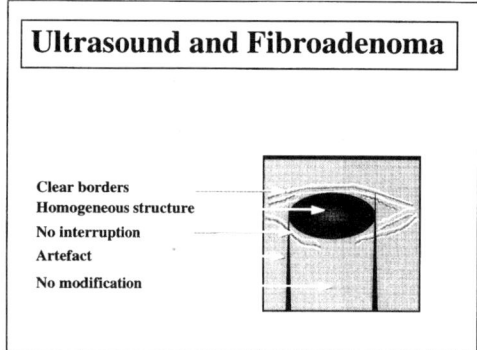

Figure 3

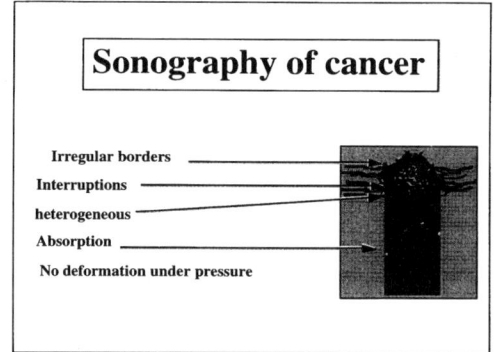

Figure 4

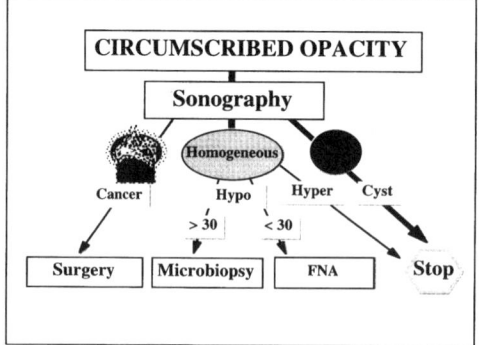

Figure 5

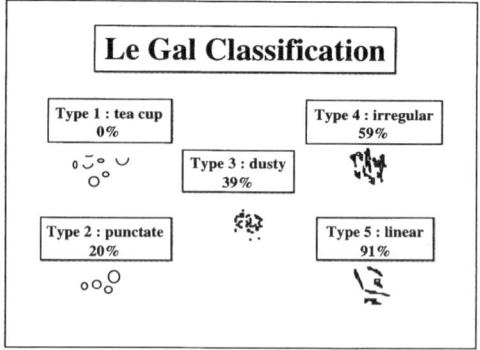

Figure 6

the conjonctive tissue by a spot compression. If the desorganisation is increased by the spot, there is a high suspiscion of breast cancer. The radial scar is the major differential diagnosis in this situation, but this benign lesion is often associated with a carcinoma (generally a tubular carcinoma). Because of the high rate of associated lesions distant from the central core detected on mammograms, it is not possible to exclude a malignant carcinoma with percutaneous fine-needle aspiration of core biopsy, even with large needles. Thus, when a stellate lesion suggestive of a radial scar is found on mammograms, surgical removal and histologic examination are mandatory in all cases, but the surgeon and the pathologist must be aware of this special pattern to avoid extensive surgery. When there is a doubt about the presence of a fibrous reaction, the follow-up is not contributive since the speed of growth of the malignant tumor in this situation is usually very slow. In this rare situation, a MRI study with Gadolinium may be usefull *(Figure 2)*.

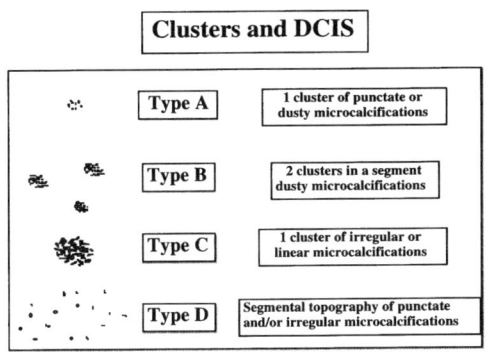

Figure 7

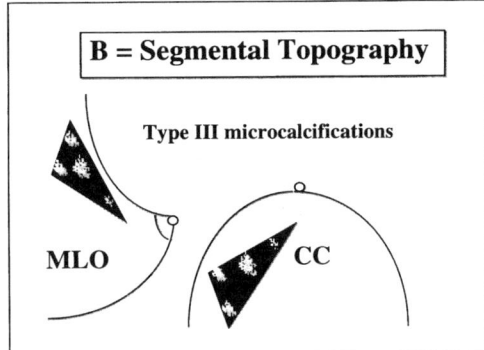

Figure 8

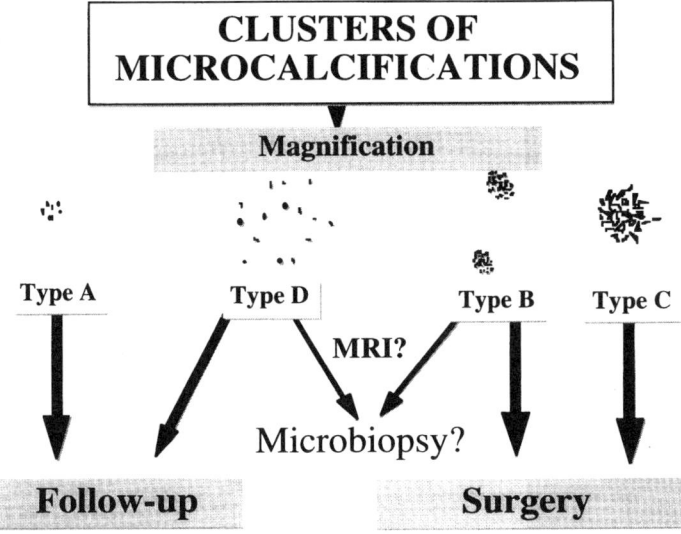

Figure 9

When a circumscribed opacity or an asymetry of density is found on mammography, the size, the border and the sonographic appearance of the lesion will allow a diagnostic in most cases. If the lesion is hyperechogenic it is usually related to normal glandular tissue. When a superficial lump is hyperechogenic it may be related to a nodular cytosteatonecrosis. When the lesion is anechogenic, it is a cyst which does not need further examination. If the cyst is painfull it may be punctionned. When the tumor is hypoechogenic three different situations are found. The first situation is the typical fibroadenoma in a young woman. In this case a fine needle biopsy may be proposed *(Figure 3)*. The second situation is the typical invasive carcinoma needing surgery *(Figure 4)*. The third situation is a probably benign nodule found in a middle age woman, in this situation fine needle and/or microbiopsy is mandatory to confirmed the diagnosis *(Figure 5)*.

Clusters of microcalcification are a highly sensitive sign of minimal breast, but their specificity is low: under 20%. Since the works of Lanyi and Le Gal, the microcalcification shape has been known to be highly suggestive of the nature of the underlying lesion *(Figure 6)*.

The characterization of microcalcifications is very difficult since there is an important overlap between their appearance on mammography in benign and malignant lesions. This is easily explained by radio-histological studies which demonstrated that irregular microcalcifications are due to intraductal necrosis highly suggestive of cancer, but regular round calcification due to a secretion can either be found in benign lesions or intraductal carcinoma *(Figure 7)*. The shape of the cluster and the segmental topography of the microcalcifications are two other elements which are important for the decision *(Figure 8)*. The place of MRI and microbiopsy is for the moment under evaluation but microbiopsy with large needles (14 G) under steretaxic guidance in selected case is promising *(Figure 9)*.

Conclusion

The diagnosis in senology will continue for a long time to be a synthesis of the different data coming from the clinical examination, ultrasounds, mammograms and cytology.

Is there now a consensus on the treatment of minimal breast cancer?

P. Rouanet, C. Charlier and H. Pujol

CRLC Val-d'Aurelle, Montpellier, France

The concept of Minimal breast cancer (MBC) is an old concept originally proposed by Gallager and Martin [1] in 1971, which associate Lobular carcinoma *in situ* (LCIS), Ductal carcinoma in situ (DCIS), Micro invasive carcinoma (µIC) and invasive carcinoma initially no greater than 0.5 cm then less than 1 cm diameter (MIC: minimal invasive carcinoma [2]). Initially, this concept was proposed to define stages of breast cancer amenable to local forms of treatment. Unity of these patients was the prognosis with an incidence rate of less than 10% node positivity.

Nowadays the evolution of the natural history of these lesions is well known. Size is not all the only determinant of biologic behavior and metastatic potential.

Lobular carcinoma *in situ*, which should be regarded as a marker of increased risk in both breast (15%) with specific therapeutic implications, rather than a precancerous lesion, has been excluded from MBC.

The current interest of MBC lies in its increasing frequency which is the result of active screening programs and a heightened public awareness.

Epidemiology of MBC

Table I. Incidence of MBC.

	DCIS	µIC	MIC
Incidence	20%	3%	5%
Mean age	50 - 56	55	55 - 60
Node positivity	0 - 1%	3 - 20%	20%
Survival at 10 years	92 - 99%	80 - 90%	80%

Screening mammography has changed the incidence of DCIS from 2% in the seventies to 20% nowadays, what Gump called in 1987 « DCIS, a revised concept » *(Table I)*.

The same findings have been reported for small breast cancer less than 1 cm. Their incidence is 5-8% for the global population but increase from 20% (Bas-Rhin) to 40% (Hérault) during screening programs. The 1990 SEER data [3] indicate that breast cancer incidence is essentially flat except for the increase in stage I (T1-NO), which has risen from 25% to almost 50% of all invasive breast cancers from 1983 to 1990.

The definitions of « microinvasion » and « minimally invasive » breast cancer are controversial and vary among different investigators. The risk of lymph node metastasis with microinvasion is reported to be 2.7 - 20%. However, the varying definitions of microinvasion and the difficulty in making this pathologic diagnosis with certainty, make the data on metastasis from MIC difficult to interpret reliably. Lagios [4] refers microinvasion to foci of invasive cancer with maximum diameters of 1 mm or less. Larger areas of invasive growth are termed MIC as defined initially by Gallagher and Martin. More generally, oncologic data for microinvasive tumor are missing for a special analysis, that is the reason why we agree to associate this form of MBC to invasive carinoma less than 1 cm. For instance, DCIS with µIC components were excluded from the EORTC prospective trial 10853.

Finally, we can individualize between DCIS and MIC, small invasive tumor with an extensive intra ductal component. Seidman [5] demonstrate that the size of only the invasive component, as determined by microscopic measurement, is a better predictor of axillary lymph nodes status than is the total tumor size. On the other hand, the total tumor size must be considered for the local prognosis.

Loco-regional therapy: surgery and radiotherapy

The various options in local therapy for patients with MBC are modified radical mastectomy, lumpectomy with or without radiation, quadrantectomy with or without radiation and simple mastectomy.

Ductal carcinoma *in situ* (DCIS)

Controversy exists concerning the natural history of DCIS, including its pathologic expression and treatment: What type of surgery is appropriate? Is adjuvant radiotherapy necessary?

For these lesions, local control is the main problem since the systemic risk does not initially exist but can appear with local recurrence.

• *Natural history of DCIS and type of surgery*
Recurrences after mastectomy for DCIS are few, averaging 3% to 5% at 5 years. If the results of mastectomy are well known, conservative surgery is a real current problem. DCIS natural history highlights the problem of multifocality of this desease which results from galatophoric branching. This anatomic pattern accounts for LR arising in the same quadrant. Breast cancer can diffuse into the gland by intra vascular, intra lymphatic or intra ductal dissemination. Faverly [6], using three dimensional imaging of DCIS, has shown that low-grade tumor has skip lesions more often than high grade DCIS. This observation suggests that wider margins

may be required for complete clearance of low-grade lesions (micropapillary and cribriform DCIS).

The prognostic significance of microscopic evaluation of the surgical margins in lumpectomy specimens has not been adequately determined. In a few studies, LR were attributed to close margins or positive margins, whereas in other studies recurrences were seen even after disease-free excision margins *(Table II)*. In a study that examined mastectomy specimens after local excision with free margins, Frazier [7] found residual disease in 26% of cases.

Table II. Average annual hazard rate of local recurrence related to margins and comedonecrosis (NSABP B-17).

Margins	Comedo necrosis	Lumpectomy (n: 274)	Lump + Irradiation (n: 299)
free	absent	1.97	1.18
free	marked	5.44	1.18
involved	absent	5.95	2.10
involved	marked	10.5	3.28

For Lagios [4], almost all recurrences were at the biopsy site or in the same quadrant. He emphasize the difficulty for a surgeon to resect a focus of microcalcifications with a margin adequate for a malignant process when this would result in overtreating 2 of every 3 patients. this point underlines the problem of frozen section for microcalcification and the reliability of free margin during a second operation for DCIS several days after the first surgery. Initially, he restricted conservative surgery to patients with areas of DCIS that measured pathologically 25 mm or less in extent, now his current practice is to accept larger foci as long as they can be adequately resected with free margins and with a cosmetic resulty acceptable to the patient. Correlative mammographic and specimen x-ray findings furthermore are not reliable. Holland [8] confirmed that the pathological extent of DCIS visualized mammographically was commonly underestimated by at least 2 cm in 16% of comedocarcinoma and 50% of micropapillary and cribriform type.

• *Effect of adjuvant radiotherapy on DCIS local control*
From 573 patients coming from the NSABP B-17 trial, Fisher [9] found two statistically significant independent parameters of LR: the presence of moderate/marked comedo necrosis and involved lumpectomy margins. He noted that the majority of LR occured within or close to the site of the initial tumor and concluded that the optimal control of LR occurs with histologically free margins and the administration of irradiation after lumpectomy regardless of tumor size or histologic type. At a median follow-up of 43 months, there was a 7% incidence of recurrence in the treated breast with the addition of radiation vs. 16.4% in patients treated with local excision alone ($p < 0.001$).

Silverstein [10] published a new prognostic classification for DCIS combining high nuclear grade and comedo-type necrosis to predict clinical recurrence. From 238 patients after breast conservation surgery, he reported no significant LR difference with or without radiotherapy, for non high nuclear grade DCIS with or without necrosis. Conversely, LR rate was significantly better (p:0.01) after radiotherapy for high grade DCIS. Yet, authors showed that high nuclear grade, even with radiation therapy, induced 30% of LR at 7 years and asked for breast excision for this subgroup. White [11] confirmed that the predominant nuclear grade was the best predictor of LR for a retrospective study of 52 DCIS treated by conservative surgery and radiotherapy. Close or positive margins were not found to be associated with local recurrence. They published an excellent local control at 8 years (94%) with this procedure but one of these recurrent patients died from metastases. There was a trend for increased LR among the cases with a higher predominant nuclear grade. Additional follow-up time will help to clarify whether this trend persists or whether the low grade lesions will merely recur at a later date. Many works documented radiotherapy's role in reducing LR, because of the relationship of LR to high risk lesions, it is conceivable that radiotherapy particularly affects high risk lesions, thus reducing the risk of local disease recurrence or delaying it.

Lagios [4] confirmed the short term benefits of radiation therapy in reducing the number of LR after CS and radiotherapy *(Table III)*. However, these benefits appear to shrink with greater follow-up. Recurrences double between 5 and 8 years and are greater still at 10 years of follow-up. He concluded that it might be more appropriate to reserve radiation therapy for invasive recurrences should they occur. Furthermore, the post irradiation LR reported by Fisher [9] at 43 months is not substantially different from that of studies using surgery alone but with careful evaluation of margins and thorough specimen examination at a comparable follow-up period.

Table III. Probability of recurrence post irradiation for DCIS (expressed as a percentage) [4].

Source	n	Follow-up (yr)			
		4	5	8	10
Bornstein - 1991	38	-	8%	27%	-
Solin - 1993	172	-	4%	9%	16%
Silverstein - 1994	118	-	8%	19%	-
Fisher - 1993	409	7%	-	-	-

The consensus on DCIS treatment doen't exist nowadays. High risk lesion are determined: mammographic size more than 2 cm, high nuclear grade, comedonecrosis. The value of free margins is discussed. Wide surgery induce easely breast deformity and seemed to be reserved to non agressive lesion. Adjuvant radiotherapy is more effective on aggressive lesion but the results must spend test of time. The value of hormonotherapy will be prouved by randomized trial.

Invasive carcinoma less than 1 cm (MIC)

Veronesi [12] analysed data from 1973 patients treated in three consecutive randomised trials in Milan. Four different radiosurgical procedures were compared: Halsted mastectomy, quadrantectomy plus radiotherapy, lumpectomy plus radiotherapy and quadrantectomy without radiotherapy. Analysis according to the size of primary carcinoma revealed that the differences in LR rate between tumor smaller and larger than 1 cm in diameter were constant across the four treatment groups. Since these studies and the NSABP B-06 study, it has been clear that less than mastectomy is an appropriate option for T1 breast cancer.

Hellman [3] analysed two series of small tumors less than 1 cm treated only with loco-regional therapy with a mean follow-up duration of 15 years. For node negative patients, 88% appeared to be cured around 10 years. The median time for recurrence is inversely related to tumor size, small tumors take a longer time to recur than do large tumors. The results from screening also document the important relation-ship of size to survival. These data suggest that MIC is usually only a locoregional process. The number of nodes involved (< 20%) is limited for such small tumors. In 50% of such patients, only one node was involved, 20% had 2 nodes, 10% had 3 nodes and 20% had four or more lymph nodes involved. Patients with one to three lymph nodes involved appeared to be cured by locoregional treatment in 70% of the cases. Analysis of twenty year data indicates that having only one node involved did not reduce survival for T1 breast cancer patients. Only when there were four or more nodes involved was there a significant reduction in survival. Conversely, Bedwani *et al.* [13] have published the American College of Surgeons' long term breast cancer survey including 16 894 patients. They concluded that tumor size alone could not be used as the only defining criterion for MIC. Only the status of axillary nodes may determine whether a small invasive tumor below 1 cm may be considered as MBC.

Risks factors for LR are: age, vascular invasion and surgical margins [14]. For the practicing surgeon, the risk factors of age and vascular invasion cannot be controlled but margins can. The use of frozen section analysis can allow the surgeon to make decisions about the adequacy of margins in the operative room with an accuracy no different from that of permanent section. This saves the patient the risk of an additional procedure and allows re-excision with more precision than a second time surgery disturbed by cytosteatonecrosis and lack of tumor topography.

For many years, the presence of an extensive intraductal component increased classically the risk of LR. Subsequently, these data have been reviewed and most centers are agreed that as long as the margins are negative the risk of LR is not increased [14]. Nevertheless, Ohtake [15] showed by a computer graphic reconstruction of the ductal lobular system, an intra ductal tumor extension from the invasive cancer through the ductal tree. Ductal anastomoses were seen and the investigators pointed out that careful attention to margins and a segmental-shaped excision seemed to be required to assure the complete excision of all the intraductal disease in these patients. Connoly [16] reinforced the concept that an understanding of the geometry of this desease would help us to further increase our local control rates and that careful attention to margins clearly allowed conservative surgery for these lesions.

The last question raises the possibility for a subgroup of MIC to be managed with lumpectomy alone without addition of radiation. LR rate varies to 9% with quadrantectomy to 19% with lumpectomy alone for T1 tumor against respectively 0.3% and 2.3% with radiotherapy. Although, LR rates have been increased, no impact on survival could be documented. To date, the standard of therapy for MIC includes whole breast irradiation.

Axilla

Treatment of axilla in patients with MBC is controversial. The risk of positive node increases from less than 1% for DCIS to 20% for small invasive carcinoma. Silverstein [17] found positive node in 0% of DCIS and the following rates for the remaining T stages: 3% T1a, 17% T1b, 32% T1c, 44% T2 and 60% T3. Avril [18] published 333 patients treated in Bordeaux for tumor less than 1 cm in post menopausal women: 78% were N-, 11% had one positive node, 5% two involved nodes and 6% more than 3 positive nodes. It adds little morbidity or time to the operative procedure to dissect the axillary contents at level I and the probability of missing a « skip » metastasis to level II or III if level I is negative is remote for this carefully selected patients.

For DCIS, the consensus would tend towards a lack of axilla sample. However, two points must be considered: high nuclear grade and comedonecrosis are risk factors for aggressivity, normality of first axillary node eliminates the systemic risk. That is the reason why, we believe that a minimal axilla sample of 2 or 3 nodes could be reasonably taken without morbidity for comedocarcinoma or DCIS with high nuclear grade.

For MIC, univariate analysis revealed node metastases to be associated with tumor size, poorly differentiated nuclear grade, high S phase fraction, presence of lymphatic and vascular invasion and age younger than 60 years. The consensus is to remove at least 10 to 12 nodes of level 1. In the future we will be able to select patients requiring axillary dissection for staging and treatment by understanding the biology of their primary tumor. Another way could be the sentinel node biopsy. Giulano [19] and Krag [20], using respectively a vital blue dye or radioisotope technique, have demonstrated the feasability and accuracy of sentinel node biopsy in breast cancer. At present, a prospective randomized trial is being carried out at the Fondation Bergonie [18] in Bordeaux, to evaluate the possibility to avoid axillary dissection for tumor less than 1 cm in post menopausal women.

Systemic therapy

Rules for breast cancer can be applied for MBC. For DCIS, this problem doesn't exist, except for LR which are invasive in 50% of cases. For μInv and MIC, axilla status make the prognosis although some authors showed independent good prognosis for tumors smaller than 1 cm.

Currently, age and tumor hormonal status are great indicators of systemic therapy in addition to nodal involvement. A consensus has been reached on chemotherapy in young women less than 30 years and on hormonotherapy in menopausal women with positive receptors.

In 1906, Cheatle said: « *In the early treatment of cancer, the saving of time means the saving of life.* » Detecting MBC has been the goal of breast cancer screening programs over the past 20 years. A better knowledge of the natural history of DCIS and MIC enables surgeons and radiotherapists for rational therapeutic indication. A consensus is not yet purchase for all types of MBC but the use of breast conservation therapy is better defined.

References

1. An orientation to the concept of minimal breast cancer. *Cancer* 1971; 28: 1505-7.
2. Hartmann WH. Minimal breast cancer. An update. *Cancer* 1984; 53: 681-4.
3. Bedwani R, Vana J, Rosner D, Schmitz RL, Murphy GP. Management and survival of female patients with « Minimal » breast cancer: as observed in the long term and short-term surveys of the american college of surgeons. *Cancer* 1981; 47: 2769-78.
4. Fisher ER, Costantino J, Fisher B, Palekar AS, Redmond C, Mamounas E. Pathologic findings from the National Surgical Adjuvant Breast Project, Protocol B-17. *Cancer* 1995; 75: 1310-9.
5. Silverstein MJ, Poller DN, Waisman JR, Colburn WJ, Barth A, Gierson ED, Lewinsky B, Gamagami P, Slamon DJ. Prognostic classification of breast ductal carcinoma *in situ*. *Lancet* 1995; 345: 1154-7.
6. Faverly D, Burgers L, Bult P, Holland R. Three dimensional imaging of mammary ductal carcinoma *in situ*: clinical implications. *Semin Diag Pathol* 1994; 11: 193-8.
7. Frazier TG, Wong WY, Rose D. Implications of accurate pathologic margins in the treatment of primary breast cancer. *Arch Surg* 1989; 124: 37-8.
8. Holland R, Hendricks JH, Verbeek AM *et al*. Extent, distribution and mammographic/histological correlations of breast ductal carcinoma *in situ*. *Lancet* 1990; 335: 519-22.
9. White J, Levine A, Gustafson G, Wimbish K, Ingold J, Pettinga J, Matter R, Martinez A, Vicini F. Outcome and prognostic factors for local recurrence in mammographically detected ductal carcinoma

in situ of the breast treated with conservative surgery and radiation therapy. *Int J Rad Oncol Biol Phys* 1995; 31: 791-7.
10. Veronesi U, Salvadori B, Luini A, Greco M, Saccozi R, Del Vezcchio M, Mariani L, Zurrida S, Rilke F. Breast conservation is a safe method in patients with small cancer of the breast. Long term results of three randomised trials on 1973 patients. *Eur J Cancer* 1995; 31: 1574-9.
11. Natural history of small breast cancers. Karnofsky memorial lecture. S Hellman. *J Clin Oncol* 1994; 12: 2229-34.
12. Bedwani R, Vana J, Rosner D, Schmitz R, Murphy G. Management and survival of female patients with « Minimal » Breast Cancer: as observed in the long term and short term survey of the american college of surgeons. *Cancer* 1981; 47: 2769-78.
13. Lagios M. Duct carcinoma *in situ*: Biological implications for clinical practice. *Seminars in Oncology* 1996; 23: 6-11.
14. Smith T. The role and extent of surgery in early invasive breast cancer. *Seminars in Oncology* 1996; 23: 12-8.
15. Giulano A, Kirgan D, Guenther J. Lymphatic mapping and sentinel lymphadenectomy for breast cancer. *Ann Surg* 1994; 220: 391-401.
16. Krag D, Weaver D, Alex J. Surgical resection and radiolocalization of the sentinel lymph node in breast cancer using a gamma probe. *Surg Oncol* 1993; 2: 335-40.

Breast Cancer. Advances in biology and therapeutics.
F. Calvo, M. Crépin, H. Magdelenat, eds. John Libbey Eurotext © 1996, pp. 105-108.

Minimal breast cancer: place of the plastic surgery

J.Y. Petit, M. Rietjens, C. Garusi and P. Veronesi

European Institute of Oncology, via Ripamonti 435, 20141 Milan, Italy

Although « minimal breast cancer » is an entity which can be discussed while giving rise to a great variety of treatment protocols, the overall good prognosis provides a special opportunity for plastic surgery indications. Howerver, there is no consensus for the cancer treatment of such tumors: diffuse ductal carcinoma *in situ* (DCIS) are best be treated by mastectomy while [1], small infiltrating carcinomas, despite a worse prognosis, can be proposed a conservative surgery (BCT). As no total agreement exists today for the extension of the cancer surgery, although there is a trend in favor of the conservative surgery, [2, 3], we shall present the panoply of the different techniques available in breast reconstructive surgery. The plastic surgery can be associated to the cancer surgery at any time of the patient follow up. The reconstruction procedure can be total or partial, and it involves in more than half of the cases a plasty procedure on the contralateral breast to improve the symmetry. Therefore, a close collaboration is mandatory between the teams in order to facilitate the operating schedule and to reduce the hospital stay and the number of procedures.

Role of the plastic surgery in case of mastectomy

The breast reconstruction can best be performed immediately at the time of the mastectomy in case of MBC. No adjuvant medical treatment is required in these cases, and the reconstruction cannot disturb the sequence of the cancer treatment even in case of delayed healing. Such tumors do not require any wide skin resection and the usual technique is a so called « skin sparing mastectomy ». Such mastectomy provides the best chances of complete removal of the ducts, including those of the nipple areolar complex since the nipple and the areola are removed. The reconstruction can be performed either with an implant or with autologous tissue.

Implant reconstruction

Different implants can be used. Since several years, the regulation of silicone prosthesis is hardly discussed and give rise to a variety of medico-legal decisions. In France, the use of gel-filled silicone implants is forbidden while in the whole Europe there is no limitations. Since the early discussions of the FDA experts in 1991, a great number of important well designed epidemiologic studies have strongly suggested the inocuity of the silicone gel. At the Gustave-Roussy Institute, we have performed a study comparing a group of breast reconstructions with gel-filled implants with a matched group of cancer patients treated by mastectomy without reconstruction that is without silicone exposure. The mean follow up time was long enough (13y) to evaluate the results. The local recurrence , the metastase and the death rates were around the half in the case of silicone exposure and no increase risk of carcinogenic effect has been observed in the group of implanted patients [4, 5].

Immediate breast reconstruction after breast sparing mastectomy consists in inserting a prosthesis (inflatable or gel-filled if allowed by the local law) behind the pectoralis major which has been previously undermind and partially detached from the costal wall. In order to complete the muscular pocket for the implant, it is required to undermind also the serratus muscle in the lower part of the reconstructed breast. Different techniques have been described to improve the shape of the reconstructed breast. But when the volume should be important it is advised to use an expander prosthesis, temporary or definitive, in order to provide a progressive tissue expansion. In other cases, it is possible to propose a reduction mammaplasty of the opposit breast which can be performed immediately or at the second stage. The interest of doing the reduction mammaplasty immediately is to obtain the histological result of the reduction specimen before the second stage in case of contralateral occult carcinoma and therefore to be able to complete the treatment earlyer.

Usually, the nipple-areolar reconstruction is performed in a second stage, when the reconstruction has reached the final cosmetic aspect. This reconstruction can generally be performed under local anesthesia, in the out patient clinic.

Autologous tissue reconstructions

The reconstruction can also be performed with autologous tissue, especially when the patient feels insecure about silicone prosthesis. The operation consists in preparing a musculo-cutaneous flap such as the rectus abdominal flap (TRAM) during the mastectomy procedure. The two team approach, again, necessitates a close collaboration between cancer and plastic surgeons.

Autologous tissue reconstructions provide the best cosmetic results. The shape can better match the contralateral breast and a certain degree of ptosis can be obtain much easier than with an implant. But the TRAM flap procedure requires a well trained plastic surgeon, and the post operative recovery is longer than the implant reconstruction. Abdominal sequelea have also to be considered when making the choice of the procedure. Free TRAM flaps using microsurgical techniques are also indicated when a microsurgery team is available.

Delayed breast reconstructions

Can be performed with the same techniques. The choice depends on the local conditions of the thoracic area. After radiotherapy, it is preferable in most cases to perform a musculocutaneous flap. Again in these cases, the autologous tissue reconstruction is the procedure of choice in what concerns the final cosmetic aspect.

Role of plastic surgery after BCT

The plastic surgeon is increasingly involved in the conservative surgery of the breast cancer. The aim of BCT is to provide the patient with a good cosmetic result while keeping the same chances of cure than with the mastectomy. MBC, when associated with an extensive DCIS component requires at least a quadrantectomy. Poor cosmetic results after quadrantectomy are observed in 10 to 20%. To avoid these cosmetic failures, different techniques of partial breast reconstruction can be proposed [6, 7]. Secondary repair of poor cosmetic results is more disappointing than immediate partial reconstruction. The risk of radio sclerosis or necrosis is higher when the surgery is performed on radiated tissue. Therefore, we suggest to develop once more a team approach and to work with the general surgeon concomitantly. The type of incision, the glandular closure with glandular flaps, the delicate skin suture are usual techniques that should be used by the general surgeon himself. More sophisticated plastic surgery techniques can be proposed when the defect is more important and when the remodelling of the gland is more difficult. Generally in these cases, it is mandatory to check the symmetry after the partial reconstruction because the remodelling can provide an important change of the position of the breast and a descrepency with the other one. The contralateral mastoplasty allows an exploration of the glandular tissue at the same time and every reduction specimen should be send to the pathologist.

Among the numerous techniques of glandular partial reconstruction, the reduction mammaplasty procedures are the most frequently used. The latissimus dorsi musculocutaneous flap can also be used in certain uncommon situations.

In our recent experience at the EIO, the percentage of BCT as compared to mastectomy indications is around 70%. Among these BCT, the number of cases requiring an immediate partial reconstruction is 25%. Such a high percentage is due to the type of quadrantectomy performed with a 3 to 4 cm free margin. The early cosmetic results of the first 70 cases, were rated as good in 70%, fair in 26% and poor in 4%. Such cases are those which were selected for concomittant plastic surgery because the expected cosmetic result was poor. Therefore we can assess that 4% poor results in such selected series of poor expected cosmetic results is very low as compared to 10 to 20% of poor results observed in the literature in unselected patients. Most of the cases of our series would have been proposed for mastectomy by surgeons inexperimented in plastic surgery.

Conclusion

The role of plastic surgery can be considered as very important and integral part of the cancer treatment, especially in case of MBC. Close collaboration of general and pastic surgeons should be developed and breast cancer should be treated with a multidisciplinary approach. Good cosmetic results after BCT or satisfactory total breast reconstructions are helping the patient to cope with the psychological distress which is frequently associated with the cancer diagnosis even in case of good prognosis cases such as MBC [8].

References

1. Fisher ER, Leeming R, Anderson S *et al*. Conservative management of intraductal carcinoma (DCIS) of the breast *J Surg Oncol* 1991; 47: 139-47.
2. Sarrazin D, Le M, Rouesse J *et al*. Conservative treatment versus mastectomy in breast cancer tumors with microscopic diameter of 20 mm or less. *Cancer* 1984; 53: 1209.
3. Veronesi U, Saccozi R, Del Vecchio M *et al*. Comparing radical mastectomy with quadrantectomy, axillary dissection and radiotherapy of patients with operable breast cancer. *N Engl J Med* 1981; 305: 6-11.
4. Petit JY, Le MG, Mouriesse H. Breast augmentation and the risk of subsequent breast cancer (Letter) *N Engl J Med* 1993; 328: 661.
5. Petit JY, Le MG, Mouriesse H. Rietjens M. *et al*. Can Breast Reconstruction with Gel-Filled Silicone Implants Increase the Risk of Death and Second Primary Cancer in Patients Treated by Mastectomy for Breast Cancer? *Plast Reconstr Surg* 1994; 115.
6. Petit JY. Chirurgie Conservatrice. In *Cancer du sein*; Medsi McGraw-Hill 1991; 86-9, 160-74.
7. Petit JY. Corrections des séquelles de traitement conservateur. In *Cancer du sein*; Medsi McGraw-Hill 1991; 142.
8. Lehmann A. Incidences psychologiques de la chirurgie du sein. In *Cancer du sein*; Medsi McGraw-Hill, JY Petit, ed, 1991.

2

Tumor biology
Prognostic factors

Molecular and clinical aspects of metalloproteases in breast cancer

Paul Basset, Akiko Okada, Rama Kannan, Jennifer Byrne, Isabelle Stoll, Agnès Noël, Vincent Dive*, Marie-Pierre Chenard, Jean-Pierre Bellocq and Marie-Christine Rio

*IGBMC, CNRS/INSERM/ULP, Illkirch, France; *CEA, DIEP, Gif/Yvette, France*

The matrix metalloproteinases (MMPs), also known as matrixins (1), are extracellular zinc-enzymes that mediate a number of tissue remodeling processes, including those associated with cancer progression [2]. The MMP family presently comprises 14 distinct members *(Figure 1)*, and most of them have been shown to cleave directly or indirectly at least one component of the extracellular matrix (ECM) [3]. This observation has led to the concept that during tumor progression, cancer cells express MMPs in order to disrupt the ECM and invade adjacent tissues [4]. However, it has been found that some MMPs implicated in the progression of human carcinomas were not expressed by the cancer cells themselves, but by stromal cells surrounding cancer cells. Thus, stromelysin-3 (ST3), gelatinase A, and more recently MT-MMP1 have been found to be specifically expressed in fibroblastic cells of human carcinomas, including those of the breast [5 and refs therein]. Furthermore, the urokinase-type plasminogen activator is also predominantly secreted by fibroblastic cells in human adenocarcinomas [6, 7].

MMPs are both produced by and acting on stromal cells

The stromal expression of MT-MMP1 in human carcinomas is of particular importance. This membrane-bound MMP is likely to be a pro-gelatinase A activator [8]. Gelatinase A is secreted as a zymogen (pro-gelatinase A) which is believed to be activated at the membrane cell-surface by binding directly or indirectly to MT-MMP1 [9, 10]. The observation that pro-gelatinase A and its membrane-bound activator are expressed by the same fibroblastic cells in human carcinomas, indicates that stromal cells are both an important source of proteolytic activities and a target for at least part of these activities *(Figure 2)*. This is also supported by observations showing that tissue inhibitors of MMPs (TIMPs) are predominantly expressed by the stromal component of human carcinomas [11-13]. In particular, TIMP-3 exhibits an expression pattern very similar to those of fibroblastic MMPs in breast carcinoma *(Figure 3)*. Taken together, these findings suggest that during human carcinoma progression, the proteolytic activities

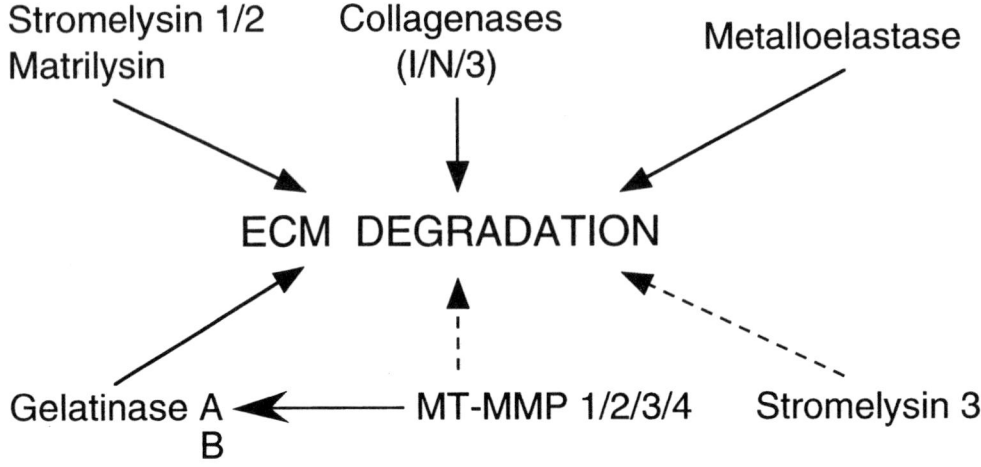

Figure 1. The matrix metalloproteinase family. Fourteen MMPs have been so far identified: one metalloelastase expressed in macrophages, three collagenases capable of cleaving native interstitial collagens, several enzymes (stromelysin 1 and 2, matrilysin, gelatinase A and B) exhibiting a broad specificity toward ECM molecules, four membrane-type (MT) MMPs, and stromelysin-3. Despite its designation, stromelysin-3 clearly differs from the other stromelysins in that it cannot cleave any of the major ECM components. Dot arrows indicate that no ECM substrate has been identified for these MMPs. Note that the ability of MT-MMPs to activate pro-gelatinase A has been so far demonstrated for MT-MMP1, 2, and 3.

generated by MMPs contribute to aspects of the malignant phenotype other than the direct promotion of cancer cell invasion. This possibility is also consistent with observations showing that MMP expression in stromal cells of human carcinomas can be detected before they become invasive [14].

MMP inhibitors as new anticancer agents

Synthetic MMP inhibitors are believed to represent a new class of potential anticancer agents [15]. Targeting proteinases produced by stromal cells rather than cancer cells may have several advantages, and would allow the identification of new anti-tumor agents capable of acting synergistically with those presently used. Although broad spectrum inhibitors have been successfully developed [16], it is currently believed that inhibitors specific for each MMP should be designed [15]. In this context, ST3 is an attractive target. ST3 has been found to be overexpressed in most human invasive carcinomas [14], and to favor tumor take of human breast cancer cells in nude mice [17]. Furthermore, it exhibits unusual functional properties. In contrast to other MMPs, ST3 cannot cleave any of the major ECM molecules [18, 19], and the proST3 activation pathway is so far unique among MMPs [20, 21].

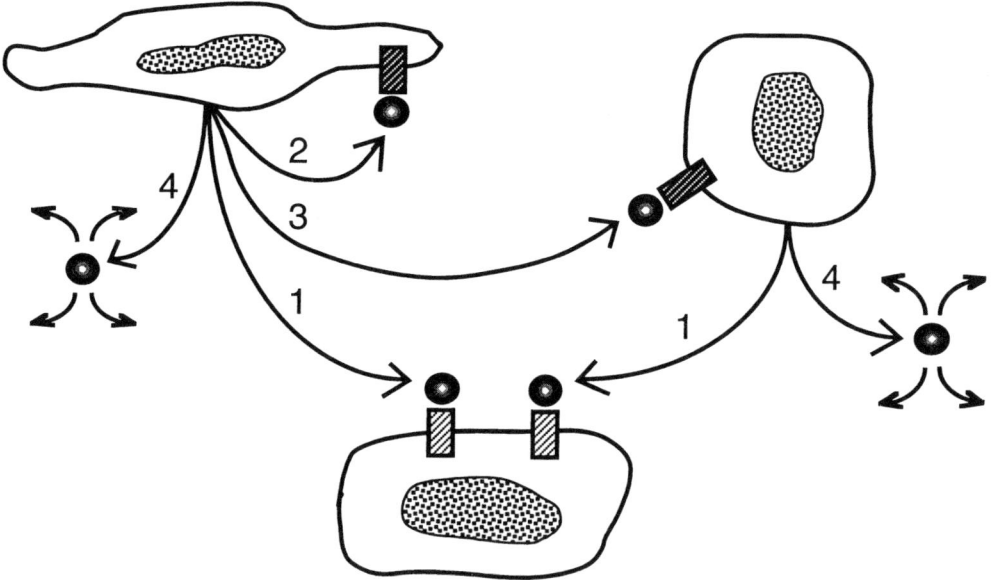

Figure 2. Delivery of stromal proteinases to epithelial and stromal compartments of human carcinomas. **1-** Proteinases secreted by fibroblastic (upper left) or inflammatory (upper right) cells may act at the cancer cell (bottom) surface where they are activated by specific membrane receptors. This has been shown for pro-urokinase which is produced by fibroblastic cells in colon carcinoma, while its receptor is found on cancer cells [6]. A similar scenario has been proposed for pro-gelatinase activation in lung-carcinoma [8]. **2-** Alternatively, pro-gelatinase A may be specifically activated at the fibroblastic cell-surface, as suggested by the observation that the RNAs for gelatinase A and MT-MMP1 (a membrane-bound pro-gelatinase A activator) were co-expressed by fibroblastic cells in several human carcinomas [5]. **3-** In breast carcinoma, pro-urokinase is secreted by fibroblastic cells [7], and activated at the surface of inflammatory cells which express the urokinase receptor [22]. **4-** Other extracellular proteinases, secreted by stromal cells may be activated in the ECM or before secretion. Thus stromelysin-3, which is specifically expressed in fibroblastic cells of human carcinomas [14], has beeen found to be secreted under an already active form having lost its N-terminal pro-domain [20, 21].

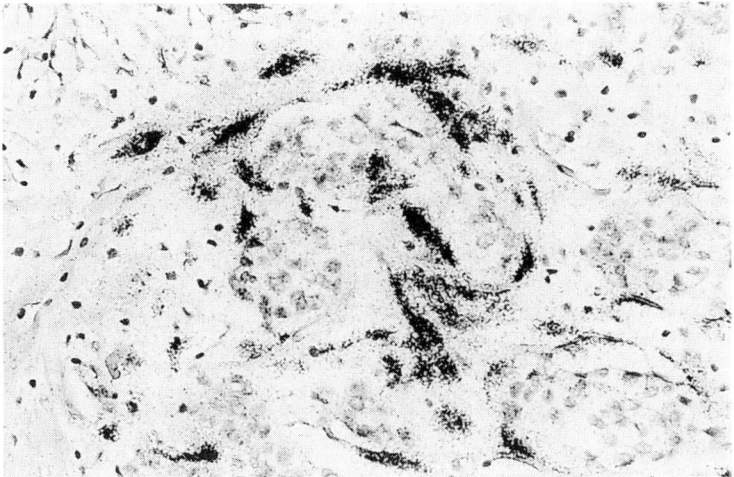

Figure 3. Expression of TIMP-3 transcripts in breast carcinoma. Bright field photomicrograph of a paraffin-embedded tissue section of an infiltrating ductal carcinoma which was stained with toluidine blue after hybridization with a ^{35}S-labeled antisense TIMP-3 riboprobe [13]. Strong labeling of fibroblastic cells surrounding cancer cells, which are not themselves labeled, is shown. Magnification 250 x.

References

1. Stöcker W, Bode W. Structural features of a superfamily of zinc-endopeptidases: the metzincins. *Curr Opin Struct Biol* 1995; 5: 383-90.
2. MacDougall JR, Matrisian LM. Contributions of tumor and stromal matrix metalloproteinases to tumor progression, invasion and metastasis. *Cancer Metastasis Rev* 1995; 14: 351-62.
3. Birkedal-Hansen H. Proteolytic remodeling of extracellular matrix. *Curr Opin Cell Biol* 1995; 7: 728-35.
4. Liotta LA. Cancer cell invasion and metastasis. *Sci Am* 1992; 266, 2: 54-63.
5. Okada A, Bellocq JP, Rouyer N, Chenard MP, Rio MC, Chambon P, Basset P. Membrane-type matrix metalloproteinase (MT-MMP) gene is expressed in stromal cells of human colon, breast, and head and neck carcinomas. *Proc Natl Acad Sci USA* 1995; 92: 2730-34.
6. Pike C, Kristensen P, Ralfkiaer E, Grondahl-Hansen J, Eriksen J, Blasi F, Dano K. Urokinase-type plasminogen activator is expressed in stromal cells and its receptor in cancer cells at invasive foci in human colon adenocarcinomas. *Am J Pathol* 1991; 138: 1059-67.
7. Wolf C, Rouyer N, Lutz Y, Adida C, Loriot M, Bellocq JP, Chambon P, Basset P. Stromelysin 3 belongs to a subgroup of proteinases expressed in breast carcinoma fibroblastic cells and possibly implicated in tumor progression. *Proc Natl Acad Sci USA* 1993; 90: 1843-7.
8. Sato H, Takino T, Okada Y, Cao J, Shinagawa A, Yamamoto E, Seiki M. A matrix metalloproteinase expressed on the surface of invasive tumour cells. *Nature* 1994; 370: 61-5.
9. Ward RV, Atkinson SJ, Reynolds JJ, Murphy G. Cell surface-mediated activation of progelatinase A: demonstration of the involvement of the C-terminal domain of progelatinase A in cell surface binding and activation of progelatinase A by primary fibroblasts. *Biochem J* 1994; 304: 263-9.
10. Strongin AY, Collier I, Bannikov G, Marmer BL, Grants GA, Goldberg GI. Mechanism of cell surface activation of 72-kDa type IV collagenase. *J Biol Chem* 1995; 270: 5331-8.
11. Polette M, Clavel C, Birembaut P. Localization by *in situ* hybridization of mRNAs encoding stromelysin 3 and tissue inhibitors of metallo-proteinases TIMP-1 and TIMP-2 in human head and neck carcinomas. *Path Res Pract* 1993; 189: 1052-7.
12. Poulsom R, Hanby AM, Pignatelli M, Jeffery RE, Longcroft JM, Rogers L, Stamp GWH. Expression of gelatinase A and TIMP-2 mRNAs in desmoplastic fibroblasts in both mammary carcinomas and basal cell carcinomas of the skin. *J Clin Pathol* 1993; 46: 429-36.
13. Byrne J, Tomasetto C, Rouyer N, Bellocq JP, Rio MC, Basset P. The tissue inhibitor of metalloproteinases-3 gene in breast carcinoma: identification of multiple polyadenylation sites and a stromal pattern of expression. *Mol Med* 1995; 1: 418-27.
14. Rouyer N, Wolf C, Chenard MP, Rio MC, Chambon P, Bellocq JP, Basset P. Stromelysin-3 gene expression in human cancer: an overview. *Invasion Metastasis* 1994-95; 14: 269-75.
15. Hodgson J. Remodeling MMPIs. *Biotechnology* 1995; 13: 554-7.
16. Brown PD, Giavazzi R. Matrix metalloproteinase inhibition: a review of anti-tumour activity. *Ann Oncol* 1995; 6: 967-74.
17. Noël A, Lefebvre O, Maquoi E, VanHoorde L, Chenard MP, Mareel M, Foidart JM, Basset P, Rio MC. *J Clin Invest* 1996; 97: in press.
18. Pei D, Majmudar G, Weiss SJ. Hydrolytic inactivation of a breast carcinoma cell-derived serpin by human stromelysin-3. *J Biol Chem* 1994; 269: 25849-55.
19. Noël A, Santavicca M, Stoll I, L'Hoir C, Staub A, Murphy G, Rio MC, Basset P. Identification of structural determinants controlling human and mouse stromelysin-3 proteolytic activities. *J Biol Chem* 1995; 270: 22866-72.
20. Pei D, Weiss SJ. Furin-dependent intracellular activation of the human stromelysin-3 zymogen. *Nature* 1995; 375: 244-7.
21. Santavicca M, Noël A, Angliker H, Stoll I, Segain JP, Anglard P, Chretien M, Seidah N, Basset P. Characterization of structural determinants and molecular mechanisms involved in pro-stromelysin-3 activation by 4-aminophenylmercuric acetate and furin-type convertases. *Biochem J* 1996; 313: in press.
22. Pyke C, Graem N, Ralfkiaer E, Ronne E, Hoyer-Hansen G, Brünner N, Dano K. Receptor for urokinase is present in tumor-associated macrophages in ductal breast carcinoma. *Cancer Res* 1993; 53: 1911-5.

Breast Cancer. Advances in biology and therapeutics.
F. Calvo, M. Crépin, H. Magdelenat, eds. John Libbey Eurotext © 1996, pp. 115-122.

Characterization of the PEA3 group of ets-related transcription factors: role in breast cancer

Yvan de Launoit*, Jean-Luc Baert, Anne Chotteau, Didier Monte, Pierre-Antoine Defossez, Laurent Coutte, Hélène Pelczar, Marie-Pierre Laget and Frauke Leenders

* Unité d'Oncologie Moléculaire, CNRS URA 1160, Institut Pasteur de Lille, 59019 Lille, France

Abstract

The PEA3 group of transcription factors belong to the Ets family and is composed of three known members, PEA3, ERM and ER81, which are more than 95% identical within the DNA-binding domain, the ETS domain, and demonstrate 50% aa identity overall. Here we present a review of the current knowledges on these transcription factors that possess two domains responsible for optimal transactivation. Recent data suggest that these factors are targets of signaling cascades such as the Ras-dependent one and may thus contribute to the nuclear response upon stimulation of cells and also to cellular transformation due to Ras. The presence of the PEA3 group members in certain breast cancer cells let suggest the involvement of these genes in the development, progression and invasion of this disease.

The *ets* gene family

The *ets* genes encode an increasingly growing family of transcription factors that includes in vertebrates *c-ets*-1, *c-ets*-2, ER71, ERF, *erg, fli*-1, SAP-1, SAP-2/ERP/*net,* elk-1, GABPα/E4TF1, *tel, elf*-1, PEA3, ER81, ERM, SPI-1 and SPI-B. These transcription factors are involved in normal development but some of these genes can become oncogenic by retroviral insertional mutagenesis [2, 3], or included in a chimeric protein as a result of a translocation event [4, 5]. The signature of the Ets family is a domain of ≈ 85 aa, the ETS domain [6], which has been widely conserved during evolution and for which the structural motif has been determined through NMR analysis [7] permitting its classification in the helix-turn-helix superfamily of DNA-binding domains. Even if most of the Ets family members bind to the core sequence 5'-AGGAAG-3', the ETS domain of all Ets proteins is, however, variable from member to member, allowing classification of Ets members in different groups with respect to their ETS domain sequence identity [1]. Moreover, the Ets proteins interacts with other factors for optimal transcription.

The PEA3 group

At the present time, the PEA3 group is composed of three members, PEA3 also called E1AF or ETV4 [8, 9], ER81 also called ETV1 [10-12] and ERM also called ETV5 [13]. As illustrated in *Figure 1*, these three proteins are more than 95% identical in the ETS domain, more than 85% in the 32 residue acidic domain (AD) which is localized in the amino-terminal part of the proteins, and almost 50% in the last 61 residues (Ct) corresponding to the carboxy-terminal tail [13].

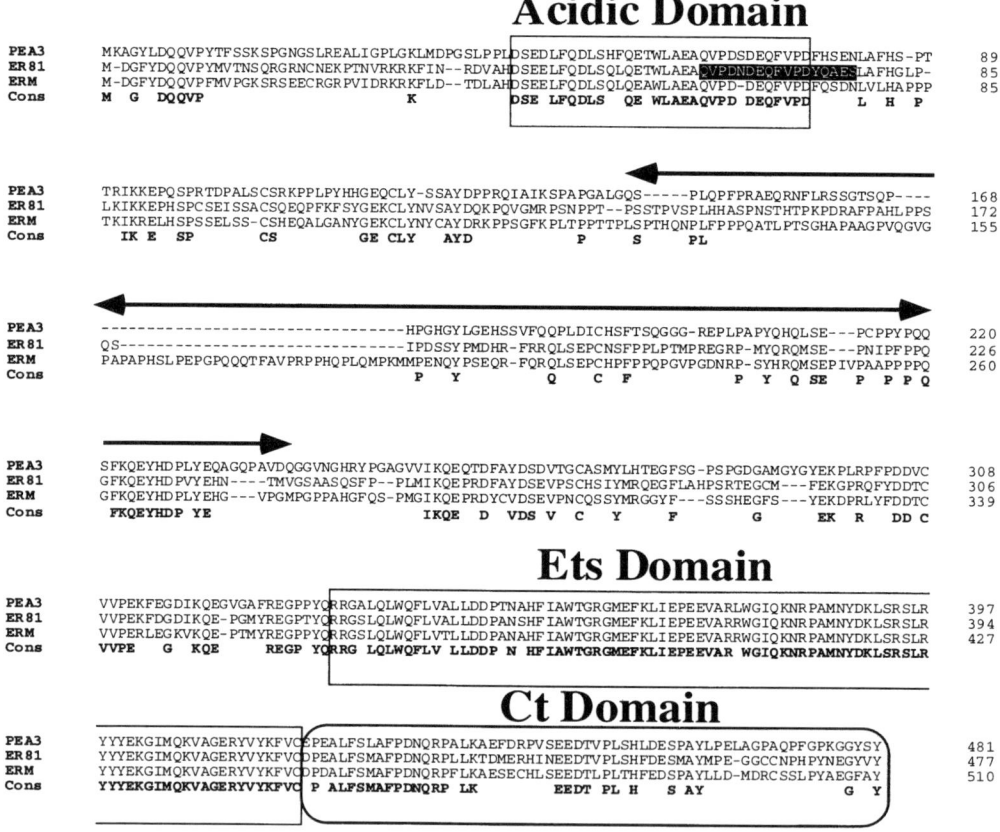

Figure 1. Sequence alignment of human PEA3 group proteins. Residues of PEA3, ER81 and ERM were aligned by computerized alignment software using the CLUSTAL package [14] relative to the first putative amino terminus methionine. Conserved for all three members are shown at the CONS line. The acidic, the ETS and the Ct domains are boxed and the glutamine rich region is indicated by an arrow. The 18 aa insertion at position aa 61 absent in human ER81 [12] present in human ETV1 [11] and corresponding to the 13 last aa of the acidic domain plus the 5 aa contiguous are black boxed.

Genomic organization and chromosomal localization

Human ERM is composed of 14 exons splited on at least 65 kb of genomic DNA *(Figure 2)* [15]. We have also characterized the human ER81/ETV1 and E1AF/PEA3/ETV4 genomic organization, and we showed that the position of the introns is highly conserved between the three genes (unpublished data). Moreover, the ETS, the Ct and the acidic domains displayed conservation of the position of the introns, thus suggesting that these three genes are probably the result of a gene duplication.

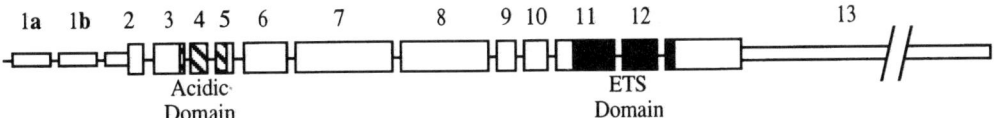

Figure 2. Schematic representation of ERM genomic DNA exons. The fourteen exons are represented by the solid rectangles and are numbered 1a, 1b and 2 to 13. The protein-coding region is represented by the large boxes, which contains the acidic (hatched box) and the ETS (black box) domains; the flanking 5'- and 3'- untranslated regions are shown as small boxes. The acidic and the ETS domains are each composed by three different exons.

Concerning the chromosomal localization ERM is situated at position 3q27-29 [15, 16] and E1AF/PEA3 [17] at position 17q21, this latter being in the vicinity of the inherited breast cancer gene BRCA1 [18]. ETV1/ER81 is located on chromosome band 7q21 and the translocation t [7, 22] (p. 22;12) is responsible for Ewing's sarcoma by fusing the EWS protein to ETV1 [11].

DNA-binding and transactivation capacities

As the other Ets family proteins, the PEA3 group members possess a DNA-binding domain responsible for their nuclear localization *(Figure 3)* and which confers to them the ability to bind to the DNA.

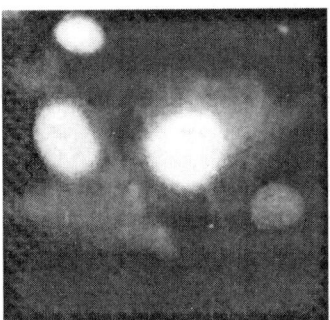

Figure 3. Nuclear localization of human ERM protein by means of immunofluorescence microscopy. The ERM-transfected Cos-1 cells were incubated with the anti-ERM$_{355-510}$ antibody directed against residues 355 to 510 of ERM containing the ETS and the Ct domains which are highly conserved between the three members of the PEA3 group.

Using gel shift analysis, it has been shown that the PEA3 group proteins bind the DNA core consensus sequence GGAA/T recognized by almost all Ets proteins [8, 10-13]. Moreover by binding site selection assay, mouse ER81 was determined to preferentially recognize the same nucleotide sequence outside the GGAA/T core sequence as did other Ets proteins such as GABPα and Ets-1 [10]. ERM contains two inhibitory domains of DNA-binding adjacent to the ETS domain, the Ct domain and a central region spanning residues 203 to 290 [19]. Point mutation at the Tyr_{419}, a conserved aa among the Ets proteins, dramatically decreased DNA-binding of the ETS domain of ERM, even if this residue is replaced by a conserved residue such as Phe, thus indicating that this residue is crucial since it is situated at the beginning of the α3 helix of the ETS domain and responsible for DNA recognition. In contrast, only mutation at position Tyr_{443} situated at the beginning of β4 sheet dramatically abolishes DNA-binding when replaced by a proline [19].

In transient cotransfection assays, these three PEA3 group proteins are able to transactivate reporter plasmids containing artificial multimerized Ets responsive elements adjacent or not to an AP1 site [9, 12, 16, 19], as well as reporter plasmids containing the functional promoter regions of the human stromelysin, the human type I and IV collagenases [20], the human vimentin (J.H. Chen, personal communication) and the human ICAM-1 (unpublished data) genes.

It has been recently shown that the 32 conserved residues of the acidic domain and the 61 conserved residues of the carboxy-terminal domains are responsible for transactivation of ERM [16, 19, 21] and ER81 [22]. Moreover, the acidic and the carboxy-terminal domains exhibit functional synergism, suggesting that they activate transcription through different mechanisms [19]. For efficient transactivation, these factors interact with other factors such as c-Jun [16], and probably with basal transcription machinery factors [19, and P. Desjardins and J. Hassell, personal communication].

Activation of PEA3 group members by several transduction pathway components

Recent studies support a model for signal transduction from activated receptor tyrosine kinases to Ras which, in turn, activates the mitogen-activated protein kinase (MAPK) pathway, which finally activate a diverse collection of nuclear transcription factors. Several Ets proteins have been demonstrated as being a target for the MAPK pathway. This is the case in vertebrates where the ternary complex factor (TCF) Ets proteins, Elk-1, Sap-1 and Erp/Net/Sap-2 are also activated by extracellular signal-regulated kinases (ERK) [23, 24] as well as by the Jun N-terminal kinase (JNK) [24], so increasing their transactivation ability on the *fos* promoter.

The transactivation capacities of mouse ER81 and human ERM have been shown to be dramatically increased by Ras, Raf-1 and the MAPK ERK-1 and ERK-2, thus concluding that these factors are a target of Ras-dependent signaling cascades and may thus contribute to the nuclear response upon stimulation of cells and also to cellular transformation due to Ras [21, 22]. The presence of MAPK phosphorylation sites conserved among ER81, ERM and PEA3 suggest that PEA3 should be also regulated by the Ras pathway. Moreover, we have shown that the protein kinase A (PKA) is also able to activate ERM transactivation [21], thus suggesting that the transactivation ability of these factors is regulated by several independent transduction signal pathways. Incidentally, a putative consensus PKA site at the the beginning of the ETS domain is conserved between ER81/ETV1 and ERM.

Expression of the PEA3 group members

Regarding at the mRNA level, ERM has been classified in adult human and mouse as a ubiquitously expressed gene with the highest expression in the brain and the lowest in the placenta [13]. In contrast, ER81 display a more restricted expression pattern with high expression levels in the human and mouse lung, heart and brain [10-12]. The mRNA of PEA3 group members are expressed in almost all the hemotapoietic cell lines tested and more particularly ERM at a relatively high level [12, 13, 25]. In a wide series of non-hematopoeitic cell lines, ERM mRNA seems to be almost ubiquitously expressed [13]. Interestingly, PEA3 whose expression is very weak in normal human tissues is expressed in these different hematopoietic cell lines [25, and unpublished data]. Concerning ER81 expression, only a few human cell lines such as teratocarcinoma Tera line expressed it [12].

The levels of ERM and ER81 mRNA expression correlate quite well with the levels of the corresponding protein expression. In fact, we have produced antibodies against these two transcription factors that specifically recognize in human cell lines the endogenous 70 kDa and 62 kDa proteins coresponding to ERM and ER81/ETV1 proteins, respectively [21, 26]. Concerning endogenous PEA3 protein, the anti-PEA3 antibody that we had prepared [26] as well as the commercial one (produced by Santa Cruz, 8), was unable to detect the endogenous PEA3 protein in several human cell types that express PEA3 mRNA. However, since this antibody recognized the overproduced PEA3 protein *in vitro (Figure 4)*, it is possible that the PEA3 translation efficiency is very low and the amount of PEA3 protein is too low to be detectable. This could be explained by the absence of an optimal translation consensus sequence around the ATG of murine and human PEA3.

The PEA3 group members in mammary cancer

A series of prognosis factors has been associated with breast cancer progression such as estrogen (ER) and progesterone (PR) receptor content, both of which determine responsiveness to antihormonal treatment. However, current antihormonal treatments are effective in only a third of the cases which has led to a search for genes responsible for loss of hormone-responsiveness or that confer autonomous growth. Several candidate genes including overexpressed, amplified and/or mutated oncogenes have been proved to be involved in mammary tumorigenesis and metastasis. A functional Ets-binding site is thus present in the HER2/ErbB-2/neu promoter in human breast cancer cells [27]. Transgenic mouse models carrying a putative oncogene under the control of a specific targeted promoter have been used to characterize the genes that, when mutated or overexpressed, induce tumors in the mammary gland [28], and transgenic animals bearing the tyrosine kinase receptor *neu* oncogene have been shown to overexpress PEA3 mRNA in mammary adenocarcinomas [29]. We recently characterized the level of mRNA and protein *(Figure 4)* expression of the three PEA3 group members in human breast cancer cell lines. We then showed that two normal epithelial breast cell lines expressed significant levels of these genes [26], thus being in good agreement with the data showing that PEA3 is expressed in the normal mouse mammary gland [8]. More particularly, we determined that ER81 expression was inversely correlated to ER and PR expression. The differential expression of these transcription factors in specific breast cancer cell lines led us to hypothesize potential roles in specific breast cancer regulation pathways. Several targets of the PEA3 proteins have been determined to be the matrix metalloproteinases. The metalloproteinases are enzymes that can degrade the extracellular matrix, thereby facilitating tumor growth, invasion, and metastasis [30]. Increased metalloproteinase expression has been associated with malignant progression in *in vivo* models of cancer development. It has recently been demonstrated that PEA3 is able to transactivate the promoters of collagenase types I and IV as well as stromelysin type I [20]. The high expression of the PEA3 group members in certain types of breast cancer cells could be linked to their metastatic potential. Moreover, it has been shown that human PEA3/E1AF, confers invasive phenotype on MCF-7 cells [31]. This hypothesis is supported by our recent data showing PEA3 group member expression in mouse mammary at different developmental stages.

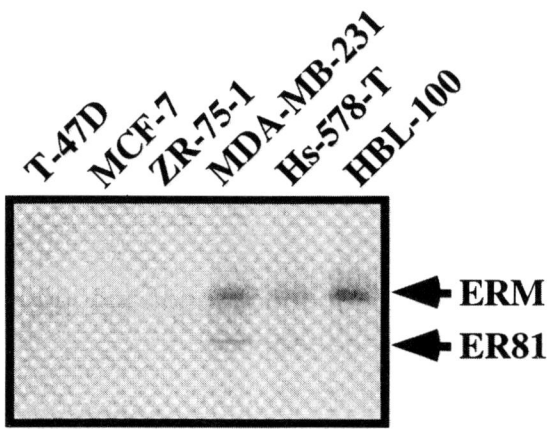

Figure 4. Immunoprecipitation of PEA3 group member proteins in human breast cancer cells. Seventy % confluent breast cancer cells were radiolabeled and twice immunoprecipitated with 1/100 of anti-ERM$_{355-510}$ antibody.

Conclusion

The demonstration that Ets responsive elements are contained within the regulatory regions of a number of genes implicated in the development, progression and invasion of breast cancer argues that these molecules may play an important role in breast cancer.

Acknowledgements

We would like to thank Agnès Bègue, Isabelle Damour, Frédérique Dewitte, Anne-Claire Flourens, Bertrand Goudeau, Daniel Lazarecki, Jean-Philippe Michalak and Laurent Pouilly for their technical assistance. This work has been carried out on the basis of grants awarded in part by the « Centre National de la Recherche Scientifique » (France), the « Fonds National de la Recherche Scientifique » (Belgium), the « Association pour la Recherche contre le Cancer » (France) and the « Ligue Contre le Cancer » (France).

References

1. Crépieux P, Coll J, and Stéhelin D. Ets family of proteins: weak modulators of gene expression in quest of transcriptional partners. *Crit Reviews Oncology* 1994; 5: 615-38.
2. Moreau-Gachelin F, Tavitian A, and Tambourin P. Spi-1 is a putative oncogene in virally induced murine erythroleukemias. *Nature* 1988; 331: 277-80.
3. Ben David Y, Giddens EB, Letwin K, and Bernstein A. Erythroleukemia induction by friend murine leukemia virus: insertional activation of a new member of the ets gene family, fli-1, closely linked to c-ets1. *Genes and Dev* 1991; 5: 908-18.
4. Delattre O, Zucman J, Plougastel B, Desmaze C, Melot T, Peter M, Kovar H, Joubert I, de Jong P, Rouleau G, Aurias A, and Thomas G. Gene fusion with an ETS DNA-binding domain caused by chromosome translocation in human tumors. *Nature* 1992; 359: 162-5.
5. Golub T, Barker GF, Lovett M, and Gililand DG. Fusion of PDGF receptor b to a novel *ets-like gene, tel*, in chronic myelomonocytic leukemia with t(5;12) chromosomal translocation. *Cell* 1994; 77: 307-16.
6. Karim FD, Urness LD, Thummel CS, Klemsz MJ, McKercher SR, Celada A, Van Beveren C, Maki RA, Gunther K, Nye JA, and Graves BJ. The ETS domain: A new DNA binding motif that recognizes a purine-rich core sequence. *Genes and Dev* 1990; 4: 1451-3.
7. Liang H, Mao X, Olejniczak ET, Nettesheim DG, Yu L, Meadows RP, Thompson CB, and Fesik SW. Solution structure of the ets domain of Fli-1 when bound to DNA. *Nature Struct Biol* 1994; 1: 871-6.
8. Xin JH, Cowie A, Lachance P, and Hassell JA. Molecular cloning and characterization of PEA3, a new member of the *Ets* oncogene family that is differentially expressed in mouse embryonic cells. *Genes and Dev* 1992; 6: 481-96.
9. Higashino F, Yoshida K, Kamio K, and Fujinaga K. Isolation of a cDNA encoding the adenovirus E1A enhancer binding protein: a new human member of the *ets* oncogene family. *Nucleic Acids Res* 1993; 21: 547-53.
10. Brown TA and McKnight SL. Specificities of protein-protein and protein-DNA interaction of GABPa and two newly defined *ets-related proteins. Genes and Dev* 1992; 6: 2502-12.
11. Jeon IS, Davis JN, Braun BS, Sublett JE, Roussel MF, Denny CT, and Shapiro DN. A variant Ewing's sarcoma translocation (7;22) fuses the EWS gene to the ETS gene ETV1. *Oncogene* 1995; 10: 1229-34.
12. Monté D, Coutte L, Baert JL, Angeli I, Stéhelin D, and de Launoit Y. Molecular characterization of the Ets-related human transcription factor ER81. *Oncogene* 1995; 11: 771-9.
13. Monté D, Baert JL, Defossez PA, de Launoit Y, and Stéhelin D. Molecular cloning and characterization of human ERM, a new member of the ETS family closely related to mouse PEA3 and ER81 transcription factors. *Oncogene* 1994; 9: 1397-406.
14. Higgins DG and Sharp PM. CLUSTAL: a package for performing multiple sequence alignment on a microcomputer. *Gene* 1988; 73: 237-44.
15. Monté D, Coutte L, Dewitte F, Defossez PA, Le Coniat M, Stéhelin D, Berger R, and de Launoit Y. Genomic organization of the human ERM (ETV5) gene, a PEA3 group member of Ets transcription factors. Submitted.
16. Nakae K, Nakajima K, Inazawa J, Kitaoka T, and Hirano T. ERM, a PEA3 subfamily of Ets transcription factors, can cooperate with c-Jun. *J Biol Chem* 1995; 270: 23795-800.
17. Isobe M, Yamagishi F, Yoshida K, Higashino F, and Fujinaga K. Assignment of the ets-related transcription factor E1A-F gene (ETV4) to human chromosome region 17q21. *Genomics* 1995; 28: 357-9.
18. Osborne-Lawrence S, Welsch PL, Spillman M, Chandrasekharappa SC, Gallardo TD, Lovett M, and Bowcock AM. Direct selection of expressed sequences within a 1-Mb region flanking BRCA1 on human chromosome 17q21. *Genomics* 1995; 25: 248-55.
19. Laget MP, Defossez PA, Albagli O, Baert JL, Dewitte F, Stéhelin D, and de Launoit Y. Two functionally distinct domains responsible for transactivation by the ETS family member ERM. *Oncogene* 1996; in press.
20. Higashino F, Yoshida K, Noumi T, Seiki M, and Fujinaga K. Ets-related protein E1A-F can activate three different matrix metalloproteinase gene promoters. *Oncogene* 1995; 10: 1461-3.

21. Janknecht R, Monté D, Baert D, and de Launoit Y. The Ets-related transcription factor ERM is a nuclear target of signaling cascades involving MAPK and PKA. Submitted.
22. Janknecht R. Analysis of the ERK-stimulated ETS-transcription factor ER81. *Mol Cell Biol* 1996; in press.
23. Janknecht R, Ernst W, Pingoud V, and Nordheim A. Activation of ternary complex factor Elk-1 by MAP kinases. *EMBO J* 1993; 12: 5097-104.
24. Whitmarsh AJ, Shore P, Sharrocks AD, and Davis RJ. Integration of MAP kinase signal transduction pathways at the serum response element. *Science* 1995; 269: 403-7.
25. Romano-Spica V, Suzuki H, Georgiou P, Chen SL, Ascione R, Papas TS, and Bhat NK. Expression of *ets* family genes in hematopoietic cells. *Int J Oncol* 1994; 4: 521-31.
26. Baert JL, Monté D, Musgrove EA, Albagli O, Sutherland RL, and de Launoit Y. Expression of the PEA3 group of Ets-related transcription factors in human breast cancer cells. Submitted.
27. Scott GK, Daniel JC, Xiong X, Maki RA, Kabat D, and Benz CC. Binding of an ETS-related protein within the DNase I hypersensitive site of the HER2/*neu* promoter in human breast cancer cells. *J Biol Chem* 1994; 269: 19848-58.
28. Cardiff RD and Muller WJ. Transgenic mouse models of mammary tumorigenesis. *Cancer Surveys* 1993; 16: 97-113.
29. Trimble MS, Xin JH, Guy CT, Muller WJ, and Hassell JA. PEA3 is overexpressed in mouse metastatic mammary adenocarcinomas. *Oncogene* 1993; 8: 3037-42.
30. Liotta LA and Stetler-Stevenson WG. Metalloproteinases and cancer invasion. *Semin Cancer Biol* 1990; 1: 99-106.
31. Kaya M, Yoshida K, Higashino F, Mitaka T, Ishii S, and Fujinaga K. A single ets-related transcription factor, E1AF, confers invasive phenotype on human cancer cells. *Oncogene* 1996; 12: 221-7.

Steroid metabolism in normal and malignant breast tissue compartments

W.R. Miller and P. Mullen

University Dept Clinical Oncology, ICRF Medical Oncology Unit, Western General Hospital, Edinburgh EH4 2XU, United Kingdom

Abstract

The stromal component of adipose tissue is a major site of oestrogen biosynthesis within the breast. In postmenopausal women this local production may maintain the growth of oestrogen dependent tumours. It is therefore relevant that, in breast cancer patients, the activity of the enzyme converting androgens into oestrogen (aromatase) is higher in quadrants bearing cancer compared with areas not involved with malignancy. Fibroblast cultures of adipose tissue from the same samples also display a similar pattern of aromatase activity, i.e. show higher activity if obtained from cancer-bearing quadrants. This relationship is observed in primary cultures but is not apparent in later passages. However, addition of tumour extracts (both benign and malignant) and breast cyst fluids to late passage cultures stimulates aromatase activity. There are quantitative differences between different extracts and fibroblasts with more pronounced effects tending to be found with extracts from malignant tissue. The factors responsible for these influences have not been fully defined but growth factors (such as IGF-1) and cytokines (such as IL-6) can mimic the effect. These results illustrate the potential for paracrine regulation of local oestrogen production within the breast and its relevance to the development and progression of breast cancer.

Introduction

The breast is a complex organ in which, apart from during pregnancy, glandular tissue comprises only a small component; elements such as stroma and adipose tissue form the bulk of the breast. Because breast cancer mainly develops in the terminal ductal-lobular units, there has been a tendency to overlook non-epithelial components. However, it is now realised that stromal and adipose tissue are not merely structural supports for glandular elements but may play more active roles and, by paracrine communication, influence both the development of normal breast and the natural history of breast cancers. Thus, stromal constituents may be abnormal or behave aberrantly in the breasts of women at high risk of breast cancer and those with established disease [11]. Fibroblasts and extracellular matrix components can enhance the take-rates and growth of breast cancer xenografts in immunocompromised mice [2, 3]. Similarly, mammary adipose tissue may be linked with the development of mammary cancer in both animals and humans [4].

Thus, only species whose glands are invested in fat develop mammary cancers and animals with experimentally-cleared fat pads have reduced incidence of spontaneous tumours and are less susceptible to carcinogen-induced neoplasia. Epidemiological evidence suggests that breast cancer incidence is substantially less in Japanese postmenopausal women compared with their counterparts in Westernized societies; there is a correspondingly reduced proportion of fat in the breasts of postmenopausal Japanese women. Japanese immigrants to Hawaii whose risk of breast cancer is now approaching that of women in USA also have increased proportions of adipose tissue within the breast. It is relevant therefore that breast adipose tissue is not metabolically inert but has the potential to synthesize and metabolise active oestrogens which might promote the development of transformed cells and stimulate the growth of hormone-dependent cancers. In this respect we have shown that (I) mammary adipose tissue from patients with breast cancer has elevated levels of aromatase activity converting androgens to oestrogens [5]; and (II) adipose tissue from the quadrants involved with breast cancer have enhanced activity compared with non-involved quadrants [6]. The present article describes further studies which explore the concept that these phenomena may result from paracrine interaction between malignant and stromal components of the breast.

Materials and methods

Breast tissues

Breast cancers were obtained either by biopsy or at mastectomy from patients with histologically confirmed malignancy of the breast. Adipose tissue was obtained at operation from the breasts of women presenting with either benign or malignant conditions of the breast. In studies directed at determining the variation of activity throughout the different quadrants of the breast, adipose tissue was obtained from each quadrant of eight mastectomy specimens, the surgical procedure being performed for breast cancer which had been confirmed histologically. Breast cyst fluids were obtained by needle puncture of palpable cysts.

Specimens from which cells were to be cultured were immediately transferred into sterile phosphate-buffered saline in universal containers. All remaining tissues were put on ice in the operating theatre and transported immediately to a laboratory.

Tissue homogenates

Homogenates which were to be added to cell cultures were prepared by disruption in MEM (minimal essential media) using a Silverson homogeniser (maximum speed, 10s x 2) and centrifuged at 1,000 g for 10 min. The resultant supernatant was sterilised through filters and added to cultures at final concentrations of 0.25 and 2.5%.

Cell lines

Gross fat was teased from breast adipose tissue and the stromal-enriched fraction was cut into small pieces with a scalpel. Aliquots (2 g) were then placed into universal containers and finely chopped with long-nose scissors. Collagenase (10 ml, 1 mg/ml) was then added and incubated for 30 min at 37 °C in a shaking water bath and the contents allowed to settle. After 10 mins the liquid phase was aspirated from below the surface lipid layer and centrifuged at 3,000 g for 10 mins. The resultant pellet was then washed (x 2) in phosphate buffer saline (PBS) and resuspended in MEM supplemented with penicillin, streptomycin and heat-inactivated fetal calf serum (15%). The suspension was then aliquoted into 60 mm petri dishes (4 ml/dish) and grown as monolayer cultures. Cells were placed in a humidified incubator in an atmosphere of 5% CO_2: 95% air for 48 h, washed thoroughly in PBS x 2, resuspended in fresh media and allowed to grow to confluence prior to assay for aromatase activity.

Aromatase assays

Particulate fractions

Tissue (2 g) was homogenised in phosphate buffer pH 7.4 (1:1 w/v) and centrifuged at 800 g for 5 min. The supernatant beneath the lipid layer was then centrifuged at 100,000 g for 1 h. The resultant pellet (particulate fraction) was re-suspended by sonication in phosphate buffer (600 µl) and assayed for aromatase activity by measuring the release of tritiated water produced during the conversion of 1β tritiated Δ 4-androstenedione to oestrone. Particulate fractions (500 µl) were added to β tritiated Δ 4-androstenedione (100 nM/l, 37 Bq) and co-factors generating nicotinamide adenine dinonucleotide phosphate (reduced form) (NADPH) in a final volume of 1.1 ml. Control incubations were performed in which particulate fractions were replaced with bovine serum albumin (1.5 mg/ml). Each sample was incubated in 37 °C for three hours with continuous shaking. Reactions were stopped by transferring aliquots into 3 mls ice cold chloroform which was thoroughly shaken and centrifuged at 2,000 g for 3 min. Duplicate aliquots from the aqueous supernatant were then transferred into 5% charcoal. After thorough mixing the charcoal was precipitated by centrifugation at 2,000 g for 15 min and the supernatant counted into a glass scintillation vial containing 10 ml NE260 scintillant (Nuclear Enterprises, Edinburgh). Counts from the control incubations were substrated from all other counts before correction for recovery losses and counting efficiency.

Aromatase assays in cultured fibroblasts were performed under two sets of conditions; (a) first generation cell lines were incubated for 4 days with dibutryl cyclic AMP (1 mM) in the absence of fetal calf serum and (b) later passages were incubated 18 h with dexamethasone (1 µM) in the presence of fetal calf serum (15%). The aromatase assay itself involved removing « spent » tissue culture media and washing the dishes with PBS. To each dish tritiated Δ 4-androstenedione (100 nM, 2 µCi) in MEM was added and incubation carried out at 37 °C for 5 hr in a humidified incubator in an atmosphere of 5% CO_2: 95% air. Blank incubations consisted of dishes containing media but no cells. After incubation all dishes were placed on ice for 15 mins, the medium aspirated, transferred to ice cold chloroform (5 ml), shaken vigorously and centrifuged for 5 min at 3,000 g. Duplicate aliquots of the aqueous phase were then mixed with 5% charcoal in phosphate buffer and centrifuged at 2,000 g for 15 min. The resultant supernatant was counted in NE260 scintillant (10 ml).

Results

Aromatase activity in adipose tissue from quadrants of cancer bearing breasts

In order to confirm our previous observation that aromatase activity was elevated in adipose tissue in quadrants that contained breast cancer, eight mastectomy specimens were studied. The adipose tissue from each quadrant was divided so that aromatase activity could be measured in both particulate fractions of tissue and cultured fibroblasts. The results from the assay of particulate fractions are shown diagrammatically in *Figure 1*.

It can be seen that the quadrant with the highest aromatase activity was involved with tumour in five of the eight cases whereas the quadrant with the lowest activity was involved with tumour in only one case.

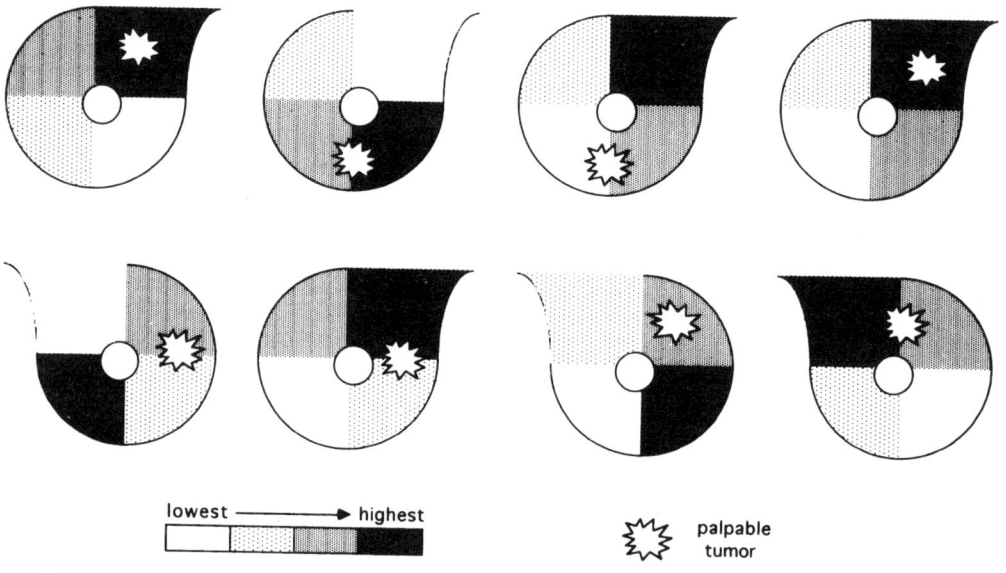

Figure 1.

Cultured fibroblasts were successfully established for each quadrant of all eight mastectomy specimens. However, two sets of culture samples became contaminated during the preincubation period with dibutryl cyclic AMP. Results are therefore only available in six of the breasts at the time of initial primary culture *(Figure 2)*. These results again show a correlation between tumour involvement in quadrants and the level of aromatase activity in the derived fibroblast cultures. Thus, the quadrant with the highest aromatase activity was involved with tumour in four cases, that with the next highest aromatase in two cases, the next lowest aromatase in a further two cases and the quadrant with the lowest aromatase activity was only involved with tumour on one occasion. In general, the level of aromatase activity in primary cultured fibroblasts correlated quantitatively with the activity found in the subcellular fraction of the adipose tissue assayed at the time of biopsy.

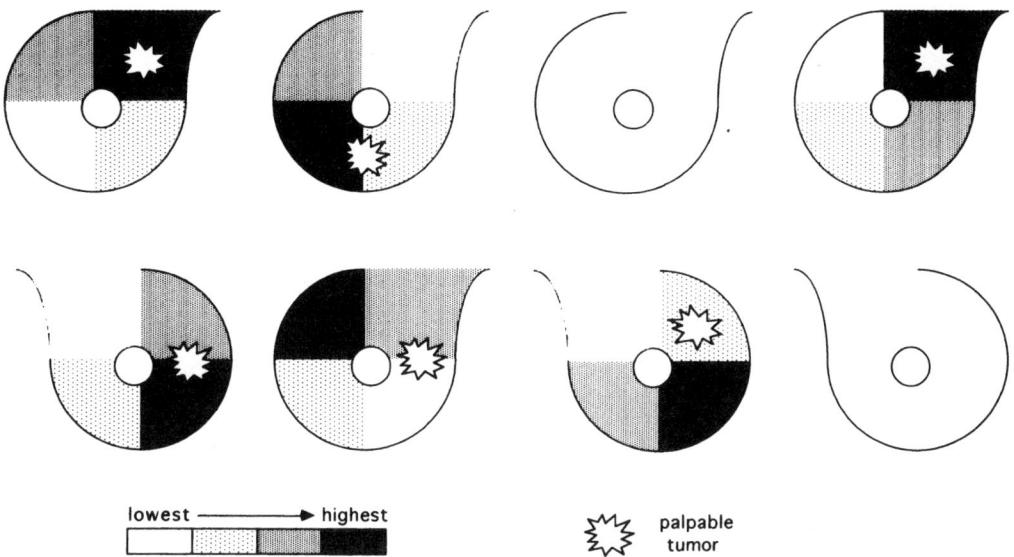

Figure 2.

Cultured fibroblasts were then passaged on for between four and six generations and assayed for aromatase activity in the presence of inducing amounts of dexamethasone (it was not possible to detect aromatase activity in the presence of dibutryl cyclic AMP, the inductive effects of this agent disappearing after only a single passage). The results of the aromatase assays of later generation fibroblasts are shown in *Figure 3*. It can be seen that there was no clear correlation between the level of aromatase in the cultured fibroblasts and the quadrant from which they were derived whether this be involved with tumour or not. The level of aromatase activity in such fibroblasts also did not correlate with that as assayed in subcellular fractions from the original adipose tissue. These results suggest that whereas the initially derived fibroblasts reflected the activity of excised adipose tissue, the factors which regulated such activity were lost on further passage or not evident in the inducing presence of dexamethasone.

The effects of adding tumour extracts and breast cyst fluids to cultured fibroblasts

Tumour homogenates were capable of inducing aromatase activity in the presence of dexamethasone in a dose-related manner. Effects were evident with both malignant and benign tumours but the magnitude of effect could differ markedly between different homogenates. However, there was a tendency for the effects of extracts from malignant tumours to be quantitatively greater than those from benign tumours. Under the same conditions the addition of breast cyst fluids produced similar effects. Whilst these were invariably stimulatory, the degree of effect varied greatly between different cyst fluids. It was evident, however, that cyst fluids classified as being Type II on the basis of electrolyte composition, as a group showed substantially greater stimulatory effects. The levels of a variety of hormones, growth factors, cytokines and proteins were measured in the cyst fluids. Although positive relationships were evident between levels of cytokines such as IL-6 and degree of stimulation, the most convincing correlation between degree of effect and any constituent was for albumin content.

The addition of exogenous factors to the medium of cultured fibroblasts

In an attempt to determine potential factors which might modulate aromatase activity in cultured fibroblasts, a series of studies were performed in which known factors were added to the cultures. IGFI added to cultures in the absence of FCS stimulated aromatase activity in a dose-related manner, an effect which could be blocked by a specific saturating antibody. However the same antibody failed to inhibit the stimulatory effects of breast cyst fluids and albumin preparation. IL-6 and soluble IL-6 receptors also had small but significant stimulatory effects on aromatase activity. However, together they produced a marked stimulatory effect which could exced 20-fold stimulation above control values. The addition of IL-6 in combination with cyst fluids to cultured fibroblasts produced no greater effect than the cyst fluid alone. Various albumin preparations were also added to the cultured fibroblast producing variable degrees of stimulation. In general, non-denatured human preparations produce substantially greater influences than either denatured or non-human preparations.

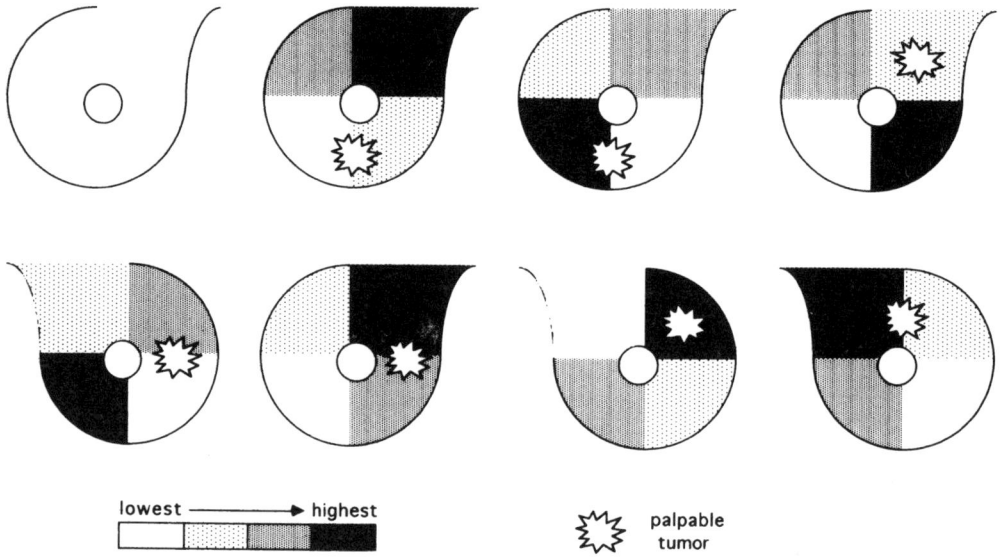

Figure 3.

Discussion

It has been confirmed that areas of the breast bearing cancer have high aromatase activity. There are several reasons for this, including (I) tumours grow preferentially in areas which possess locally high aromatase activity; (II) fat adjacent to tumours is inherently different or may disproportionately contain populations of cells which possess high aromatase activity; (III) tumours secrete factors into their local environment which induce aromatase activity. In order to understand better the basic observation we have performed more detailed studies and shown that fibroblasts derived from breast quadrants which are involved with malignancy also display higher aromatase activity in culture. The number of fibroblasts in such cultures do not vary according to the quadrants from which they were derived and therefore the differences in aromatase are unlikely to be due to the original biopsies having variable proportions of fibroblasts. It seems more likely therefore that either the fibroblasts are inherently different when derived from cancer-bearing quadrants or that they have been influenced by the close proximity of tumour. In the case of the latter scenario it might be expected that any tumour influences might disappear after long-term culture. This would be compatible with the observation in the present studies which indicates that the differences in fibroblasts derived from tumour bearing and non-tumour bearing areas are not seen in later passages. However, in order to demonstrate aromatase activity in these fibroblasts, it is necessary to culture in the presence of the corticoids. Whether the results are a feature of early versus late passage or the change in inducing agent from dibutryl cyclic AMP to dexamethasone is still to be resolved.

The dexamethasone cultures have also been used as model system in which to test the ability of breast-derived extracts and fluids to induce aromatase activity. These studies show the clear potential of such extracts and fluids to potentiate aromatase activity. The tendency for homogenates of malignant tumours to produce quantitatively greater effects would be consistent with such cancers being able to produce factors which can induce aromatase activity in the surrounding stroma. In this respect it is relevant that some but not all studies have shown that aromatase within breast cancers themselves may immuno-localise to the stromal component [7, 8]. The identity of inducing factors remains to be definitively determined. Growth factors and cytokines, such as IGF-I, IL-6 and IL-8, may be stimulatory [9-12]. However blocking antibodies do not necessarily attenuate effects in tumour extracts and breast fluids; neither do concentrations of individual cytokines with breast extracts and fluids always correlate well with quantitative effects on aromatase. There may be confounding factors like the need to measure both cytokines and their receptors - synergic effects of IL-6 and its soluble receptor are spectacular in comparison with the modest effects of either agent alone [13].

There are already precedents for the compartmentalisation of oestrogen biosynthesis and its regulation by soluble factors - this appears to be the case in the placenta, ovary and testis. Similarly others have shown that other aspects of steroid metabolism within the breast may be regulated by a paracrine manner, soluble factors from one tissue compartment influencing enzyme activity in another [14, 15]. Given the unusual profiles of steroid hormones within the breast it will be important to define more precisely regulatory factors - their control could be used therapeutically to influence the natural history of breast cancer.

References

1. Schor SL, Schor AM, Howell A, Crowther D. Hypothesis: the persistent expression of fetal-like phenotypic characteristics by fibroblasts is associated with an increased susceptibility to neoplastic disease. *Exp Cell Biol* 1987; 55: 11.
2. Horgan K, Jones DL, Mansel RE. Mitogenicity of human fibroblasts in vivo for human breast cancer cells. *Br J Surg* 1987; 74: 227-9.
3. Noel A, De-Pauw-Gillet MC, Purnell G, Nusgens B, Lapiere CM, Foidart JM. Enhancement of tumorigenicity of human breast adenocarcinoma cells in nude mice by matrigel and fibroblasts. *Br J Cancer* 1993; 68: 909-15.
4. Miller WR. Intra-mammary steroid transformation: implications for tumorigenesis and natural progression. In: Krey LC, Gulyas BJ, McCracken JA eds. *Autocrine and Paracrine Mechanisms in Reproductive Endocrinology*. Plenum Publishing Corp, New York 1989: 185-99.
5. O'Neil JS, Miller WR. Aromatase activity in breast adipose tissue from women with benign and malignant breast disease. *Br J Cancer* 1987; 56: 601-40.
6. O'Neil JS, Elton RA, Miller WR. Aromatase activity in adipose tissue from breast quadrants: a link with tumour site. *Br Med J* 1988; 296: 741-3.

7. Esteban JM, Warsi Z, Haniu M, Hall P, Shiveley JE, Chen S. Detection of intratumoral aromatase in breast carcinomas. *Am J Pathol* 1992; 140: 337-43.
8. Santen RJ, Martel J, Hoagland M *et al*. Stromal spindle cells contain aromatase in human breast tumors. *J Clin Endocrinol Metab* 1994: 79: 627-32.
9. Reed MJ, Topping L, Coldham NG, Purohit A, Ghilchik M, James VHT. Control of aromatase activity in breast cancer cells: the role of cytokines and growth factors. *J Steroid Biochem Molec Biol* 1993; 4: 589-96.
10. Miller WR, Mullen P. Factors influencing aromatase activity in the breast. *J Steroid Biochem Mol Biol* 1993; 44: 597-604.
11. Purohit A, Ghilchik MW, Duncan V, Wang DY, Singh A, Walker MM, Reed MJ. Aromatase activity and interleukin-6 production by normal and malignant breast tissues. *J Clin Endocrinol Metab* 1995; 80: 3052-8.
12. Macdiarmid F, Wang D, Duncan LJ, Purohit A, Ghilchik MW, Reed MJ. Stimulation of aromatase activity in breast fibroblasts by tumour necrosis factor alpha. *Mol Cell Endocrinol* 1994; 106: 17-21.
13. Singh A, Purohit A, Wang DY, Duncan LJ, Ghilchik MW, Reed MJ. IL-6sR: Release from MCF-7 breast cancer cells and role in regulating peripheral oestrogen synthesis. *J Endocrinol* 1995; 147: R9-R12.
14. McNeill JM, Reed MJ, Beranek PA, Newton CJ, Ghilchik MW, James VHT. The effect of epidermal growth factor, transforming growth factor and breast tumour homogenates on the activity of oestradiol 17β hydroxysteroid dehydrogenase in cultured adipose tissue. *Cancer Letts* 1986; 31: 213-9.
15. Adams EF, Newton CJ, Tait GH, Braunsberg H, Reed MJ, James VHT. Paracrine influence of human breast stromal fibroblasts on breast epithelial cells: secretion of a polypeptide which stimulates reductive 17-beta-oestradiol dehydrogenase activity. *Int J Cancer* 1988; 42: 119-22.

Breast Cancer. Advances in biology and therapeutics.
F. Calvo, M. Crépin, H. Magdelenat, eds. John Libbey Eurotext © 1996, pp. 131-137.

Signal transduction of prolactin and cytokine receptors

Vincent Goffin, Christine Bole-Feysot, Fatima Ferrag, Ronda Maaskant, Valérie Vincent, Edda Weimann and Paul A. Kelly

Inserm Unité 344 - Endocrinologie Moléculaire, Faculté de Médecine Necker, 75015 Paris, France

Introduction

Prolactin (PRL) and growth hormone (GH) receptors are members of a larger family known as Cytokine Receptors. Cytokines are chemical mediators that include interleukins, polypeptide hormones and other growth factors. They regulate growth, differentiation and specific cellular functions by interacting with their cognate receptors. Cytokine receptors, which contain no tyrosine kinase domain in their cytoplasmic regions, have been grouped into different classes. The hematopoietic or cytokine/GH/PRL receptor family (Class I) and the interferon receptor family (Class II) share both structural features and newly identified common signal transduction pathways. It has been demonstrated recently that both classes of receptors are associated with various members of the Janus (JAK) family of tyrosine kinases and activate a new family of transcription factors that couple ligand binding to the activation of gene expression and are thus termed STAT proteins, for signal transducers and activators of transcription.

Structure of cytokine receptors

Class I and Class II cytokine receptors appear to derive from an ancestral gene from which multiple duplications and modifications have occurred [1]. There are over twenty members of Class I cytokine receptors. These include the receptors for interleukins (IL)-2, IL-3, IL-4, IL-5, IL-6, IL-7, IL-9, IL-11, IL-12, IL-13, IL-15, G-CSF, GM-CSF, leukemia inhibitory factor (LIF), ciliary neurotrophic factor (CNTF), oncostatin M (OSM), erythropoietin (EPO), growth hormone (GH) and prolactin (PRL), the ligand of c-mpl, known as thrombopoietin (TPO), and the obesity factor, leptin. The major region of homology of Class I receptors lies in the extracellular, ligand-binding domain and is formed of ~ 200 amino acids [2]. With the exception of the CNTFR which is membrane-anchored *via* a glycosyl-phosphatidylinositol linkage, all receptors have a single transmembrane domain of 22-28 amino acids. No consensus catalytic domain, and only limited sequence similarity has been found in the cytoplasmic domains of these receptors. However, two motifs, Box 1 and Box 2, are relatively conserved in the cytoplasmic membrane-proximal region of most receptors [3]. Box 1 comprises a Pro-X-Pro sequence and a preceding cluster of hydrophobic amino acids. The Box 1 region is encoded by an exon just after the one encoding the transmembrane domain for all members of the Class I receptor genes [1]. Box 2 is conserved in approximately 50% of the members of the receptor family; it begins with a cluster of hydrophobic amino acids, followed by negatively charged residues and ends with one or two positively charged amino acids. Soluble forms of some receptors, that can function as agonists or antagonists, have also been described [4]. This is the case for receptors for IL-4, IL-5, IL-7, IL-9, G-CSFR, LIF, GH, PRL and CNTF.

Activation of PRL and GH receptors by ligand-induced homodimerization

One of the first remarkable discoveries made possible by the availability of the GHR cDNA was that crystals of recombinant hGH-hGH binding protein (bp) complexes were composed of a single molecule of hormone bound to two molecules of binding protein, suggesting the occurrence of ligand-induced receptor [5]. Mutational and structural analysis of hGH identified two regions - referred to as binding sites 1 and 2 - involved in contacts with the hGHbp [6]. It was further demonstrated that membrane-bound GHR is activated by ligand-induced dimerization which occurs sequentially, hGH-receptor binding through site 1 being required before interaction can occur through site 2. Receptor activation by oligomerization of membrane components is a general rule in the cytokine receptor superfamily [7, 8] and the multiple similarities between data obtained from studies of hGH and hPRL, such as the localization of functional regions, the comparable behavior of equivalent analogs mutated at either binding site, or the PRL-like effects of divalent but not monovalent anti-PRLR antibodies [9] strongly suggest that the PRLR is also activated by ligand-induced homodimerization.

Receptor antagonists

One major interest of these molecular studies in view of potential clinical application is the development of potent PRL or GH antagonists [10, 11], designed by blocking binding site 2, which prevents receptor dimerization and subsequent activation. Pathologies linked to hyperprolactinemia are usually treated with the dopamine analog bromocriptine, which blocks the pituitary synthesis of PRL. In some cases, however, such therapy can not used due to side effects. Moreover, it has recently been shown that the human breast cancer cell line T-47D secretes hPRL which, in turn, exerts an autocrine effect on cell proliferation [12]. If such *in vitro* observations are relevant to the situation found *in vivo* in human breast tumors, the availability of hormone antagonists, acting at the receptor level, might be an alternative clinical approach to bromocriptine therapy which is ineffective on peripheral (extra-pituitary) PRL synthesis.

Signalling pathways of PRL and GH receptors

Signalling cascades activated by cytokine receptors have been and continue to be extensively studied and deciphering the connections between tyrosine kinases, serine/threonine kinases, phosphatases, Stat proteins and other transducers has become a major challenge of modern molecular biology. In the following sections, we will focus on the involvement of JAK2, Stat proteins, Src tyrosine kinases, tyrosine phosphatases and the MAP kinase pathway in PRLR and GHR signalling.

The receptor-associated JAK2 tyrosine kinase

Although cytoplasmic domains of the PRLR and GHR are devoid of any intrinsic enzymatic activity [2], hormonal stimulation leads to tyrosine phosphorylation of several cellular proteins, including the receptors themselves. The first major step in the understanding of PRLR/GHR signalling was the identification of JAK2, a member of the Janus tyrosine kinase family, as (one of) the tyrosine kinase responsible for these phosphorylations [13-15]. In the murine lymphoid pre-B BaF3 cell line, involvement of JAK1, another Janus kinase, has also been proposed in PRLR signalling [16]. It has been shown that JAK2 is constitutively associated with the PRLR [14, 15], whereas it is recruited by GHR only upon ligand activation [13]. For both receptors, there is strong evidence that box 1 is the site of interaction with JAK2 [17-19]. Although the mechanism by which the kinase is activated remains poorly understood, it is usually assumed that receptor clustering upon ligand binding brings two JAK2 molecules close to each other, which allows trans-phosphorylation and subsequent activation of the enzyme [8]. JAK2, whose activation occurs very rapidly after hormonal stimulation (within less than 1 min for PRLR), is thought to be the initial element upstream of several signalling pathways of both PRLR or GHR. Receptor analogs appropriately mutated within box 1 to disturb the association with and/or activation of JAK2, have been reported inactive in almost all *in vitro* biological responses analyzed so far (see below). One of the likely substrates of JAK2 is the receptors themselves and phosphorylated tyrosine residues have been identified on both GHR and PRLR [18, 20, 21]. Presumably, there are a multitude of other substrates, such as Stat proteins and receptor-associated phosphatases.

Stat proteins

Stat proteins are a family of latent cytoplasmic proteins recently described as involved in cytokine receptor signalling [8]. Stats are assumed to associate through their SH2 domains with phosphotyrosines of activated receptors, where they become phosphorylated, presumably by the receptor-associated Janus kinases [22]. They then dissociate from the receptor through a mechanism that remains unknown, homo- or hetero-dimerize and translocate to the nucleus where they interact with and activate specific DNA elements found in the promoters of target genes [8, 23]. Three members of the Stat family have been thus far clearly identified as transducer molecules of PRL/GH receptors: Stat5, previously referred to as mammary gland factor (MGF) [20, 22], Stat3 [20, 24-26], and Stat1 [26, 27]. It has been demonstrated that the DNA binding activity of Stat5 requires phosphorylation of a single tyrosine residue (Tyr 694) which is mediated by JAK2, but not by Src kinases [22] confirming Stat proteins as Janus kinase substrates. In agreement, Stat1 is not phosphorylated in cells transfected with cDNA encoding a box 1-deleted mutant of the PRLR, unable to associate with JAK2 [19].

The activation of identical Stat proteins by different cytokine receptors questions the mechanisms by which specificity of signalling pathways is achieved in response to a particular hormonal stimulation. For example, although several cytokines (EPO, GM-CSF, GH, PRL, IL-2, IL-3, IL-5) activate the DNA binding ability of Stat5 and/or transactivate the β-casein-luciferase reporter gene *in vitro*, it is unlikely that all these cytokines stimulate the synthesis of milk proteins in vivo. This suggests that different Stat combinations and/or involvement of other signal transducers direct the specificity of the final response.

Src kinases

Fyn, a member of the Src family of tyrosine kinases, is associated with the PRLR and activated by PRL stimulation in the rat T lymphoma Nb2 cell line [28]. Preliminary studies performed in our laboratory suggest that this association involves the membrane proximal region of the PRLR. Recently, association of the PRLR with Src has also been reported after PRL stimulation in lactating rat hepatocytes [29]. Although a role in the promotion of cell growth has been suggested [29], the involvement of Src kinases in signal transduction by these receptors remains unknown.

Tyrosine phosphatases

Involvement of tyrosine phosphatase in PRLR/GHR signalling has been suggested [20, 30], although such associations remain poorly documented. Since many intracellular signalling steps require tyrosine phosphorylation (of receptors, Janus kinases, Stats, etc.), one would anticipate that tyrosine phosphatases would be negative regulators of signal transduction. In fact, it has recently been reported that the phosphatase PTP-1D (now renamed SHP-2), identified as a JAK2 substrate, acts as a positive regulator of PRLR-dependent induction of b-casein gene transcription [30]. Recent results obtained in our laboratory strongly suggest participation of phosphatases in GHR signalling also, since the time-course of JAK2 dephosphorylation is retarded when the C-terminal tail of the receptor is truncated [20]. Investigation of cytokine receptor signalling also argues for correlation between phosphatase activity and Stat activation [31].

Ras/Raf/MAP kinase pathway

Signalling through the mitogen-activated protein kinase (MAPK) kinase pathway involves a series of interactions, the Shc/SOS/Grb2/Ras/Raf/MAPK. Activation of the MAPK pathway has been reported in different biological systems following PRL [32] and GH [18] stimulation. Whether activation of the MAP cascade requires JAK2, Fyn (or another Src kinase) or some other pathway is currently unknown.

Structure-function relationships of GH and PRL receptors

Which cytoplasmic sub-domain for different bioactivities?

Although participation of all the above-mentioned molecules in PRLR/GHR signalling has been reported, the exact mechanisms involved in specific pathways leading to the expression of a particular biological activity remain poorly understood. Classically, two categories of hormone-induced biological effects are considered, whether hormonal activation leads to transcription of immediate early genes, leading to cell proliferation, or involves transcription of specific genes associated with cell differentiation [8, 23]. Functional analysis of serial truncated mutants of the hGHR have shown that the 54 membrane-proximal amino acids of the cytoplasmic tail are sufficient to transmit, albeit submaximally, a proliferative signal in the promyeloid FDC-P1 cell line, and that proliferation of this cell line (as well as MAPK stimulation) does not depend on presence of phosphorylated tyrosines. Similarly, studies performed with the PRLR showed that the 94 membrane-proximal residues are sufficient to transduce a proliferative signal in murine 32D cells and that proliferation of NIH-3T3 fibroblasts, but not of FDC-P1 and BaF-3 hematopoietic cells, can be induced by the short form of the rat PRLR, whose cytoplasmic domain contains only 57 residues and no phosphorylated tyrosine. At least in some cell types, proliferative signals seem thus to only require region(s) of the cytoplasmic domain restricted to the membrane-proximal portion (including box 1). In contrast, several signals of differentiation analyzed thus far (e.g. activation of Spi or β-casein promoters) require in addition the C-terminal region of the receptors and presence of phosphorylated tyrosines. Finally, is has been reported that mutations preventing PRL or GH receptor association with or activation of JAK2 are detrimental to effects on proliferation as well as on differentiation, strengthening the central role of JAK2 in PRLR/GHR signalling (8 and references therein).

Physiological significance of different receptor isoforms?

Different forms of membrane and soluble PRL and GH receptors have been reported, although their role and physiological significance remain poorly understood. In rats, three isoforms of membrane PRLR have been cloned (reviewed in 2), which only differ by the length and composition of the cytoplasmic (signalling) domain. The inability of the short form to activate transcription of genes involved in differentiation questions the physiological significance of this isoform, which in some tissues such as the liver, represents as much as 90% of the total PRLR population. Its involvement in proliferation of some cell types has been suggested but remains controversial (see above). In man, recent reports brought some evidence for an unexpected heterogeneity of the PRLR in both normal and tumor tissues [33-35]. The role of soluble GH and PRL binding proteins remains unclear. By protecting bound hormones from clearance, they have been proposed to increase half-life of their ligands. Moreover, if binding proteins have no intracellular signalling potency per se, it has been proposed that ligand-mediated interaction of these binding proteins with membrane PRLR receptors (or other transducer molecule) could initiate signal transduction in cells [36].

References

1. Nakagawa Y, Kosugi H, Miyajima A, Arai KI, Yokota T. Structure of the gene encoding the a subunit of the human granulocyte-macrophage colony stimulating factor receptor. *J Biol Chem* 1994; 269: 10905-12.
2. Kelly PA, Djiane J, Postel-Vinay MC, Edery M. The prolactin/growth hormone receptor family. *Endocr Rev* 1991; 12: 235-51.
3. Murakami M, Narazaki M, Hibi M, Yawata H, Yazukawa K, Hamaguchi M, Taga T, Kishimoto T. Critical cytoplasmic region of the IL-6 signal transducer, gp 130, is conserved in the cytokine receptor family. *Proc Natl Acad Sci USA* 1991; 88: 11349-53.
4. Rose-John S, Heinrich PC. Soluble receptors for cytokines and growth factors: generation and biological function. *Biochem J* 1994; 300: 281-90.
5. De Vos AM, Ultsch M, Kossiakoff AA. Human growth hormone and extracellular domain of its receptor: crystal structure of the complex. *Science* 1992; 255: 306-12.
6. Wells JA. Binding in the growth hormone receptor complex. *Proc Natl Acad Sci USA* 1996; 93: 1-6.
7. Kitamura T, Ogorochi T, Miyajima A. Multimeric cytokine receptors. *Trends Endocrinol Metab* 1994; 5: 8-14.
8. Finidori J, Kelly PA. Cytokine receptor signalling through two novel families of transducer molecules: Janus kinases, and signal transducers and activators of transcription. *J Endocrinol* 1995; 147: 11-23.
9. Goffin V, Shiverick KT, Kelly PA, Martial JA. Sequence-function relationships within the expanding family of prolactin, growth hormone, placental lactogen and related proteins in mammals. *Endocr Rev* 1996; in press.
10. Fuh G, Cunningham BC, Fukunaga R, Nagata S, Goeddel DV, Wells JA. Rational design of potent antagonists to the human growth hormone receptor. *Science* 1992; 256: 1677-79.
11. Goffin V, Kinet S, Ferrag F, Binart N, Martial JA, Kelly PA. Antagonistic properties of human prolactin analogs that show paradoxical agonistic activity in the Nb2 bioassay. *J Biol Chem* 1996; in press.
12. Ginsburg E, Vonderhaar BK. Prolactin synthesis and secretion by human breast cancer cells. *Cancer Res* 1995; 55: 2591-5.
13. Argetsinger LS, Campbell GS, Yang X, Witthuhn BA, Silvennoinen O, Ihle JN, Carter-Su C. Identification of Jak2 as a growth hormone receptor-associated tyrosine kinase. *Cell* 1993; 74: 237-44.
14. Campbell GS, Argetsinger LS, Ihle JN, Kelly PA, Rillema JA, Carter-Su C. Activation of JAK2 tyrosine kinase by prolactin receptors in Nb2 cells and mouse mammary gland explants. *Proc Natl Acad Sci USA* 1994; 91: 5232-6.
15. Lebrun JJ, Ali S, Sofer L, Ullrich A, Kelly PA. Prolactin induced proliferation of Nb2 cells involves tyrosine phosphorylation of the prolactin receptor and its associated tyrosine kinase. *J Biol Chem* 1994; 269: 14021-6.
16. Dusanter-Fourt I, Muller O, Ziemiecki A, Mayeux P, Drucker B, Djiane J, Wilks A, Harper AG, Fischer S, Gisselbrecht S. Identification of Jak protein tyrosine kinases as signaling molecules for prolactin. Functional analysis of prolactin receptor and prolactin-erythropoietin receptor chimera expressed in lymphoid cells. *EMBO J* 1994; 13: 2583-91.
17. DaSilva L, Howard OMZ, Rui H, Kirken RA, Farrar WL. Growth signaling and Jak2 association mediated by membrane-proximal regions of prolactin receptors. *J Biol Chem* 1994; 269: 18267-70.
18. Sotiropoulos A, Perrot-Applanat M, Dinerstein H, Pallier A, Postel-Vinay MC, Finidori J, Kelly PA. Distinct cytoplasmic regions of the growth hormone receptor are required for activation of Jak2, mitogen-activated protein kinase, and transcription. *Endocrinology* 1994; 135: 1292-8.
19. Lebrun JJ, Ali S, Ullrich A, Kelly PA. Proline-rich sequence-mediated JAK2 association to the prolactin receptor is required but not sufficient for signal transduction. *J Biol Chem* 1995; 270: 10664-70.
20. Sotiropoulos A, Moutoussamy S, Renaudie F, Clauss M, Kayser C, Gouilleux F, Kelly PA, Finidori J. Differential activation of Stat3 and Stat5 by distinct regions of the growth hormone receptor. *Mol Endocrinol* 1996; in press.
21. Lebrun JJ, Ali S, Goffin V, Ullrich A, Kelly PA. A single phosphotyrosine residue of the prolactin receptor is responsible for activation of gene transcription. *Proc Natl Acad Sci USA* 1995; 92: 4031-5.

22. Gouilleux F, Wakao H, Mundt M, Groner B. Prolactin induces phosphorylation of Tyr694 of Stat5 (MGF), a prerequisite for DNA binding and induction of transcription. *EMBO J* 1994; 13: 4361-9.
23. Horseman ND, Yu-Lee LY. Transcriptional regulation by the helix bundle peptide hormones: growth hormone, prolactin, and hematopoietic cytokines. *Endocr Rev* 1994; 15: 627-49.
24. Gronowski AM, Zhong Z, Wen Z, Thomas MJ, Darnell Jr JE, Rotwein P. *In vivo* growth hormone treatment rapidly stimulates the tyrosine phosphorylation and activation of STAT3. *Mol Endocrinol* 1995; 9: 171-7.
25. Sotiropoulos A, Moutoussamy S, Binart N, Kelly PA, Finidori J. The membrane proximal region of the cytoplasmic domain of the growth hormone receptor is involved in the activation of Stat 3. *FEBS Lett* 1995; 369: 169-72.
26. DaSilva L, Rui H, Erwin RA, Zack Howard OM, Kirken RA, Malabarba MG, Hackett RH, Larner AC, Farrar WL. Prolactin recruits STAT1, STAT3 and STAT5 independent of conserved receptor tyrosines TYR402, TYR476, TYR515 and TYR580. *Mol Cell Endocrinol* 1996; 117: 131-40.
27. Meyer DJ, Campbell GS, Cochran BH, Argetsinger LS, Larner AC, Finbloom DS, Carter-Su C, Schwartz J. Growth hormone induces a DNA binding factor related to the interferon-stimulated 91-kDa transcription factor. *J Biol Chem* 1994; 269: 4701-4.
28. Clevenger CV, Medaglia MV. The protein tyrosine kinase p59fyn is associated with prolactin (PRL) receptor and is activated by PRL stimulation of T-lymphocytes. *Mol Endocrinol* 1994; 8: 674-81.
29. Berlanga JJ, Fresno Vara JA, Martin-Perez J, Garcia-Ruiz JP. Prolactin receptor is associated with c-src kinase in rat liver. *Mol Endocrinol* 1995; 9: 1461-7.
30. Ali S, Chen Z, Lebrun JJ, Vogel W, Kharitonenkov A, Kelly PA, Ullrich A. PTP1D is a positive regulator of the prolactin signal leading to b-casein promoter activation. *EMBO J* 1996; 15: 135-42.
31. Stahl N, Farruggella TJ, Boulton TG, Zhong Z, Darnell JE Jr, Yancopoulos GD. Choice of STATs and other substrates specified by modular tyrosine-based motifs in cytokine receptors. *Science* 1995; 267: 1349-53.
32. Erwin RA, Kirken RA, Malabarba MG, Farrar WL, Rui H. Prolactin activates Ras *via* signaling proteins SHC, growth factor receptor bound 2, and son of sevenless. *Endocrinology* 1995; 136: 3512-8.
33. Nagano M, Chastre E, Choquet A, Bara J, Gespach C, Kelly PA. Expression of prolactin and growth hormone receptor genes and their isoforms in the gastrointestinal tract. *Am J Physiol* 1995; 268: G431-G442.
34. Fuh G, Wells JA. Prolactin receptor antagonists that inhibit the growth of breast cancer cell lines. *J Biol Chem* 1995; 270: 13133-7.
35. Clevenger CV, Chang WP, Ngo W, Pasha TLM, Montone KT, Tomaszewski JE. Expression of prolactin and prolactin receptor in human breast carcinoma. *Am J Pathol* 1995; 146: 695-705.
36. Lesueur L, Edery M, Paly J, Kelly PA, Djiane J. Roles of the extracellular and cytoplasmic domains of the prolactin receptor in signal transduction to milk protein genes. *Mol Endocrinol* 1993; 7: 1178-84.

Breast Cancer. Advances in biology and therapeutics.
F. Calvo, M. Crépin, H. Magdelenat, eds. John Libbey Eurotext © 1996, pp. 139-146.

Targeting the product of the HER2/*neu* protooncogene for therapy

Paul Carter

Department of Molecular Oncology, Genentech Inc, 460 Point San Bruno Boulevard, South San Francisco, CA 94080, USA

Introduction

The protooncogene HER2/*neu* (also known as c-*erb*B2) encodes a receptor tyrosine kinase, $p185^{HER2}$, which is homologous to the EGF receptor [1-3]. HER2/neu amplification has been found in ~ 30% of primary human breast cancers and prognosticates decreased overall survival and time to relapse [4]. HER2/neu amplification and/or overexpression has subsequently been correlated with poor clinical prognosis in several other cancers including: ovarian, endometrial, gastric and lung adenocarcinoma [reviewed in Ref. 5-7]. This has encouraged the development of a plethora of potential therapeutics targeting the product of HER2/neu [reviewed in Ref. 8]. Here we focus on the humanized anti-$p185^{HER2}$ antibody, huMAb4D5-8 [9] and the development of technologies that allow its use as building block for immunotherapeutic design.

Murine anti-$p185^{HER2}$ antibody has therapeutic potential

The murine anti-$p185^{HER2}$ monoclonal antibody, 4D5 [10], has several properties which give it therapeutic potential [reviewed in Ref. 7, 11]. Firstly, 4D5 retards the growth of a variety of human tumor cell lines overexpressing $p185^{HER2}$ in monolayer culture. 4D5 also down regulates $p185^{HER2}$ from the surface of cells and inhibits colony formation in soft agar suggesting that it may be reverse the transformed phenotype. 4D5 localizes to $p185^{HER2}$-overexpressing tumor xenografts in nude mice and furthermore inhibits their growth. 4D5 enhances the sensitivity of some human cell lines to cisplatin both *in vitro* and *in vivo*. Finally, 4D5 reverses the TNF-α resistant phenotype which appears to be characteristic of breast tumor cells overexpressing $p185^{HER2}$.

Humanization of anti-p185^{HER2} antibody

« Humanization » has been a widely adopted strategy to increase the clinical potential of rodent-derived monoclonal antibodies by reducing their likely immunogenicity and recruiting secondary immune functions [reviewed in Ref. 12, 13]. In humanizing 4D5 its six antigen-binding loops and a few judiciously chosen additional residues were grafted into a human IgG$_1$. The most potent humanized variant, huMAb4D5-8, binds to the extracellular domain of p185^{HER2} about 3-fold more tightly than the murine parent antibody and is almost as potent in inhibiting the proliferation of SK-BR-3 breast tumors cells [9]. As anticipated from its IgG$_1$ isotype, huMAb4d5-8 supports antibody-dependant cellular cytotoxicity (ADCC) against tumor cells overexpressing p185^{HER2} in the presence of human effector cells whereas the parent antibody, a murine IgG$_1$, does not [9]. The efficiency of ADCC correlates with the extent of p185^{HER2} expression [14]: low level of cytotoxicity were observed with cell lines expressing normal levels of p185^{HER2}, whereas efficient ADCC was observed with tumor cell lines expressing high levels of p185^{HER2}. This bodes well for on-going clinical trials using huMAb4d5-8 since the highest level of p185^{HER2} overexpression correlates with the poorest clinical prognosis [4, 15]. The minimal cytotoxicity observed against normal cell lines [14] is fortunate since low levels of p185^{HER2} are observed on a variety of normal epithelial cells [16].

Clinical trials with humanized anti-p185^{HER2} antibody

The humanized anti-p185^{HER2} antibody, huMAb4D5-8, entered a phase I clinical trial in June 1992 and subsequently has completed two phase I and two phase II trials. In one phase II trial patients with metastatic breast cancer received weekly intravenous doses of the humanized antibody [17]. Objective responses were observed in five out of forty three assessable patients: one complete remission and four partial remissions. The antibody had minimal toxicity and no antibody response has been detected against the humanized antibody. This is in striking contrast to the immunogenicity of many murine antibodies which frequently precludes repeated dosing [18, 19]. The synergistic anti-tumor activity of huMAb4D5-8 and cisplatin demonstrated both *in vitro* and *in vivo* [20] encouraged a second phase II trial to evaluate treatment with antibody in combination with cisplatin (results to be reported elsewhere). A double-blind phase III trial was initiated in June 1995 in breast cancer patients with previously untreated metastatic disease.

Humanized anti-p185^{HER2} antibody: building block for immunotherapeutic design

Successful treatment of human tumors with murine monoclonal antibodies has been broadly stymied by a combination of antibody, antigen, tumor and host related problems [reviewed in Ref. 21]. Regarding the choice of antigen, the HER2/*neu* product is a favorable target since the titer of shed antigen is rarely sufficient to compromise the level of free antibody in serum [17]. Furthermore, tumor cells evading antibody therapy by loss of antigen expression may be less of problem with HER2/*neu* than for some tumor antigens since antigenic modulation (*in vitro* at least) reverses the transformed phenotype [7, 11]. As for the antibody itself, humanization has apparently overcome the immunogenicity [17] and lack of effector functions [9] of the murine parent antibody, 4D5.

Two major problems in treating solid tumors with antibodies that are not addressed by humanization are the small fraction of antibody which reaches its target (typically ≤ 0.01% injected dose / g tumor [21]) and heterogeneous antibody distribution with a tendency to accumulate close to the vasculature [22]. This has motivated us to use the humanized anti-p185^{HER2} antibody, huMAb4D5-8 [9], as a building block to design potentially more potent immunotherapeutics. These include humanized bispecific F(ab')$_2$ [23-26] and diabody [27] fragments (anti-p185^{HER2}/anti-CD3) for retargeting cytotoxic T cells against tumor cells, a disulfide-stabilized Fv-b-lactamase fusion protein for activation of cephem prodrugs of doxorubicin and taxol [28, 29] and so called « stealth » immunoliposomes for targeted drug delivery [30] *(Figure 1)*.

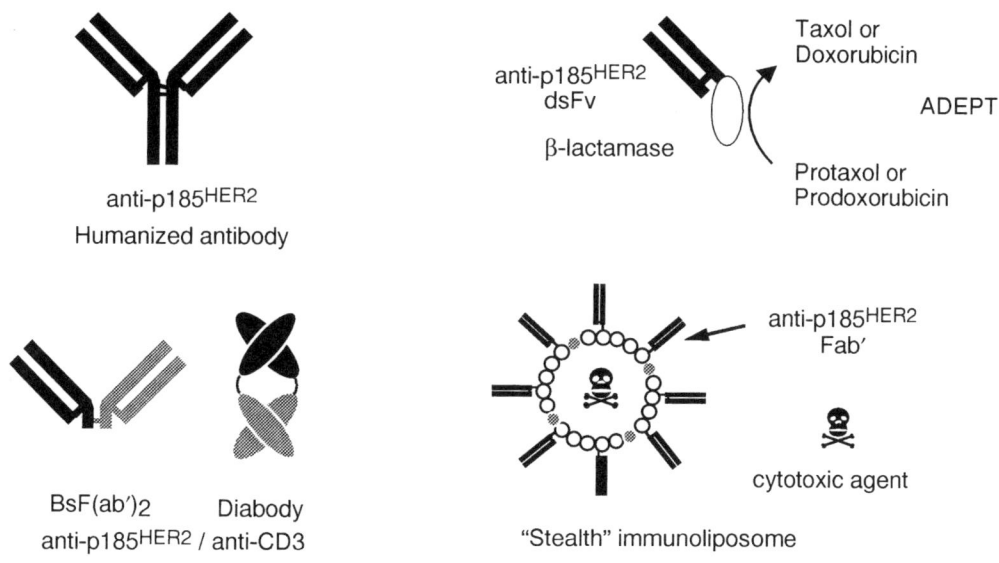

Figure 1. Humanized anti-p185^{HER2} antibody: a building block for immunotherapeutic design. The humanized bispecific F(ab')$_2$ [23-26] and diabody [27] fragments (anti-p185^{HER2}/anti-CD3) efficiently retarget cytotoxic T cells to kill tumor cells overexpressing p185^{HER2} *in vitro*. The disulfide-stabilized (ds) Fv-β-lactamase fusion protein was constructed for targeted delivery of cephem prodrugs including for doxorubicin and ted variant, huMAb4D5-8, binds to the extracellular domain of p185^{HER2} about 3-fold more tightly than the murine parent antibody and is almost as potent in inhibiting the proliferation of SK-BR-3 breast tumor cells [9]. As anticipated from its IgG1 isotype, huMAb4D5-8 supports antibody-dependent cellular cytotoxicity (ADCC) against tumor cells overexpressing p185^{HER2} in the presence of human effector cells whereas the parent antibody, a murine IgG1, does not [9]. The efficiency of ADCC correlates with the extent of p185^{HER2} expression [14]: low levels of cytotoxicity were observed with cell lines expressing normal levels of p185^{HER2}, whereas efficient ADCC was observed with tumor cell lines expressing high levels of p185^{HER2}. This bodes well for on-going clinical trials using huMAb4D5-8 since the highest level of p185^{HER2} overexpression correlates with the poorest clinical prognosis [4, 15]. The minimal cytotoxicity observed against normal cell lines [14] is fortunate since low levels of p185^{HER2} are obseaxol [28, 29]. Fab' fragments have been used to target cytotoxic agents such as doxorubicin encapsulated in sterically stabilized (« stealth ») immunoliposomes [30].

Development of anti-p185^{HER2}/anti-CD3 bispecific antibodies

Clinical evaluation of bispecific antibodies (BsAb) has been significantly curtailed by the difficulty of preparing them in sufficient quantity and purity using non-recombinant methods. Despite the limited availability of BsAb, a few small scale clinical trials have been conducted and yielded some promising results [reviewed in Ref. 31]. This has encouraged us to develop novel recombinant methods for preparing BsAb fragments using a humanized anti-p185^{HER2}/anti-CD3 BsAb as a driving problem.

Our first strategy for preparing BsAb fragments relied upon high level secretion of humanized Fab' fragments from E. coli [32]. Traditional directed-chemical coupling of Fab' fragments was then used to efficiently form BsF(ab')$_2$ fragments *in vitro* [23, 24]. The humanized anti-p185^{HER2}/anti-CD3 BsF(ab')$_2$ is exceedingly potent in retargeting the cytotoxicity of IL-2 activated human T cells against tumor cells overexpressing p185^{HER2} [23, 25, 26]. The limitations of this route to BsF(ab')$_2$ from a biotechnology perspective are that it uses two separate E. coli hosts, the coupling yields are relatively low (~ 50%) and the chemical linker used to link Fab' arms is potentially immunogenic.

An alternative technology for preparing BsAb fragments that circumvents these limitations is the « diabody » [33]. The construction of single-chain (sc) Fv fragments with short linkers ($\leq$ 10 residues) greatly restricts intra-chain pairing of variable domains. Inter-chain pairing of such scFv may occur to form a bivalent (scFv)$_2$ - the diabody. A bispecific diabody may be formed by the coexpression of two cross-over scFv fragments in which the V$_L$ and V$_H$ domains for the two antibodies are present on different polypeptide chains [33]. After secretion of these two chains from *E. coli* they can associate to form a non-covalent heterodimer which may reconstitute both antigen binding specificities.

We designed, expressed and characterized an anti-p185^{HER2}/anti-CD3 diabody thereby extending this technology in two major ways [27]. Firstly, we demonstrate that a diabody can be secreted from *E. coli* cultured in the fermentor and recovered in very high yield (> 900 mg/L). Secondly we demonstrate that a diabody can simultaneously bind antigen on two different cells and direct the efficient lysis of target tumor cells in the presence of IL-2 activated T cells. Indeed the anti-p185^{HER2}/anti-CD3 diabody has similar potency to the corresponding BsF(ab')$_2$ in retargeted cellular cytotoxicity [27]. Approximately 60% of diabody preparations are functional heterodimers as judged by titration with antigen and gel filtration [27]. « Knobs-into-holes » engineering of antibody domain interfaces [34] was to used to enhance diabody formation to yield > 85% functional heterodimer (Z. Zhu, PC, unpublished data). Knob-into-hole diabodies appear to be the most promising route currently available to prepare BsAb fragment for clinical applications.

Targeted prodrug therapy

The use of enzyme activatable prodrugs in conjunction with antibody enzyme fusion proteins or conjugates is a promising strategy for enhancing the anti-tumor efficacy of antibodies and minimizing the toxicity of chemotherapeutics [reviewed in Ref. 35, 36]. Indeed targeted prodrugs have proved to be much more efficacious than corresponding free drugs against human tumor xenografts in nude mice [37-40] including one example targeting p185^{HER2} [41].

We developed a fusion protein comprising a disulfide-stabilized Fv fragment of humAb4D5¤8 fused to β-lactamase for use in targeted prodrug therapy in conjunction with cephem-based prodrugs [28]. β-lactamase is an attractive choice of enzyme for prodrug activation because of its high catalytic efficiency and broad substrate specificity. Furthermore, there are no known similar activities, competing substrates or inhibitors endogenous to man. Cephalosporins have proved to be highly versatile triggers in the construction of enzyme-activatable prodrugs including for vinca alkaloids nitrogen mustard drugs, a carboplatin analog, doxorubicin, and taxol [reviewed in Ref. 42]. The cephem moiety is attached to a group on the chemotherapeutic agent judiciously chosen so that the prodrug is less toxic than the drug. Fully active drug (or drug analog) is released after β-lactamase-mediated cleavage of the β-lactam ring. In the case of our cephem taxol prodrug, β-lactamase releases an intermediate which undergoes a self-immolation reaction to release free taxol [29].

Repeated clinical use of fusion proteins for ADEPT will likely be confounded by an immune response mounted against the xenogeneic components. This limitation has long been recognized and the use of humanized anti-tumor and catalytic antibodies has been proposed as a possible solution [43]. The advent of large human antibody phage libraries [44, 45] together with advances in the development of catalytic antibodies [46] and efficient diabody production [27] significantly enhance the feasibility of such an approach. Human enzymes offer an alternative to human catalytic antibodies, albeit with potential drawbacks of unwanted activation of prodrug by endogenous enzyme, interference from endogenous substrates or inhibitors, and potential immunogenicity if intracellular enzymes are selected. Nevertheless a humanized anti-CEA antibody fused to a human enzyme, glucuronidase, in conjunction with a glucuronide prodrug of doxorubicin was found to be efficacious in tumor-bearing nude mice [38], which augurs well for this approach.

Conclusions and perspectives

Our humanized anti-p185^{HER2} antibody, huMAb4D5-8 [9], has shown some promise in patients [17] and currently is in phase III clinical trials for metastatic breast cancer. In parallel with this clinical effort, huMAb4D5-8 is being used to drive the development of the next generation of therapeutic antibodies technologies. In addition, two bispecific antibodies for effector cell retargeting developed are now being clinically evaluated (anti-p185^{HER2}/anti-FcγRI [47]) and (anti-p185^{HER2}/anti-FcγRIII [48]). These efforts *in toto* are indicative of significant past and on-going progress toward developing an effective therapy for human malignancies involving overexpression of the product of the HER2/*neu* protooncogene.

References

1. King CR, Kraus MH, Aaronson SA. Amplification of a novel v-*erb*B-related gene in a human mammary carcinoma. *Science* 1985; 224: 974-6.
2. Coussens L, Yang-Feng TL, Liao YC, Chen E, Gray A, McGrath J, Seeburg PH, Libermann TA, Schlessinger J, Francke U, Levinson A, Ullrich A. Tyrosine kinase receptor with extensive homology to EGF receptor shares chromosomal location with *neu* oncogene. *Science* 1985; 230: 1132-9.
3. Semba K, Kamata N, Toyoshima K, Yamamoto T. A v-*erb*B-related protooncogene, c-erbB-2, is distinct from the c-erbB-1/epidermal growth factor-receptor gene and is amplified in a human salivary gland adenocarcinoma. *Proc Natl Acad Sci USA* 1985; 82: 6497-501.

4. Slamon DJ, Clark GM, Wong SG, Levin WJ, Ullrich A, McGuire WL. Human breast cancer: correlation of relapse and survival with amplification of the HER-2/*neu* oncogene. *Science* 1987; 235: 177-82.
5. Dougall WC, Qian X, Peterson NC, Miller MJ, Samanta A, Greene MI. The neu-oncogene: signal transduction pathways, transformation mechanisms and evolving therapies. *Oncogene* 1994; 9: 2109-23.
6. Hynes NE. Amplification and overexpression of the erbB-2 gene in human tumors: its involvement in tumor development, significance as a prognostic factor, and potential as a target for cancer therapy. *Cancer Biol* 1993; 4: 19-26.
7. Park JW, Carter P, Shalaby R, Maneval D, Shepard HM. Targeting the c-erbB-2 proto-oncogene with monoclonal antibodies. In: Lemone, N, Epenetos, A, eds. *Mutant oncogenes: targets for therapy.* London: Chapman and Hall Medical, 1993: 3-14.
8. Carter P, Rodrigues ML, Lewis GD, Figari I, Shalaby MR. Towards an immunotherapy for p185^{HER2} overexpressing tumors. In: Ceriani, RL, ed. *Antigen and antibody molecular engineering in breast cancer diagnosis and treatment.* New York: Plenum Publishing, 1994: 83-94.
9. Carter P, Presta L, Gorman CM, Ridgway JBB, Henner D, Wong WLT, Rowland AM, Kotts C, Carver ME, Shepard HM. Humanization of an anti-p185^{HER2} antibody for human cancer therapy. *Proc Natl Acad Sci USA* 1992; 89: 4285-9.
10. Hudziak RM, Lewis GD, Winget M, Fendly BM, Shepard HM, Ullrich A. p185^{HER2} monoclonal antibody has antiproliferative effects *in vitro* and sensitizes human breast tumor cells to tumor necrosis factor. *Mol Cell Biol* 1989; 9: 1165-72.
11. Shepard HM, Lewis GD, Sarup JC, Fendly BM, Maneval D, Mordenti J, Figari I, Kotts CE, Palladino Jr MA, Ullrich A, Slamon D. Monoclonal antibody therapy of human cancer: taking the *HER2* protooncogene to the clinic. *J Clin Immunol* 1991, 11: 117-27.
12. Winter G, Harris WJ. Humanized antibodies. *Immunol Today* 1993; 14: 243-6.
13. Adair JR, Bright SM. Progress with humanised antibodies - an update. *Exp Opin Invest Drugs* 1995; 4: 863-70.
14. Lewis GD, Figari I, Fendly B, Wong WL, Carter P, Gorman C, Shepard HM. Differential responses of human tumor cells lines to anti-p185^{HER2} monoclonal antibodies. *Cancer Immunol Immunother* 1993; 37: 255-63.
15. Slamon DJ, Godolphin W, Jones LA, Holt JA, Wong SG, Keith DE, Levin WJ, Stuart SG, Udove J, Ullrich A, Press MF. Studies of the HER-2/neu proto-oncogene in human breast and ovarian cancer. *Science* 1989; 244: 707-12.
16. Press MF, Cordon-Cardo C, Slamon DJ. Expression of the HER-2/*neu* proto-oncogene in normal human adult and fetal tissues. *Oncogene* 1990; 5: 953-62.
17. Baselga J, Tripathy D, Mendelsohn J, Baughman S, Benz CC, Dantis L, Sklarin NT, Seidman AD, Hudis CA, Moore J, Rosen PP, Twaddell T, Henderson IC, Norton L. Phase II study of weekly intravenous recombinant humanized anti-p185^{HER2} monoclonal antibody in patients with HER2/*neu*-overexpressing metastatic breast cancer. *J Clin Oncol* 1996; 14: 737-44.
18. Miller RA, Oseroff AR, Stratte PT, Levy R. Monoclonal antibody therapeutic trials in seven patients with T-cell lymphoma. *Blood* 1983; 62: 988-95.
19. Schroff RW, Foon KA, Beatty SM, Oldham RK, Morgan Jr, AC. Human anti-murine immunoglobulin responses in patients receiving monoclonal antibody therapy. *Cancer Res* 1985; 45: 879-85.
20. Pietras RJ, Fendly BM, Chazin VR, Pegram MD, Howell SB, Slamon DJ. Antibody to HER-2/*neu* receptor blocks DNA repair after cisplatin in human breast and ovarian cancer cells. *Oncogene* 1994; 9: 1829-38.
21. Sedalacek H-H, Seemann G, Hoffmann D, Czech J, Lorenz P, Kolar C, Bosslet K, eds. In: *Antibodies as carriers of cytotoxicity. Contributions to oncology Vol. 43,* Munich: Karger, 1992.
22. Juweid M, Neumann R, Paik C, Perez-Bacete MJ, Sato J, van Osdol W, Weinstein JN. Micropharmacology of monoclonal antibodies in solid tumors: direct experimental evidence for a binding site barrier. *Cancer Res* 1992; 52: 5144-53.
23. Shalaby MR, Shepard HM, Presta L, Rodrigues ML, Beverley PCL, Feldmann M, Carter P. Development of humanized bispecific antibodies reactive with cytotoxic lymphocytes and tumor cells overexpressing the *HER2* protooncogene. *J Exp Med* 1992; 175: 217-25.

24. Rodrigues ML, Shalaby MR, Werther W, Presta L, Carter P. Engineering a humanized bispecific F(ab')₂ fragment for improved binding to T-cells. *Int J Cancer Suppl* 1992; 7: 45-50.
25. Shalaby MR, Carter P, Maneval D, Giltinan D, Kotts C. Bispecific HER2 x CD3 antibodies enhance T-cell cytotoxicity *in vitro* and localize to *HER2*-overexpressing xenografts in nude mice. *Clin Immunol Immunopath* 1995; 74: 185-92.
26. Zhu Z, Phillips G, Carter P. Engineering high affinity humanized anti-p185^{HER2} / anti-CD3 bispecific F(ab')₂ for efficient lysis of p185^{HER2} overexpressing tumor cells. *Int J Cancer* 1995; 62: 319-24.
27. Zhu Z, Zapata G, Shalaby MR, Snedecor B, Chen H, Carter P. High level secretion of a humanized bispecific diabody from *Escherichia coli*. *Bio/Technol* 1996; 14: 192-6.
28. Rodrigues ML, Presta LG, Kotts CE, Wirth C, Mordenti J, Osaka G, Wong WLT, Nuijens A, Blackburn B, Carter P. Development of a humanized disulfide-stabilized anti-p185^{HER2}Fv-β-lactamase fusion protein for activation of a cephalosporin doxorubicin prodrug. *Cancer Res* 1995; 55: 63-70.
29. Rodrigues ML, Carter P, Wirth C, Mullins S, Lee A, Blackburn BK. Synthesis and characterization of a cephalosporin-taxol prodrug. *Chem Biol* 1995; 2: 223-7.
30. Park JW, Hong K, Carter P, Asgari H, Guo LY, Keller GA, Wirth C, Shalaby R, Kotts C, Wood WI, Papahadjopoulos D, Benz CC. Development of anti-p185^{HER2} immunoliposomes for cancer therapy. *Proc Natl Acad Sci USA* 1995; 92: 1327-31.
31. Carter P, Ridgway J, Zhu Z. Toward the production of bispecific antibody fragments for clinical applications. *J Hematother* 1995; 4: 463-70.
32. Carter P, Kelley RF, Rodrigues ML, Snedecor B, Covarrubias M, Velligan MD, Wong WLT, Rowland AM, Kotts CE, Carver ME, Yang M, Bourell JH, Shepard HM, Henner D. High level *Escherichia coli* expression and production of a bivalent humanized antibody fragment. *Bio/Technology* 1992; 10: 163-7.
33. Holliger, P, Prospero, T, Winter, G. « Diabodies »: small bivalent and bispecific antibody fragments. *Proc Natl Acad Sci USA* 1993; 90: 6444-8.
34. Ridgway JBB, Presta LG, Carter P. « Knobs-into-holes » engineering of antibody C$_H$3 domains for heavy chain heterodimerization. *Protein Eng* 1996 (in the press).
35. Senter PD, Wallace PM, Svensson HP, Vrudhula VM, Kerr DE, Hellström I, Hellström KE. Generation of cytotoxic agents by targeted enzymes. *Bioconjug Chem* 1993; 4: 3-9.
36. Bagshawe KD. Antibody-directed enzyme prodrug therapy. *Clin Pharmacokinet* 1994; 27: 368-76.
37. Meyer DL, Jungheim LN, Law KL, Mikolajczyk SD, Sheperd TA, Mackensen DG, Briggs SL, Starling JJ. Site-specific prodrug activation by antibody-β-lactamase conjugates: regression and long-term growth inhibition of human colon carcinoma xenograft models. *Cancer Res* 1993; 53: 3956-63.
38. Bosslet K, Czech J, Hoffmann D. Tumor-selective prodrug activation by fusion protein-mediated catalysis. *Cancer Res* 1994, 54, 2151-9.
39. Svensson HP, Vrudhula VM, Emswiler JE, MacMaster JF, Cosand WL, Senter PD, Wallace PM. *in vitro* and *in vivo* activities of a doxorubicin prodrug in combination with monoclonal antibody β-lactamase conjugates. *Cancer Res* 1995; 55: 2357-65.
40. Kerr DE, Schreiber GJ, Vrudhula VM, Svensson HP, Hellström I, Hellström KE, Senter PD. Regressions and cures of melanoma xenografts following treatment with monoclonal antibody β-lactamase conjugates in combination with anticancer prodrugs. *Cancer Res* 1995; 55: 3558-33.
41. Eccles SA, Court WJ, Box GA, Dean CJ, Melton RG, Springer CJ. Regression of established breast carcinoma xenografts with antibody-directed enzyme prodrug therapy against c-*erb*B2 p185. *Cancer Res* 1994; 54: 5171-7.
42. Jungheim LN, Sheperd TA. Design of antitumor prodrugs: substrates for antibody targeted enzymes. *Chem Rev* 1994; 94: 1553-66.
43. Bagshawe KD, Sharma SK, Springer CJ, Antoniw P, Rogers GT, Burke PJ, Melton R, Sherwood R. Antibody-enzyme conjugates can generate cytotoxic drugs from inactive precursors at tumor sites. *Antibody Immunoconj Radiopharm* 1991; 4: 915-22.
44. Griffiths AD, Williams SC, Hartley O, Tomlinson IM, Waterhouse P, Crosby WL, Kontermann R, Jones PT, Low NM, Allison TJ, Prospero TD, Hoogenboom HR, Nissim A, Cox JPL, Harrison JL, Zaccolo M, Gherardi E, Winter G. Isolation of high affinity human antibodies directly from large synthetic repertoires. *EMBO J* 1994; 13: 3245-60.
45. Vaughan TJ, Williams AJ, Pritchard K, Osbourn JK, Pope AR, Earnshaw JC, McCafferty J, Hodits

RA, Wilton J, Johnson KS. Human antibodies with sub-nanomolar affinities isolated from a large non-immunized phage display library. *Nature Bio/Technol* 1996; 14, 309-14.
46. Schultz PG, Lerner RA. From molecular diversity to catalysis: lessons from the immune system. *Science* 1995; 269: 1835-42.
47. Valone FH, Kaufman PA, Guyre PM, Lewis LD, Memoli V, Deo Y, Graziano R, Fisher JL, Meyer L, Mrozek-Orlowski M, Wardwell K, Guyre V, Morley TL, Arvizu C, Fanger MW. Phase Ia/Ib trial of bispecific antibody MDX-210 in patients with advanced breast or ovarian cancer that overexpresses the proto-oncogene HER-2/neu. *J Clin Oncol* 1995; 13: 2281-92.
48. Weiner LM, Clark JI, Davey M, Li WS, de Palazzo IG, Ring DB, Alpaugh RK. Phase I trial of 2B1, a bispecific monoclonal antibody targeting the c-erbB-2 and FcγRIII. *Cancer Res* 1995; 55: 4586-93.

Targeting of EGF receptors: approaches and clinical results

Christopher Dean, Helmout Modjtahedi, Suzanne Eccles, Elizabeth Jackson, Gary Box, Tamas Hikish, Ian Smith and Martin Gore

Section of Immunology, Institute of Cancer Research and The Royal Marsden Hospital Trust, Sutton, Surrey, UK

Abstract

In breast cancer, expression of the receptor for EGF (EGFR) and its ligands is correlated with resistance to endocrine therapy and poorer relapse-free survival. The EGFR, a receptor tyrosine kinase (RTK), is a potential target for therapy of breast and other cancers and drugs which prevent its activation such as tyrosine kinase inhibitors and monoclonal antibodies are currently under investigation. Monoclonal antibodies which selectively target the receptor have been found to be potent inhibitors of signal transduction via *the EGFR and to induce regression of xenografted tumours growing in nude mice. Clinical trials in cancers other than those of the breast have shown promising results and point to the use of antibodies in an adjuvant setting for the elimination of residual disease.*

Introduction

The EGF receptor is a glycoprotein of 170 kDa with an external ligand binding domain and a cytoplasmic kinase containing domain [1, 2]. Following binding of peptide ligand, the receptors dimerize either with each other or with a related receptor and this is followed by phosphorylation of tyrosine residues in the cytoplasmic domain by the receptor kinase [3]. The mechanism of signal transduction *via* this receptor has been the subject of intensive research over the last two decades and much is now known about the pathways involved in cellular activation [reviewed in 3].

Three related receptors have been identified on the basis of the similarity of their kinase domains namely c-erbB-2 [4], c-erbB-3 [5] and c-erbB-4 [6]. Interestingly, c-erbB-2, which is overexpressed by some 1,620% of breast cancers has been found to be a marker of poor prognosis [7]. The more recently described c-erbB-3 and c-erbB-4 gene products have been found to be receptors for growth factors known collectively as neuregulins which include heregulin, neu differentiation factor and glial growth factor [8-10]. In some cases, the effects of the neuregulins appear to involve heterodimer formation with the c-erbB-2 receptor. In breast cancers and other tumours, expression of the EGFR and the three other receptors varies and the combinations differ from one tumour cell type to another. However, it is becoming increasingly apparent that crosstalk between the receptors may occur and this is important in determining the pathway(s) for signal transduction.

The finding that the EGF receptor is overexpressed in certain cancers has pointed to its potential as a target for therapy [11, 12], a suggestion indicated by the early finding that tumour cell proliferation could be inhibited by certain antibodies to the EGFR which prevented ligand binding [reviewed in 13]. Also, there is currently a considerable effort being made to identify smaller molecules that will inhibit signal transduction via the receptor by blocking the kinase or interfering with downstream signalling [14, 15]. Recently, three mutant EGF receptors have been reported in brain tumours which have lost part or most of the extracellular domain [16]. The type III mutants (EGFRvIII) are the most common and have a deletion of 267 amino acids near the Nterminus with the result that the mutant receptor contains a novel peptide sequence at the junction. Antibodies have been made to this peptide which bind to the mutant but not the normal receptor [17]. The mutant receptor, which does not bind EGF, has been reported to be expressed also in breast and lung cancers [18]. It would appear that many of the type III mutant receptors are expressed in the cytoplasm but if sufficient were present at the cell surface they could form useful tumour specific targets for antibodydirected therapies.

EGFR expression in breast cancer

Despite the very large number of investigations relating to the expression of the EGFR in breast cancer there remains confusion in the literature as to whether the EGFR is overexpressed by malignant compared with normal breast tissue [19, 13]. Certainly gene amplification is rare in breast cancer (< 3%). What is clear, however is that there is an inverse correlation between expression of the EGFR and oestrogen receptors [20, 21]. As a consequence patients with tumours which express higher levels of the EGFR tend to be poorly responsive to endocrine therapy. Also, while the usefulness of EGFR expression as a prognostic indicator remains controversial there is a consensus of opinion that EGFR expression is associated with poor relapsefree survival [21].

Activation of the EGFR

A number of peptide growth factors have been discovered which can activate the EGFR [13]. In addition to EGF, these include transforming growth factor alpha (TGFα), heparin binding EGF (HBEGF), amphiregulin (AR) and betacellulin (BTC). One or more of these peptide growth factors may be produced constitutively by the tumours and activation can occur either by interaction of the EGF receptors with growth factors secreted by the same cell (autocrine), expressed on adjacent cells (juxtacrine) or produced at a distance (paracrine). Clearly treatments which target ligand binding must be effective in blocking activation by any of these ligands.

Ligand binding leads to phosphorylation of tyrosines in the cytosolic tails of the receptor and these phosphotyrosine containing peptides are recognised and bound by the SH2 domains of various effector molecules such as phospholipase C gamma [22]. Also, the peptide residues may bind adaptor molecules such as grb2 which can then initiate the important ras -> raf -> MAP kinase -> transcription factor pathway resulting in mitogenesis and cell proliferation [3].

Importantly, the EGFR may be activated following heterodimer formation with other receptor tyrosine kinases. For example, it has been found that binding of heregulin to c-erbB-4 can lead to trans-phosphorylation of the EGFR [23]. Indeed it was shown earlier that, following ligand binding, the EGFR can transphosphorylate c-erbB-2 [24, 25] or c-erbB-3 [26] and evidence is accumulating to show that interactions between different members of the Type 1 family of growth factor receptors are important in controlling the proliferation, transformation or differentiation of cells. Again, to inhibit signal tranduction *via* the EGFR it may be necessary to develop treatments which block the activity of other receptor kinases since drugs which are specific inhibitors of the EGFR kinase may not prevent its trans-activation.

Inhibitors of receptor tyrosine kinases and signal transduction

A number of tyrosine kinase inhibitors have been shown to block the activation of the EGFR and to inhibit the growth *in vitro* of cells expressing these receptors. Of these, the tyrphostins [27] and erbstatin [28] were the forerunners of the many new drugs that are currently being evaluated. A number of these also appear to have specificity for the EGFR or c-erbB-2 kinases [29] and to prevent the growth of a human squamous cell carcinoma in nude mice [30]. Dianilino-phthalimides were found to be potent EGFR and c-erbB-2 kinase inhibitors *in vitro* and were shown to inhibit EGFR or c-erbB-2 driven tumour growth in nude mice [31]. Other broad spectrum kinase inhibitors have been developed but these may prove to be toxic *in vivo*. In the ras pathway, postranslational modification by farnesylation is essential for its localisation to the cell membrane and inhibitors of the enzyme farnesyl protein transferase are being investigated as inhibitors of the ras pathway. The development of these and other potential drugs for signal transduction therapy has been reviewed recently [14].

Monoclonal antibodies to the EGFR

It was demonstrated more than a decade ago that some mouse monoclonal antibodies (mAbs) could prevent the binding of EGF to the extracellular domain of the receptor [32] and inhibit the growth *in vitro* of tumours which overexpressed the EGFR [33, reviewed in 13]. There are two important advantages in the use of antibodies for targeting the EGFR. The first is that antibodies which block ligand binding prevent signal transduction via the receptor and this may be important where the tumour cell growth is driven by overexpression of the receptor and/or autocrine stimulation. Second, certain antibodies can activate complement and recruit Fc receptor-bearing host effector cells to initiate tumour cell destruction. In each case high affinity antibodies will be more effective than those of lower affinity. In general rat monoclonal antibodies have higher affinities for antigen than their murine counterparts.

In the last decade we have developed a number of rat monoclonal antibodies against the EGF receptor using three different carcinoma cell lines as immunogen [reviewed in 13] and we have used these mAbs to investigate their effects on receptor function and their usefulness for therapeutic application. Competitive inhibition studies showed that the mAbs could be separated topographically on their binding into one of four (AD) epitope clusters. MAbs binding to epitope A would appear to be nearest the Nterminus of the receptor and include the rat ICR9 and also the murine EGFR1. Interestingly, treatment of EGFR expressing cells with ICR9 but not EGFR1 promotes the binding to the receptor of the EGF family of ligands and this in turn stimulates proliferation of these cells. MAbs which belong in epitope cluster B (*e.g.* ICR10 and ICR15) are poor inhibitors of ligand binding and may recognise a sequential determinant since we find that ICR10 can also bind to the receptor in Western blots. The mAbs in epitope clusters C and D were the best inhibitors of ligand binding *(Figure 1)* and some of these *e.g.* ICR16 and ICR62 (cluster C) and ICR64 (cluster D) were the most effective inhibitors of both ligand binding [34] and cell proliferation both *in vitro (Figure 2)* and *in vivo* as xenografts in nude mice [35]. These antibodies neither bind to formalin fixed tissues nor Western blot and we conclude that they all recognize conformational determinants on the receptor.

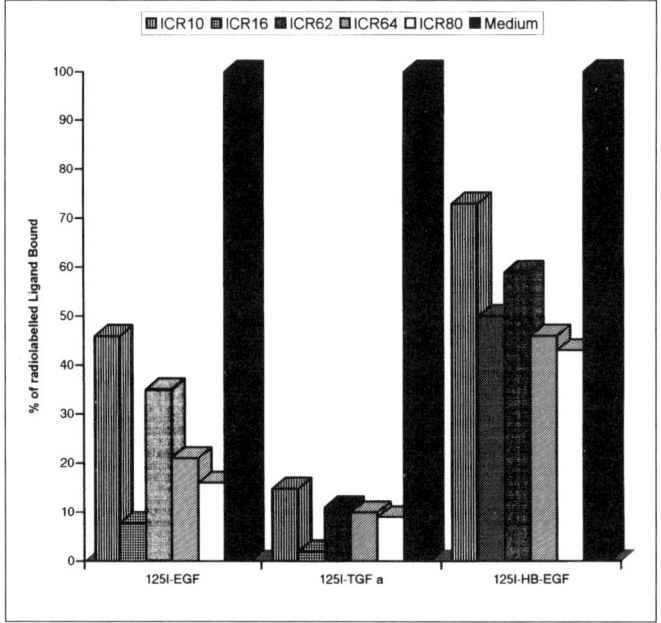

Figure 1. Effect of co-incubation with rat monoclonal antibodies to the EGFR on the binding of ^{125}I-labelled ligand to MDA-MB 468 cells.

Mechanism of action of antibodies that alter EGF receptor function

Bivalency does not appear to be necessary for antibody to induce the alterations in EGF receptor function since we find that Fab fragments of ICR9 and ICR62 are as good as the intact antibodies in promoting (ICR9) or preventing (ICR62) the binding of EGF or TGFα to

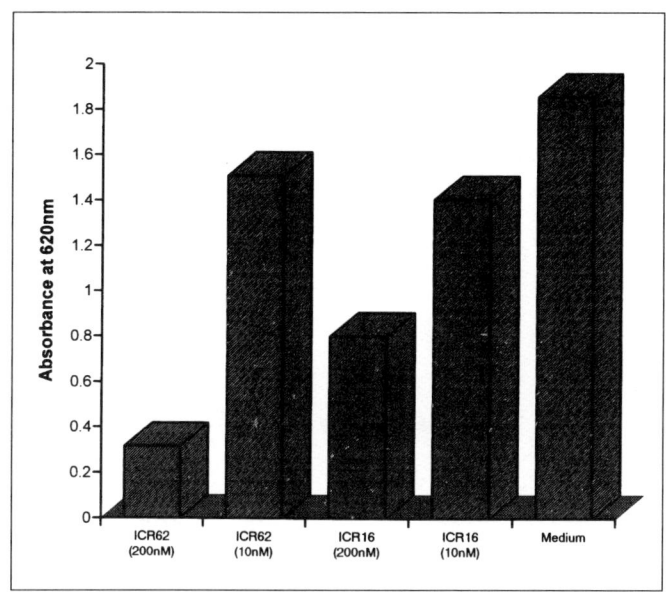

Figure 2. Effect of treatment with rat mAbs ICR16 or ICR62 on the growth *in vitro* of MDA-MB 468 cells. Cells were incubated until those in the medium control were nearly confluent when the number of cells were determined as described in [34].

the EGFR [36]. Both ICR62 and its Fab fragment block phosphorylation of the EGFR induced by treatment with EGF, TGFα, HBEGF, or betacellulin [37], which is illustrated in *Figure 3* for the breast cancer cell line MDAMB 468. This shows that ICR62 inhibits activation of the receptor by the ligands most commonly produced by tumours. Our data is consistent with the idea that antibodies which block ligand binding do so by preventing the conformational change(s) in the extracellular domain of the EGFR that would normally occur during or subsequent to ligand binding which then permits the receptor to undergo dimerization with another receptor. This suggestion is consistent with the findings that a) monovalent Fab fragments of the antibodies are as effective as the divalent mAbs and b) the truncated EGFR encoded by verbB is constitutively activated *i.e.* it is the conformational status of the extracellular domain that determines whether or not the receptor can dimerize with and be activated by other receptor tyrosine kinases (RTK). If transactivation (*i.e.* EGFR -> EGFR, EGFR -> RTK or RTK -> EGFR) not auto-phosphorylation were common events then this conclusion could have important implications for the therapeutic application of monoclonal antibodies which prevent changes in conformaton of the EGFR.

Preclinical studies with antibodies that block ligand binding

Experiments carried out in several laboratories have shown that treatment of nude mice bearing xenografted human tumours with mAbs to the EGFR can restrict the growth of the tumours [reviewed in 13]. Our experience with the rat mAbs suggests that the effectiveness of the antibodies is related not only to their blockade of EGFR function but also to their ability to interact with host immune effector cells and to activate complement [38]. While ICR16 (rat IgG2a) and ICR64 (rat IgG1) were the most effective antibodies at inhibiting cell proliferation

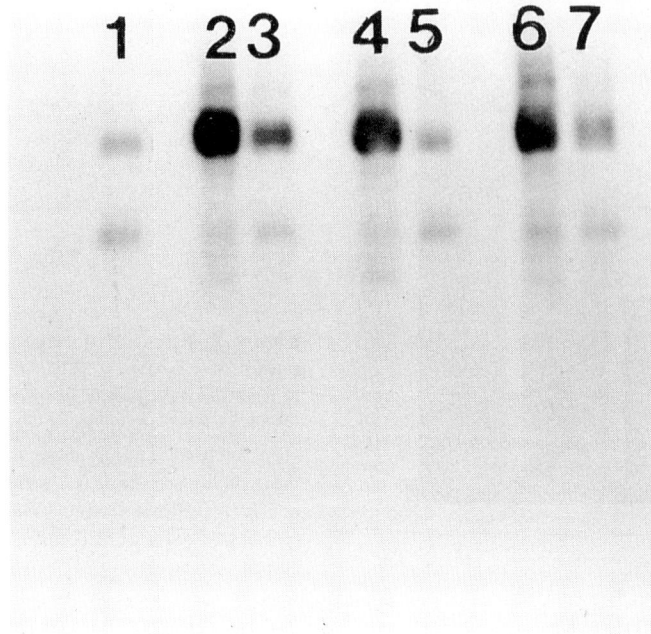

Figure 3. Effect of co-incubation with ICR62 on ligand-induced phosphorylation of the EGFR in MDA-MB468 cells. Lysates were immunoprecipitated with anti-EGFR mab, separated on 6% SDS-containing gels then blotted and probed with the anti-phosphotyrosine mAb PY20 [37]. Lanes: 1, medium control; 2, 10 nM EGF; 3, 10 nM EGF + 400 nM ICR62; 4, 10 nM TGFα; 5, 10 nM TGFα + 400 nM ICR62; 6, 10 nM HB-EGF; 7, 10 nM HB-EGF + 400 nM ICR62.

in vitro [35], ICR62 (rat IgG2b) was superior *in vivo* probably because this isotype activates complement and recruits FcRbearing host effector cells. Indeed, the results obtained with mice bearing the head and neck cancer HN5 were particularly striking and evidence for infiltration of the tumours by host lymphocytes could be seen in those treated with ICR62 [39]. Of particular significance was the finding that when HN5 tumours growing in nude mice were treated with each of the three antibodies the tumours displayed clear evidence of terminal differentiation. The development of keratin whorls during tumour regression was a characteristic feature with this head and neck tumour. It was subsequently found that induction of terminal differentiation of HN5 cells was also induced *in vitro* by treatment with these antibodies. The cells were arrested in G1 and synthesised the differentiation markers involucrin and cytokeratin 10 [39].

Treatment of mice bearing xenografts of the breast cancer MDAMB 468 with 11 doses of 200 mg of ICR16 (day 023) or ICR62 (day 725) were also effective in inhibiting the outgrowth of the tumours *(Figure 4)* but no evidence for induction of differentiation was found during treatment. Instead histological examination provided suggestive evidence that the tumour cells were undergoing apoptosis. This may reflect the differing tissue origins of the head and neck and breast cancers and their responses to growth factor deprivation. Interestingly, even lower doses of these antibodies were effective antitumour agents and treatment of mice bearing MDAMB 468 xenografts with 11 doses of 40 mg of ICR62 from day 018 inhibited tumour growth completely *(Figure 5)*.

The therapeutic effectiveness of antibodies which block activation of the EGF receptor is dependent on the levels of expression of receptor and ligand. The most sensitive tumours were those with the highest levels of expression *e.g.* MDAMB 468 (3×10^5 EGFR/cell), A431 ($2,6 \times 10^6$ EGFR/cell) and HN5 (1.4×10^7 EGFR/cell) whereas tumours with expression levels nearer to those of normal cells *i.e.* 10^4 10^5 receptors/cell (*e.g.* SKOV3) were less responsive to antibody treatment. This may reflect their dependence on other signal transduction pathways for maintaining proliferation. While this may suggest that effective treatment of all EGFR expressing tumours may not be achievable it implies that normal tissues expressing this level of EGFR may be spared damage.

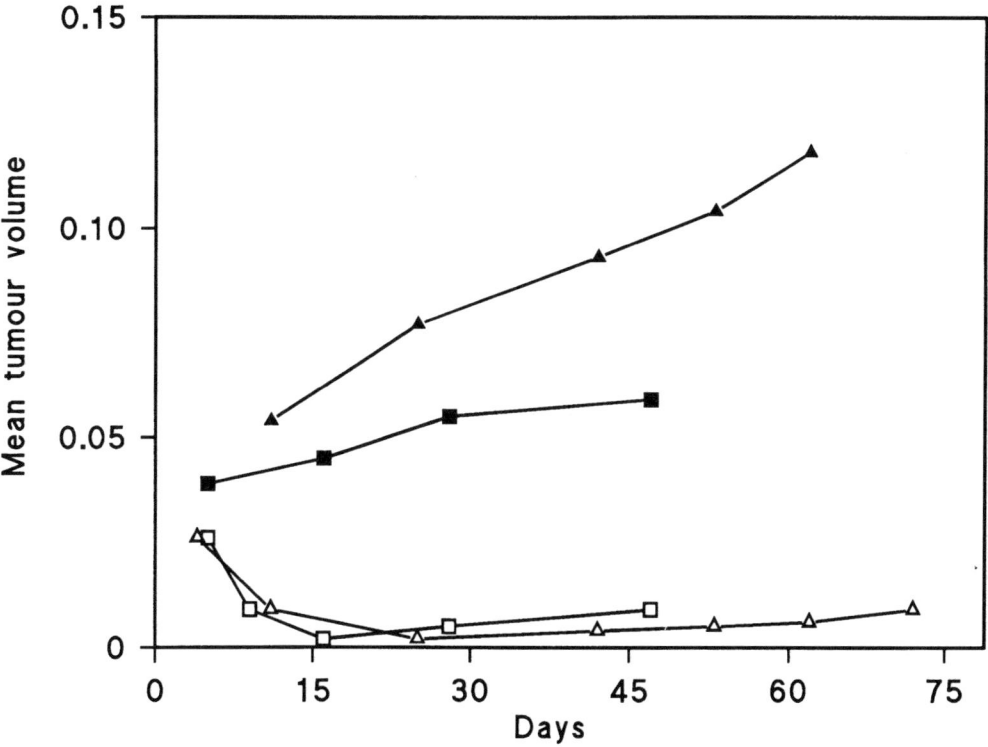

Figure 4. Inhibitory effects of anti-EGFr mAbs on growth of MDA-MB 468 breast carcinoma xenografts. Mice were treated with 11 doses of 200 µg of: ICR62 on days 7-25 (△); ICR16 on days 0-23 (□); control IgG2b mAb (■) or control IgG2a mAb (n). Results are expressed as mean tumour volume (cm^3).

Clinical studies with antibodies to the EGFR

The encouraging results obtained during preclinical testing has prompted several groups to initiate clinical studies. To date, no clinical trials using antibodies to the EGFR have been carried out in patients with breast cancer. This is in part due to the ambivalent results reported for receptor expression in breast cancer and the apparently higher levels of expression in other cancers such as squamous cell carcinoma of the lung or head and neck. On the other hand, the good response of the breast carcinoma MDAMB 468 to treatment with rat mAb ICR62 during preclinical testing should encourage us to test this antibody in breast cancer patients whose tumours express higher levels of the EGFR and are likely to be unresponsive to endocrine therapy.

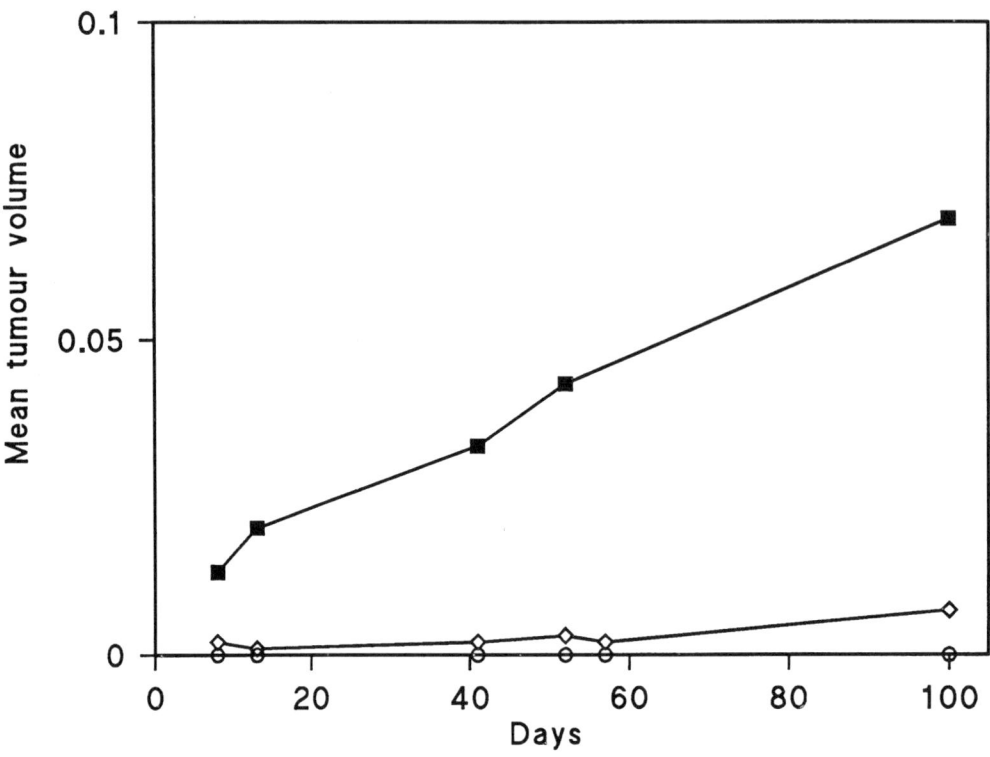

Figure 5. Inhibitory effects of anti-EGFR mAbs on growth of MDA MB 468 breast carcinoma xenografts. Mice were treated during days 0-18 with 11 doses of 40 µg of: ICR62 (o); ICR16<z14> (◊) or control mAb (■).

The first clinical study was in patients with head and neck cancer and utilised the murine mAb EGFR1 and the results obtained by radioimmunoscintigraphy demonstrated uptake of radiolabel by the tumours [40]. Using the mouse mAb 225, Mendelsohn and colleagues gave lung cancer patients single doses of up to 300 mg of antibody labelled with Indium^{111}. No adverse effects were reported and good tumour lcalisation was observed with doses above 40 mg [41]. In this investigation, high uptake in the liver was reported so that only at doses above 25 mg/patient was significant uptake seen in the tumours. Radioimaging and radioimmunotherapy trials using the mouse antibodies EGFR1, or 425 have also been conducted in patients with glioma [42, 43] or malignant astrocytomas [44] with promising results.

We have investigated the effect of treatment of patients with head and neck or lung cancer with unlabelled ICR62 in single doses of up to 100 mg of antibody. In no case was any serious toxicity noted and biopsies of tumours taken from patients given either 40 mg or 100 mg of antibody showed good antibody localisation to the tumour cells [45]. At these higher doses antibody could be detected in the blood at 24 hours; only 4/20 patients showed HARA responses and only two of these were anti-idiotypic in nature. A phase I/II therapy trial using multiple doses of ICR62 is planned in patients with head and neck or squamous cell lung cancer. In a similar study, also in patients with head and neck or non-small cell lung cancer, but using the mouse antibody RG83852, tumour localisation was only detected with doses of

400 mg/m^{-2} or greater [46]. It is not clear why a higher dose was needed to obtain immunohistochemical staining of the receptor but lower antibody affinity may be the explanation.

Concluding remarks

There are two important obstacles to successful therapy using monoclonal antibodies directed against the EGFR. The first is the host immune response against the mouse or rat protein, the severity of which varies from antibody to antibody. The use of humanized antibodies may overcome this problem but sometimes at a cost because the affinity for the receptor may change. More important is the tumour load. It is unlikely that late stage, bulky tumours can be eradicated by antibody treatment alone. The most promising role for antibody is for the treatment of minimal residual disease following debulking by either surgery or chemotherapy. Clinical trials using combined chemo- and immunotherapy are already in progress [47]. Indeed, the very promising results reported recently in patients with Dukes' C colorectal cancer would support this view [48]. In this trial, following surgery, 189 patients were given adjuvant treatment with 500 mg of mouse antibody 17-1A (which recognises a 37-40 kDa cell surface glycoprotein present on normal and tumour cells) followed by four 100 mg infusions at monthly intervals. Despite HAMA responses in 80% of the patients the treatment reduced the overall 5 year death rate by 30% and the recurrence rate by 27%. These results should encourage us to persue treatment with antibodies to the EGFR in an adjuvant setting.

References

1. Yamamoto T, Nishida T, Miyajima, N, Kawai S, Ooi T, Toyashima K. The *erbB gene of avian erythoblastosis virus is a member of the src* gene family. *Cell* 1983; 35: 71-8.
2. Downward J, Yarden Y, Mayes E, Scrace G, Totty N, Stockwell P, Ullrich A, Schlessinger J, Waterfield M. Close similarity of epidermal growth factor receptor and v-*erb*B oncogene protein sequences. *Nature* 1984; 307: 521-7.
3. Schlessinger J, Ullrich A. Gowth factor signalling by receptor tyrosine kinases. *Neuron* 1992; 9: 383-91.
4. Cousens L, Yang Feng T, Liao Y, Chen E, Gray A, McGrath J, Seeburg P, Liberman T, Schlessinger J, Francke U, Levinson A, Ullrich A. Tyrosine kinase receptor with extensive homology to EGF receptor shows chromosomal location with *neu* oncogene. *Science* 1985; 230: 1132-9.
5. Kraus M, Issing W, Miki T, Popescu N, Aaronson S. Isolation and characterization of ERBB3, a third member of the ERRB/epidermal growth factor receptor family: evidence for overexpression in a subset of human mammary tumours. *Proc Natl Acad Sci USA* 1989; 86: 9193-7.
6. Plowman G, Culouscou J, Whitney G, Green J, Carlton G, Foy L, Neubauer M, Shoyab M. Ligand-specific activation of HER4/p180*erb*B4, a fourth member of the epidermal grwth factor receptor family. *Proc Natl Acad Sci USA* 1993; 90: 1746-50.
7. Slamon D, Clark G, Wong S, Levin W, Ullrich A, McGuire W. Human breast cancer: correlation of relapse and survival with amplification of the HER-2/*neu* oncogene. *Science* 1987; 235: 177-82.
8. Holmes W, Sliwkowski M, Akita R, Henzel W, Lea J, Park J, Yansura D, Abodi S, Raab H, Lewis G, Shepard H, Kwang WJ, Wood W, Goeddel D, Vandlen R. Identification of heregulin, a specific activator of p185^{erbB2}. *Science* 1992; 256: 1205-10.
9. Wen D, Peles E, Cupples R, Suggs S, Bacus S, Luc Y, Trail G, Hu S, Silbiger S, Levy R, Koski R, Lu H, Yarden Y. Neu differentiation factor: a transmembrane glycoprotein containing an EGF domain and an immunoglobulin homology unit. *Cell* 1993; 69: 559-72.
10. Marchionni M, Goodearl A, Chen M, Bermingham-McDonogh O, Kirk C, Hendricks M, Danehy F, Misumi D, Sudhalter J, Kobayachi K, Wroblewski D, Lynch C, Baldassare M, Hiles I, Davis J,

Hsuan J, Totty N, Otsu M, McBurney R, Waterfield M, Stroobant P, Gwynne D. Glial growth factors are alternatively spliced erbB-2 ligands expressed in the nervous system. *Nature* 1993; 362: 312-8.
11. Cowley G, Smith J, Gusterson B, Hendler F, Ozanne B. The amount of EGF receptor is elevated on squamous cell carcinomas. *Cancer Cells* 1984; 1: 5-10.
12. Gullick W. Prevelence of aberrant expression of the epidermal growth factor receptor in human cancers. *Br Med Bull* 1991; 47: 87-98.
13. Modjtahedi H, Dean C. The receptor for EGF and its ligands: Expression, prognostic value and target for therapy in cancer (Review). *Int J Oncol* 1994; 4: 277-96.
14. Levitzki A. Signal-transduction therapy: a novel approach to disease management. *Eur J Biochem* 1994; 226: 1-13.
15. Workman P. Cell proliferation, cell cycle and apoptosis targets for cancer drug discovery: strategies, strengths and pitfalls. In: Thomas N, ed. *Apoptosis and cell cycle control in cancer Oxford: Bios-Scientific Publishers*, 1996: 205-32.
16. Humphrey P, Gangarosa L, Wong A, Archer G, Lund-Johansen M, Bjerkvig R, Laerum OD, Friedman H, Bigner D. Deletion-mutant epidermal gowth factor receptor in human gliomas: effect of type II mutations on receptor function. *Biochem Biophys Res Commun* 1991; 178: 1413-20.
17. Humphrey P, Wong A, Vogelstein B, Zalutsky M, Fuller G, Archer G, Friedman H, Kwatra M, Bigner S, Bigner D. Anti-synthetic peptide antibody reacting at the fusion junction of deletion-mutant epidermal growth factor receptors in human glioblastoma. *Proc Natl Acad Sci USA* 1990; 87: 4207-11.
18. Wickstrand C, Hale L, Batra S, Hill M, Humphrey P, Kurpad S, McLendon R, Moscatello D, Pegram C, Reist C, Traweck S, Wong A, Zalutsky M, Bigner D. Monoclonal antibodies against EGFRvIII are tumour specific and react with breast and lung carcinomas and malignant gliomas. *Cancer Res* 1995; 55: 3140-8.
19. Harris A. What is the biological, prognostic and therapeutic role of the EGF receptor in human breast cancer? *Breast Cancer Research and Treatment* 1994; 29: 1-2.
20. Fox S, Smith K, Hollyer J, Greenall M, Hastrich D, Harris A. The epidermal growth factor receptor as a prognostic marker: Results of 370 patients and review of 3,009 patients. *Breast Cancer Research and Treatment* 1994; 29: 41-9.
21. Nicholson R, Mclelland R, Gee J, Manning D, Cannon P, Robertson J, Ellis I, Blamey R. Epidermal growth factor receptor expression in breast cancer: Association with response to endocrine therapy. *Breast Cancer Research and Treatment* 1994; 29: 117-25.
22. Meissenhelker J, Suh PG, Rhee S, Hunter T. Phospholipase C-gamma is a substrate for the PDGF and EGF receptor tyrosine kinases *in vivo* and *in vitro*. *Cell* 1989; 57: 1109-22.
23. Zhang K, Sun J, Liu N, Wen D, Chang D, Thomason A, Yoshinga S. Transformation of NIH3T3 cells by HER3 or HER4 receptors requires the presence of HER1 or HER2. *J Biol Chem* 1996; 271: 3884-90.
24. Kokai Y, Dobashi K, Weiner D, Myers J, Nowell P, Greene M. Phosphorylation process induced by epidermal growth factor alters the oncogenic and cellular *neu* (NGL) gene products. *Proc Natl Acad Sci USA* 1988; 85: 5389-93.
25. Spivak Kroizman T, Rotin D, Pinchassi D, Ullrich A, Schlessinger J, Lax I. Heterodimerization of c-erbB2 with different epidermal growth factor receptor mutants elicits stimulatory or inhibitory responses. *J Biol Chem* 1992; 267: 8056-63.
26. Soltoff S, Carraway K, Prigent S, Gullick W, Cantley L. ErbB3 is involved in activation of phosphatidoinositol 3-kinase by epidermal growth factor. *Mol Cell Biol* 1994; 14: 3550-8.
27. Gazit A, Yaish P, Gilon C, Levitzki A. Tyrphostins 1: synthesis and biological activity of protein tyrosine kinase inhibitors. *J Med Chem* 1989; 32: 2344-52.
28. Taketura N, Yasui W, Kyo E, Yoshita K, Kamedo T, Kitadai P, Abe K, Umezawa K, Tahara E. Effects of tyrosine kinase inhibitor erbstatin on cell growth and growth factor receptor gene expression in human gastric carcinoma cells. *Int J Peptide Res* 1991; 38: 204-11.
29. Osherov N, Gazit A, Gilon C, Levitzki A. Selective inhibition of the EGF and HER2/*neu* receptors by tyrphostins. *J Biol Chem* 1993; 268: 11134-42.
30. Yoneda T, Lyall R, Alsine M, Pearsons P, Spada A, Levitzki A, Zilberstein A, Mundy G. The anti-proliferative effects of tyrosine kinase inhibitor tyrphostin on a human squamous cell carcinoma *in vitro* and in nude mice. *Cancer Res* 1991; 51 4430-5.

31. Buchdunger E, Trinks U, Mett H, Regenass U, Müller M, Meyer T, McGlyn E, Pinna L, Traxler P, Lydon N. 4,5-Dianilinophathalimide: a protein tyrosine kinase inhibitor with selectivity for the epidermal growth-factor receptor signal transduction pathway and potent *in vivo* anti-tumour activity. *Proc Natl Acad Sci USA* 1993; 91: 2334-8.
32. Sato J, Kawamoto T, Le A, Mendelsohn J, Polikoff J, Sato J. Biological effects *in vitro* of Mabs to human EGF receptors. *Mol Biol Med* 1983; 3: 929-37.
33. Masui H, Kawamoto T, Sato J, Wolf B, Sato G, Mendelsohn J. Growth inhibition of human tumour cells in athymic mice by anti-epidermal growth factor receptor monoclonal antibodies. *Cancer Res* 1984; 44: 1002-7.
34. Modjtahedi H, Styles J, Dean C. The human EGF receptor as a target for cancer therapy: six new rat mAbs against the receptor on the breast carcinoma MDA-MB 468. *Br J Cancer* 1993; 67: 247-53.
35. Modjtahedi H, Eccles S, Box G, Styles J, Dean C. Immunotherapy of human tumour xenografts overexpressing the EGF receptor with rat antibodies that block growth factor-receptor interaction. *Br J Cancer* 1993; 67: 254-61.
36. Modjtahedi H, Jackson E, Dean C. Monovalent antibodies to the EGF receptor: effects on proliferation and differentiation of tumours overexpressing the EGF receptor. *Tumour Targeting* 1995; 1: 99-106.
37. Modjtahedi H, Dean C. Binding of betacellulin to the EGF receptor is blocked by antibodies which act as EGF, TGFα and HB-EGF antagonists. *Biochem Byophys Res Commun* 1996 (in press).
38. Eccles S, Modjtahedi H, Court W, Box G, Dean C. Preclinical studies with human tumour xenografts using rat monoclonal antibodies directed against the epidermal growth factor receptor. In EGF receptor in tumour growth and progression, *Ernst Schering Research Foundation Workshop 19*, 1996; in Press.
39. Modjtahedi H, Eccles S, Sandle J, Box G, Titley J, Dean C. Differentiation or immune destruction: two pathways for therapy of squamous cell carcinomas with antibodies to the epidermal growth factor receptor. *Cancer Research* 1994; 54: 1695-701.
40. Soo K, Ward M, Roberts K, Keeling F, Carter R, McCready R, Ott R, Powell E, Ozanne B, Westwood J, Gusterson B. Radioimmunoscintigraphy of squamous carcinomas of the head and neck. *Head Neck Surg* 1987; 9: 349-52.
41. Divgi C, West S, Kris M, Real F, Yeh D, Gralla R, Merchant B, Schweighart S, Unger M, Larson S, Mendelsohn J. Phase 1 and imaging trial of Indium 111-labelled anti-EGF receptor antibody 225 in patients with squamous cell lung carcinomas. *J Natl Cancer Inst* 1991; 83: 97-104.
42. Kalofonos H, Pawlikowska T, Hemingway A, Courtnay-Luck N, Dhokia B, Snook D, Sivalapenko G, Hooker G, McKenzie C, Lavender P, Thomas D, Epenetos A. Antibody guided diagnosis and therapy of brain gliomas using radiolabelled antibodies against epidermal growth factor receptor and placental alkaline phosphatase. *J Nucl Med* 1989; 30: 1636-45.
43. Dadparvar S, Krishna L, Miyamoto C, Brady L, Brown S, Bender H, Slizofkii w, Chevres A, Woo D. Indium-111-labelled anti-EGFr-425 scintigraphy in the detection of malignant gliomas. *Cancer Suppl* 1994; 73: 884-9.
44. Brady L, Miyamoto C, Woo D, Rackover M, Emrich J, Bender H, Dadparvar S, Steplewski Z, Koprowski H. Malignant astrocytomas treated with iodine-125 labelled monoclonal antibody 425 against epidermal growth factor receptor: a phase II trial. *Int Rad Oncol Biol Phys* 1991; 22: 225-30.
45. Modjtahedi H, Hickish T, Nicolson M, Moore J, Styles J, Eccles S, Jackson E, Salter J, Sloane J, Spencer L, Priest K, Smith I, Dean C, Gore M. Phase I trial and tumour localisation of the anti-EGFR monoclonal antibody ICR62 in head and neck or lung cancer. *Br J Cancer* 1996; 73 : 228-35.
46. Perez-Soler R, Donato N, Shin D, Rosenblum M, Zhang H, Tornos G, Brewer H, Chang J, Lee J, Hough K, Murray J. Tumour epidermal growth factor receptor studies in patents with non-small-cell lung cancer or head and neck cancer treated with monoclonal antibody RG 83852. *J Clin Oncol* 1994; 12: 730-9.
47. Mendelsohn J. EGF receptor blockade as anti-cancer therapy. *Proc Amer Ass Cancer Res* 1996; 37: 647-8.
48. Reithmüller G, Schneider-Gadicke E, Schlimok G, Schmiegel W, Raab R, Pichlmair H, Hirche H, Pichlmayr R, Buggisch P, Witte J and the German Cancer Aid 17-1A Study Group. Randomised trial of monoclonal antibody for adjuvant therapy of resected Dukes'C colorectal carcinoma. *Lancet* 1994; 343: 1177-83.

Pharmacological targeting of signal transduction processes

Paul T. Kirschmeier, Joseph J. Catino, Ronald J. Doll, F. George Njoroje, Donna M. Carr, Linda J. James, Kimberly Grey, Louise M. Perkins, David Whyte, Fang Zhang and W. Robert Bishop

Departments of Tumor Biology and Chemistry, Schering Plough Research Institute, 2015 Galloping Hill Rd, Kenilworth, N.J. 07033

Abstract

Oncogenic activated forms of ras proteins are associated with a broad range of human cancers. The post-translational modification of this protein by the 15 carbon isoprenoid lipid farnesyl is obligatory for ras induced cellular transformation. We describe the activity of a novel series of potent farnesyl transferase (FTP) inhibitors (FTI)[1], represented by SCH44342. This compound inhibits FPT with an IC50 of approximately 250 nM, while it is only weakly active against geranylgeranyl transferase type 1 (IC50 > 114 µM). It inhibits the post-translational C-terminal processing of H-ras in ras transformed rat fibroblasts and in Cos cells in a transient expression assay with IC50's ranging from 1 to 3 µM. SCH44342 suppresses the growth in agar phenotype of rat2 cells transformed by ras CVLS, farnesylated ras, with an IC50 of 8-10 µM but not of rat2 cells transformed by ras CVLL, a geranylgeranyled mutant form of the protein. Compounds in this chemical series also suppress the growth in agar phenotype of several human breast and lung cancer cell lines. Surprisingly, not all of the cell lines that are sensitive to FTI's harbor activated ras mutations. This is especially true of the breast cancer lines where the frequency of ras mutation is < 10%. The mechanism of action of the compounds in these cell lines is not well understood. However, the targeting of cellular signal transduction pathways has led to the discovery of potentially useful anticancer therapeutics.

Introduction

Signal transduction processes govern cell proliferation and differentiation. Genetic analysis has shown that the misfunctioning of proteins that comprise the signal transduction pathways provide a molecular basis for understanding the development of neoplastic disease [1]. The ras family of small GTP binding proteins are central to the process of normal signal transduction and the development of malignancies. The ras proteins receive proliferative signals that originate from activation of growth factor receptors or other tyrosine kinases [1, 2]. The ras protein is then converted from a GDP bound form to a GTP bound form. When bound to GTP, the ras proteins undergo a conformational change, and are capable of stimulating signal transmission through interaction with downstream protein targets. These interactions result in a pleiotropic response characterized by the activation of the MAP kinase cascade, gene induction, and cytoskeletal changes. The ras proteins can become constitutively activated by mutations that impair their intrinsic GTPase activity. Additionally signaling through normal ras can be augmented by constitutive activation of signals upstream of ras. These two molecular events can also contribute to the maintenance of the neoplastic phenotype in tumor cells.

The ras protein must be localized to the plasma membrane to fulfill its biological function [3]. Targeting of the ras proteins to the plasma membrane is achieved by the addition of the 15 carbon isoprenoid lipid, farnesyl to the protein *via* a thioether linkage to the cysteine four residues from the carboxy terminus. The enzyme responsible for this modification is farnesyl protein transferase [4]. Substrates for this enzyme are proteins whose carboxy termini end with a « CaaX » motif, where X is methionine or serine and « a » is an aliphatic amino acid. Mutants of ras where the cysteine in the « CaaX » motif was replaced by a serine cannot activate the downstream kinase signaling cascades and cannot transform normal rodent fibroblasts. Ras proteins that are not farnesylated are not localized to the cell membrane. The unmodified proteins remain cytoplasmic and lack normal biological function. Inhibitors of FPT would therefore be expected to block the lipid modification of mutationally activated ras proteins and suppress or revert the malignant phenotype caused by expression of those proteins [5].

We developed a unique series of non peptidomimetic farnesyl transferase inhibitors that lack the free sulfhydryl group found on other compounds in this inhibitor class [6]. We explored their biochemical mechanism and their activity in fibroblast cell systems. In addition, we found that the anchorage independent growth of a number of human tumor cell lines, including breast cancer cell lines, was inhibited by farnesyl transferase inhibitors. However, the sensitivity of a cell line did not necessarily correlate with the presence of an activating mutation of one of the isoforms of ras. Therefore the biochemical mechanism for the sensitivity observed in some cell lines is not well understood and is the subject of current investigations.

Materials and methods

Plasmids and cell lines

Rat-2 cells expressing either [val12]H-Ras-CVLS or [val12]H-Ras-CVLL were constructed by transfecting pOPRSV [val12]H-Ras-CVLS or pOPRSEU [val12]H-Ras-CVLL into Rat2 fibroblasts (ATCC # CRL-1764). Transfected cells were selected in DMEM containing 10% FBS and 250 µg/ml G418. Human tumor cell lines were obtained from the ATCC and cultured in the suggested medium.

Determination of enzyme activity

Methodology for assaying farnesyl and geranylgeranyl transferase activity and determining the IC50 values for compounds is described in Bishop *et al.*

Growth in agar

The ability of cells to grow in agar was assessed as described by Nagasu *et al.* [7].

Results and discussion

SCH44342 is a potent, selective inhibitor of farnesyl transferase

The tricyclic compound SCH44342 *(Figure 1)* inhibits the activity of farnesyl protein transferase with an IC50 of 0.25 µM [6] . This compound inhibited the activity on a related protein prenyl transferase, geranylgeranyl transferase 1, with an IC50 > 114 µM [6]. SCH44342 therefore has the desirable characteristics of potency and selectivity. A kinetic analysis of the mechanism of inhibition by this compound showed it to be competitive with the p21 ras protein substrate [6]. SCH44342 was not derived from modification of peptide inhibitors nor does this compound have a free sulfhydryl group found in other members of this class of inhibitors. Still it shows remarkable selectivity for the inhibition of farnesyl protein transferase and behaves as a competitive inhibitor with the protein substrate.

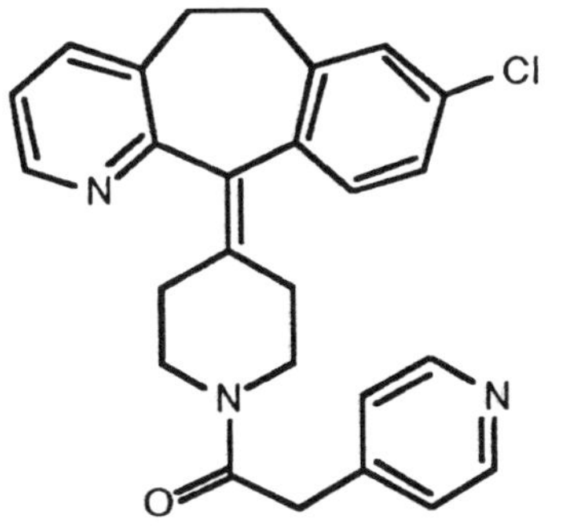

Figure 1. Structure of SCH 44342. SCH 44342 is a representative compound in the tricyclic series of non-peptide inhibitors of farnesyl transferase. These compounds appear to be competitive with the ras p21 substrate.

The processing of ras p21 is inhibited by SCH44342

Figure 2 shows that p21 ras processing is inhibited in cells treated with SCH44342. The ras proteins from cells that were metabolically labeled in presence of increasing concentrations of SCH44342 were separated on 15% SDS polyacrylamide gels. This system reveals two species of ras protein distinguished by their electrophoretic mobility. The more rapidly migrating form is fully processed ras and the more slowly migrating form is the nonprenylated precursor form of the protein. In the presence of this compound we observed a dose dependent inhibition of p21 ras processing with an IC50 of 2-3 µM. As a control the carboxy terminal amino acid of the ras protein was mutated from S to L, making the resultant protein a substrate for the geranylgeranyl transferase. In Rat 2 cells transformed by this protein, SCH44342 was unable to block processing and protein at a compound concentrations migrated as the fully processed species. These results show that SCH44342 is able to get into cells, inhibits farnesyl transferase activity in cells and retains its selectivity for FT over GGT.

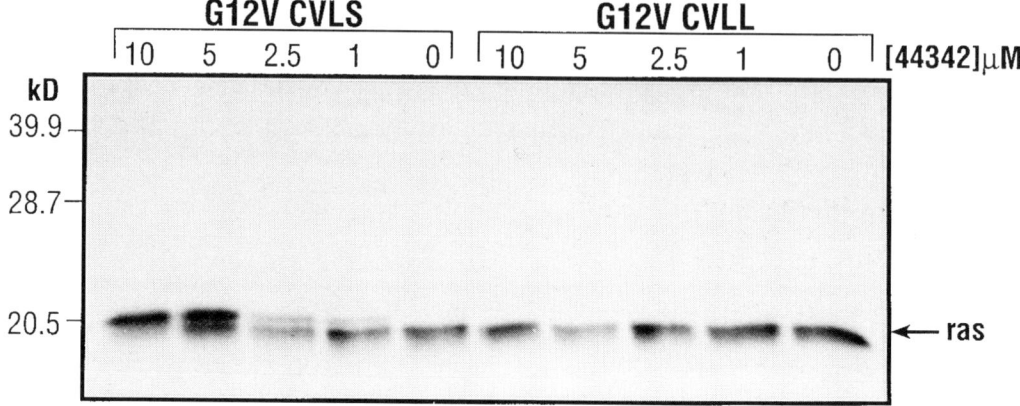

Figure 2. SCH 44342 inhibits processing of H-Ras-CVLS but not H-Ras-CVLL, in Rat-2 fibroblasts. Rat 2 fibroblasts expressing a [val[12]] activated form of either H-Ras-CVLS or H-Ras-CVLL were labeled with [^{35}S] methionine in the presence of the indicated concentration of SCH 44342. Ras proteins were immunoprecipitated using agarose-conjugated Y13-259, an anti-Ras rat monoclonal antibody. Immunoprecipitates were run on 14% acrylamide SDS-PAGE gels and autoradiographed.

SCH44342 suppresses anchorage independent growth of ras transformed fibroblasts

Rat2 fibroblast cell lines transformed by ras CVLS or ras CVLL were constructed. SCH44342 suppressed the growth of the cell lines transformed by ras CVLS in a dose dependent manner with an IC50 of approximately 10 μM *(Figure 3)*. However, the growth in agar phenotype of the Rat2 cells transformed by ras CVLL remained unaffected by the compound *(Figure 3)*. There is a marked selectivity of the compound for the cells that are transformed by a farnesylated ras protein suggesting that inhibition of the postranslational modification of this oncoprotein would potentially useful clinical therapeutics.

Inhibition of FTP suppresses anchorage independent growth of human tumor cell lines

The sensitivity of human breast and lung cancer cell lines to farnesyl transferase inhibitors was determined. The results of these studies are shown in *Table I*. Two of the lung cancer lines, A549 and NCI-H460, harbor a mutated K-ras gene. Both of these lines were sensitive to an analog of SCH44342. Interestingly, many of the other lung cancer lines examined also showed sensitivity to the inhibitors, even though they were wild-type ras. These results confirm those reported for a farnesyl transferase inhibitor belonging to a different structural type [7, 8]. Furthermore, the results in *Table I* show that 4/7 breast cancer lines were also sensitive to the farnesyl transferase inhibitors. None of these lines tested harbors a mutated ras oncogene. These results confirm and extend those from other laboratories.

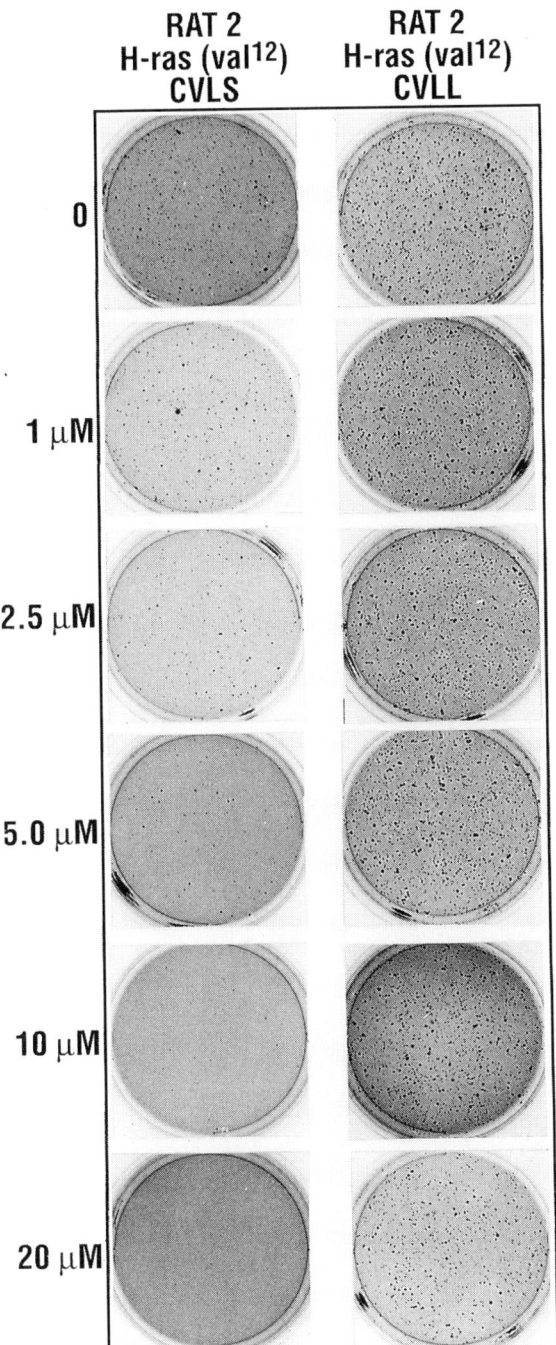

Figure 3. Effect of SCH 44342 on soft agar growth of Rat-2 fibroblasts transformed with [val[12]] H-Ras-CVLS or [val[12]] H-Ras-CVLL. Rat 2 fibroblasts transformed with the [val[12]] activated form of H-Ras-CVLS or CVLL were plated in soft agar in the presence of the indicated concentration of SCH 44342 as described in experimental procedures. Colonies were photographed after 14 days.

The mechanism of action that explains the sensitivity of the cell lines that lack a ras mutation is not known. One possibility is that these cell lines depend on another farnesylated protein for growth. That protein has not yet been identified although there are some 30-40 farnesylated proteins in the cell and their role in cell growth remains uncharacterized [9]. Farnesylation of prelamin A and lamin B was considered essential for cell growth. Recent studies, however, have shown that these proteins can be assembled into the nuclear lamina in the presence of farnesyl transferase inhibitors [6, 10]. Our results have also shown that inhibition of lamin farnesylation does not correlate to growth in agar sensitivity to the FT inhibitors.

Table I. Cell lines derived from human tumors are sensitive to farnesyl transferase inhibitors. Cell lines were plated in agar as described in Materials and methods. Plates were incubated for 12-15 days at 37 C and colonies were stained and counted. The sensitivity of cell lines to the FTI does not depend on the presence of a mutated ras isoform.

Cell line	Tissue of origin	ras mutation	Sensitivity to FT inhibition
MCF-7	Breast	WT	S
HBL-100	Breast	WT	S
DU4475	Breast	WT	S
MDA MB 468	Breast	WT	S
SK-Br3	Breast	WT	R
MDA MB 453	Breast	WT	R
T47D	Breast	WT	R
NCI-H460	Lung	Q61H (K ras)	S
A549	Lung	G12S (K ras)	S
NCI-H146	Lung	WT	S
NCI-H69	Lung	WT	S
LoVo	Colon	G12D (K ras)	S
HCT 116	Colon	G13D (K ras)	S

Another possibility explaining the sensitivity of cell lines lacking activating ras mutations to FT inhibition may be the presence of constitutive growth promoting signals upstream of ras. While this cannot be completely ruled out, it likely does not provide a complete explanation. The breast cancer cell lines, SK BR3 and BT 474 harbor amplification of HER-2, a growth factor receptor tyrosine kinase, that transmits signals through ras are relatively resistant to the FT inhibitors. This suggests either a ras independent mechanism of cell signaling by the growth factor receptor or a mechanism that abrogates the effect of the FT inhibitor. One mechanism for this possibility was suggested by the observation that the K-ras4B protein could be geranylgeranylated [11]. The biological consequences of alternative prenylation are not completely understood. Evidences suggests that gerenylgeranylation of wild type H-ras interferes with normal function and is growth inhibitory [12]. Such a mechanism could conceivably provide an explanation for the sensitivity of cell lines that lack an activated ras protein but express significant levels of K-ras 4B. This and other mechanisms of tumor cell sensitivity to farnesyl transferase inhibitors needs to be explored. However, the sensitivity of many tumor cell lines suggests that the FT inhibitors may be more broadly useful as cancer chemotherapeutics than originally proposed.

---

(1) The abbreviations used are: FT, farnesyl transferase; GGT, geranylgeranyl transferase; FTI, farneysl transferase inhibitor.

References

1. Bishop JM. Molecular themes in oncogenesis. *Cell* 1991; 64 (2): 235-48.
2. Medema RH, Bos JL. The role of p21ras in receptor tyrosine kinase signaling. *Crit Rev Oncog* 1993; 4 (6): 615-61.
3. Hancock JF, Cadwallader K, Paterson H, Marshall CJ. A CAAX or a CAAL motif and a second signal are sufficient for plasma membrane targeting of ras proteins. *Embo J* 1991; 10 (13): 4033-9.
4. Casey PJ, Solski PA, Der CJ, Buss JE. p21ras is modified by a farnesyl isoprenoid. *Proc Natl Acad Sci USA* 1989; 86 (21): 8323-7.
5. Gibbs JB, Oliff A, Kohl NE. Farnesyltransferase inhibitors: Ras research yields a potential cancer therapeutic. *Cell* 1994; 77 (2): 175-8.
6. Bishop WR, Bond R, Petrin J, Wang L, Patton R, Doll R, Njoroge G, Catino J, Schwartz J, Windsor W, Syto R, Schwartz J, Carr D, James L, Kirschmeier P. Novel tricyclic inhibitors of farnesyl protein transferase. Biochemical characterization and inhibition of Ras modification in transfected Cos cells. *J Biol Chem* 1995; 270 (51): 30611-8.
7. Nagasu T, Yoshimatsu K, Rowell C, Lewis MD, Garcia AM. Inhibition of human tumor xenograft growth by treatment with the farnesyl transferase inhibitor B956. *Cancer Res* 1995; 55 (22): 5310-4.
8. Sepp-Lorenzino L, Ma Z, Rands E, Kohl NE, Gibbs JB, Oliff A, Rosen N. A peptidomimetic inhibitor of farnesyl protein transferase blocks the anchorage-dependent and -independent growth of human tumor cell lines. *Cancer Res* 1995; 55 (22): 5302-9.
9. James GL, Goldstein JL, Pathak RK, Anderson RG, Brown MS. PxF, a prenylated protein of peroxisomes. *J Biol Chem* 1994; 269 (19): 14182-90.
10. Dalton MB, Fantle KS, Bechtold HA, DeMaio L, Evans RM, Krystosek A, Sinensky M. The farnesyl protein transferase inhibitor BZA-5B blocks farnesylation of nuclear lamins and p21ras but does not affect their function or localization. *Cancer Res* 1995; 55 (15): 3295-304.
11. James GL, Goldstein JL, Brown MS. Polylysine and CVIM sequences of K-RasB dictate specificity of prenylation and confer resistance to benzodiazepine peptidomimetic *in vitro*. *J Biol Chem* 1995; 270 (11): 6221-6.
12. Cox AD, Hisaka MM, Buss JE, Der CJ. Specific isoprenoid modification is required for function of normal, but not oncogenic ras protein. *Mol Cell Biol* 1992; 12 (6): 2606-15.

Breast Cancer. Advances in biology and therapeutics.
F. Calvo, M. Crépin, H. Magdelenat, eds. John Libbey Eurotext © 1996, pp. 167-173.

The role of angiogenesis in tumour progression of breast cancer

M.D. Giampietro Gasparini

Department of Oncology, St. Bortolo Hospital, I, 36100 Vicenza, Italy

Abstract

The characteristics and the degree of neovascularization in pre-invasive and invasive breast cancer, the role of angiogenesis in breast cancer progression, its prognostic and predictive significance and the potential targets for a pharmacologic modulation of angiogenesis will here be presented and discussed

Background on the biologic and clinical significance of angiogenesis in solid tumours

There is compelling evidence that, in general, angiogenesis is necessary for tumour progression. The acquisition of the angiogenic phenotype is accompanied by rapid growth and invasiveness of primary tumours and facilitates metastasis.
The angiogenic activity of a tumour is the result of the net balance between angiogenic stimuli and inhibitory pathways which, in turn, are regulated by complex cellular, genetic and biochemical mechanisms. Ultimately, the onset of neovascularization facilitates tumour progression and metastasis through three main mechanisms: I) the « perfusion effect ». An adequate neovascularization is necessary for an appropriate delivery of nutrients and oxygen for the expansion of tumour growth; II) the neoformation of microvessels within the stroma of solid tumours facilitates the penetration and the transport in the bloodstream of tumour cells that may colonize distant sites and; III) the « paracrine effect ». Endothelial cells produce some cytokines (*e.g.* IL-6, granulocyte colony-stimulating factor) and growth factors (*e.g.* angiogenic peptides and others) that directly stimulate tumour cells to grow [1, 2].
Several methods have been developed to determine the angiogenic activity of human tumours. They include the immunohistochemical assessment of intratumoral microvessel density, the

expression of some markers involved in neovascularization such as integrin $\alpha_v\beta_3$, tissue metalloproteinases and the serum/urine levels of angiogenic factors [3, 4]. An optimal technique has not yet been developed, however, the above methods have permitted to quantify the angiogenic activity of human tumours of different histologic type and to understand its clinical significance.

Several angiogenesis inhibitors, which may act with different mechanisms of action have been developed and some are presently under early clinical evaluation [5]. It has been proposed a new anticancer therapeutic paradigm that consists of the inhibition of the two-cell compartments, *i.e.* the parenchyma and the stroma, because both contribute to the biological aggressiveness of a solid tumour [6]. Anti-angiogenesis agents administered together with conventional cytotoxic treatments in experimental models have confirmed the importance of such an approach [7, 8].

Histopathologic and experimental studies on breast cancer angiogenesis

Gimbrone and Gullino [9] first, twenty years ago, studied neovascularization of breast cancer. They assessed the angiogenic response induced in the rabbit iris by the transplantation of xenografts of normal, hyperplastic and neoplastic mouse mammary tissues. Neovascularization was induced by most of the carcinomas and only by 30% of the hyperplasias. Furthermore, papillary hyperplasias chemically induced in mice, after serial transplantation, gave origin to invasive carcinomas, after having acquired angiogenic activity [10]. Using similar methods these observations were reproduced also in human breast diseases: all the fragments of invasive carcinomas induced a strong neovascularization versus a minority of hyperplastic lobules when transplanted into rabbit iris [11]. Jensen *et al.* [12] compared the angiogenic activity of normal breast lobules from benign tissues and from invasive ductal carcinomas and found that the latter induced angiogenesis twice as often as the lobules from non-cancerous breasts. Overall, these studies suggest that angiogenesis may be a potential marker for precancerous breast lesions and that neovascularization may be an early step in breast cancer progression.

More recently, Weidner *et al.* [13] developed an immunohistochemical method to identify microvessels by using a specific endothelial marker (a polyclonal antibody to factor VIII-RA, von Willebrand factor) and to assess the degree of microvessel density in human breast carcinoma.

In a pilot study they found that *in situ* carcinomas may be in the prevascular as well as in the vascular phase, and that invasive carcinomas presented a heterogeneous distribution of microvessels. A statistically significant association was observed between the degree of angiogenesis, at the vascular « hot spot » of the invasive carcinomas, with the presence of metastasis [13].

Guidi *et al.* [14] extended this preliminary observation and described the presence of two distinct patterns of neovascularization in ductal *in situ* carcinomas. The majority of these lesions showed a diffuse pattern of stromal microvessels surrounding involved spaces. This pattern was prominent in comedo-type lesions with marked stromal desmoplasia and was associated with high tumour cell proliferative index and expression of the oncoprotein c-erbB-2. The second pattern, present in 38% of the lesions, is a microvessel cuffing in direct opposition to the basement membrane of involved spaces. The clinical significance of the two patterns of vascularization is not yet known.

Two independent studies assessed the pattern of vascularization in benign breast lesions. Fregene *et al.* [15] compared the degree of microvessel density of proliferative or non-proliferative benign lesions in pre and postmenopausal women. The highest member of intralesional microvessels was observed among postmenopausal patients with proliferative breast diseases. Guinebretiere *et al.* [16] found that the risk of developing invasive breast cancer increases significantly in the women with high intralesional microvessel density. Several other authors have determined the degree of intratumoral microvessel density in invasive breast cancer and its relationship with the conventional pathologic features and other biologic markers. The most important findings of these studies are that neovascularization tends to be higher in larger primaries and in node-positive tumours and that microvessel density seems to be independent of other biological markers such as: markers of tumour cell proliferation, p53 protein expression, c-erbB-2 oncoprotein, epidermal growth factor receptor and bcl-2 expression [5]. Furthermore, McCulloch *et al.* [17] studied intratumoral vascular density and cell shedding of tumour cells into the bloodstream in 16 women operated of invasive breast carcinoma. They found a significant correlation between intratumoral vascularization with the detection of circulating tumour cells during surgery.

More recently, some groups have determined angiogenesis in breast cancer using alternative immunohistochemical techniques. Bianchi *et al.* [18] studied the expression of the urokinase receptor (u-PAR). They observed a positive expression in endothelial cells, macrophages and breast cancer cells, but not in normal breast tissue. The expression of the u-PAR system has been correlated to neovascularization, so the determination of u-PAR is an evaluable alternative method to assess angiogenesis. Brooks *et al.* found that the integrin $\alpha_v\beta_3$ is actively involved in angiogenesis and they determined its expression in experimental and human breast cancers. Most breast cancer tumours with activated angiogenesis showed high levels of expression of $\alpha_v\beta_3$ integrin, which seems to play a significant role both in angiogenesis and tumour growth [4].

Contrino *et al.* [19] detected *in situ* the expression of the tissue factor (TF), a regulator of the activation of coagulation in mammary cells, and found it is specific for vascular endothelial cells and that its expression correlates with the malignant phenotype of human breast disease. The authors suggested that TF may be a useful marker to identify the switch to the angiogenic phenotype and to assess the degree of neovascularization in human pathology.

Several experimental studies performed in recent years support the above histopathologic studies demonstrating that angiogenesis plays a relevant role in breast cancer progression. Kurebayashi *et al.* [20] and Zhang *et al.* [21] performed *in vivo* studies with transfectants of MCF-7 human breast cancer cells with fibroblast growth factor 4 (FGF4) or vascular endothelial growth factor (VEGF 121), respectively. They found that both the angiogenic peptides facilitate tumour growth, with enhanced neovascularization [21] and metastasis [20]. The study of Zajchowski *et al.* [22] provided a further demonstration on the role played by angiogenesis in breast cancer growth. Overexpression of the natural angiogenic inhibitor thrombospondin (TSP) was associated, in their experimental model, with the suppression of the development of invasive tumours in nude mice.

Researches performed by the group of Tuszynski *et al.* [23, 24] have shown the pattern of localization of TSP and its receptor in human breast cancer and that TSP is associated to an increased expression of urokinase-type plasminogen activator and plasminogen activator inhibitor-1 in human MDA-MB-231 breast cancer cells.

The Folkman group [25] recently found that systemic administration of angiostatin, a specific endothelial cell proliferation inhibitor, potently suppresses growth of several human cancers transplanted in immunocompromised SCID mice. In particular, growth of human breast carcinomas was inhibited by angiostatin up to 95%. Histologic studies showed that after the treatment the tumours regressed to dormant foci in which tumour cell proliferation is balanced by enhanced apoptosis (« dormancy therapy »).

Clinical significance of angiogenesis

Angiogenic activity of human invasive breast cancer, determined using diverse methods, appears to be heterogeneous. For example, a high difference in the degree of microvessel density of each single breast cancer has been found with a range from a few microvessels per mm^2 at the « hot spot » of low vascularized tumours to more than 250 microvessels per mm^2 in highly angiogenic tumours [5]. The results of most studies indicate that vascular density is a powerful and independent prognostic indicator in breast cancer patients [26]. Furthermore, preliminary findings suggest that in high-risk operable breast cancer patients treated with adjuvant anticancer treatments, the degree of intratumoral vascularization identifies subgroups of patients with different likelihood to gain benefit from both adjuvant hormone therapy [27] and chemotherapy [28]. Overall, the patients with low vascularized tumours are those who have a more favourable outcome, whilst those with highly angiogenic tumours have a poorer prognosis.

Similarly, a variable expression of the genes of the FGF family has been found in samples of human breast cancer. FGF4 is overexpressed in one-third of the invasive tumours, whilst FGF1 RNA expression was detected in most of the cases [29].

Toi *et al.* [30] observed that approximately 50% of invasive breast carcinomas express VEGF and that its positivity is significantly associated to microvessel density.

In some breast cancer patients angiogenic peptides are abnormally elevated in the serum or urine. In 29% of 144 patients with breast cancer, basic FGF presented high urine levels [31] and about 10% of breast cancer patients had elevated bFGF levels in their serum [32]. Both the determinations predicted clinical outcome of the patients.

It seems appropriate to speculate that the knowledge of the angiogenic activity of each single tumour may be used as a target for the identification of the patients whose tumours are likely to be more responsive to angiogenesis inhibitors.

Several specific inhibitors of angiogenesis have been developed and some are already in clinical evaluation [5]. Some molecules besides being markers of angiogenesis may be themselves targets for therapeutic intervention. For example, Burrows *et al.* [33] and Brooks *et al.* [4] found that the antibody TEC-11 to endoglin, a proliferative protein expressed by proliferating endothelial cells, linked to ricin and the antibody LM609 to the vascular integrin $\alpha_v\beta_3$, may provide an effective antiangiogenic approach for the treatment of solid tumours.

Future research should be devoted to identifying specific markers related to the mechanisms of action of different angiogenesis inhibitors that may be useful for monitoring their therapeutic efficacy. It should be determined whether the expression of specific markers of activated endothelial cells (for example antibodies TEC-11, E9 [33]) is a potential target for responsiveness to drugs that inhibit proliferating endothelium (AGM-1470, angiostatin) [5, 25]. The expression of tissue-metalloproteinases may represent a potentially useful target of efficacy of metalloproteinases inhibitors (e.g. BB-94). The determination of tissue expression or serum/urine levels of angiogenic peptides may be related to the effect of agents neutralizing these growth factors [34].

In conclusion, our present knowledge on angiogenesis in breast carcinoma suggests that the acquisition of angiogenic activity is necessary in the multi-step mechanisms of breast cancer progression and metastasis.

From a clinical point of view, the determination of angiogenic activity seems to be a useful prognostic and predictive tool to predict outcome of patients with early-stage breast cancer. However, since any technique to assess angiogenesis has yet to be completely standardized and validated in prospective controlled clinical trials, at present, these determinations may be recommended for applied research but not for routine clinical use [5, 26].

Finally, pharmacologic modulation of angiogenesis represents a new, promising therapeutic strategy for chemoprevention and therapy of breast cancer.

Approximately one-half of the patients operated of invasive breast carcinoma are at risk, mainly if node-positive, and ultimately most of these die of metastasis.

Angiogenesis is a necessary step in the cascade of events leading to metastasis [35, 36], so inhibition of neovascularization may represent a new potential approach to prevent the development of metastasis [36, 37-39]. Controlled clinical trials are warranted to prove this therapeutic strategy once certain angiogenesis inhibitors will be found to be safe and active and will be approved for clinical use [40].

References

1. Gasparini G. Angiogenesis in preneoplastic and neoplastic lesions. *Cancer J* 1995; 8: 91-3.
2. Folkman J. Angiogenesis in cancer, vascular rheumatoid and other disease. *Nature Med* 1995; 1: 27-31.
3. Barbareschi M, Gasparini G, Morelli L, Forti S, Dalla Palma P. Novel methods for the determination of the angiogenic activity of human tumors. *Breast Cancer Res Treat* 1995; 36: 205-17.
4. Brooks PC, Stromblad S, Klemke R, Visscher D, Sarkar FH and Cheresh DA. Anti-integrin $\alpha_v\beta_3$ blocks human breast cancer growth and angiogenesis in human skin. *J Clin Invest* 1995; 96: 1815-22.
5. Gasparini G and Harris AL. Clinical importance of the determination of tumor angiogenesis in breast carcinoma: Much more than a new prognostic tool. *J Clin Oncol* 1995; 13: 765-82.
6. Folkman J. Clinical applications of research on angiogenesis. *New Engl J Med* 1995; 333: 1757-63.
7. Teicher BA, Holden SA, Ara G, Alvarez-Sotomayor E, Huang Zdm Chen YN and Brem H. Potentiation of cytotoxic cancer therapies by TNP470 alone and with other anti-angiogenic agents. *Int J Cancer* 1994; 57: 920-5.
8. Gasparini G and Harris AL. Does improved control of tumour growth require an anti-cancer therapy targetting both neoplastic and intratumoral endothelial cells? *Eur J Cancer* 1994; 30A: 201-6.
9. Gimbrone MA and Gullino PM. Neovascularization induced by intraocular xenografts of normal, preneoplastic, and neoplastic mouse mammary tissues. *J Natl Cancer Inst* 1976; 56: 305-18.
10. Brem S, Gullino PM and Medina D. Angiogenesis: a marker for neoplastic transformation of mammary pappillary hyperplasia. *Science* 1997; 195: 880-1.
11. Brem SS, Jensen HM and Gullino PM. Angiogenesis as a marker of preneoplastic lesions of the human breast. *Cancer* 1978; 41: 239-44.
12. Jensen AM, Chen I, DeValut MR and Lewis AE. Angiogenesis induced by « normal » human breast tissue: a probable marker for precancer. *Science* 1982; 218: 293-5.
13. Weidner N, Semple JP, Welch WR and Folkman J. Tumor angiogenesis and metastasis - correlation in invasive breast carcinoma. *N Engl J Med* 1991; 324: 1-8.
14. Guidi AJ, Fisher L, Harris JR and Schnitt SJ. Microvascular density and distribution in ductal carcinoma *in situ* of the breast. *J Natl Cancer Inst* 1994; 86: 614-9.
15. Fregene TA, Kellog CM and Pienta KJ. Microvessel quantification as a measure of angiogenic activity in benign breast tissue lesions: a marker for precancerous disease? *Int J Oncol* 1994; 4: 1199-202.
16. Guinebretiere JM, Monique GL, Govoille A, Bahi J and Contesso C. Angiogenesis and risk of breast cancer in women with fibrocystic disease. *J Natl Cancer Inst* 1994; 86: 635-6.
17. McCulloch P, Choy A and Martin L. Association between tumour angiogenesis and tumour cell shedding into effluent venous blood during breast cancer surgery. *The Lancet* 1995; 346: 1334-5.

18. Bianchi E, Cohen RL, Thor AT, Todd III RF, Mizukami IF, Lawrence DA, Ljung BM, Shuman MA and Smith HS. The urokinase receptor is expressed in invasive breast cancer but not in normal breast tissue. *Cancer Res* 1994; 54: 861-6.
19. Contrino J, Hair G, Kreutzer DL and Rickles FR. *In situ* detection of tissue factor in vascular endothelial cells: Correlation with the malignant phenotype of human breast disease. *Nature Med* 1996; 2: 209-15.
20. Kurebayashi J, McLeskey SW, Johnson MD, Lippman ME, Dickson RB and Kern FG. Quantitative demonstration of spontaneous metastasis by MCF-7 human breast cancer cells cotransfected with fibroblast growth factor 4 and LacZ. *Cancer Res* 1993; 53: 2178-87.
21. Zhang HT, Craft P, Scott PAE, Ziche M, Welch HA, Harris AL, Bicknell R. Enhancement of tumor growth and vascular density by transfection of vascular endothelial cell growth factor into MCF-7 human breast carcinoma cells. *J Natl Cancer Inst* 1995; 87: 213-9.
22. Zajchowski DA, Band V, Trask DK, Kling D, Connolly JL and Sager R. Suppression of tumor-forming ability and related traits in MCF-7 human breast cancer cell by fusion with immortal mammary epithelial cells. *Cell Biol* 1990; 87: 2314-8.
23. Tuszynski GP and Nicosia RF. Localization of thrombospondin and its cysteine-serine-valine-threonine-cysteine-glycine specific receptor in human breast carcinoma. *Lab Invest* 1994; 70: 228-33.
24. Arnoletti JP, Albo D, Granick MS, Solomon MP, Castiglioni A, Rothman VL and Tuszynski GP. Thrombospondin and transforming growth factor-beta 1 increase expression of urokinase-type plasminogen activator and plasminogen activator inhibitor-1 in human MDA-MB-231 breast cancer cells. *Cancer* 1995; 76: 998-1005.
25. O'Reilly MS, Holmgren L, Chen C and Folkman J. Suppression of angiogenesis by angiostatin induces and sustains dormancy of human primary tumors in mice. *Nature Med* 1996; 2: in press.
26. Gasparini G. Prognostic and predictive value of intratumoral microvessel density in human solid tumours. In: *Tumor Angiogenesis*. Eds: Lewis CE, Bicknell R and Ferrara N. Oxford: Oxford University Press, 1996; in press.
27. Gasparini G, Fox SB, Verderio P, Bonoldi E, Bevilacqua P, Boracchi P, Dante S, Marubini E and Harris AL. The determination of angiogenesis adds information to estrogen receptor status in predicting the efficacy of adjuvant tamoxifen in node-positive breast cancer patients. *Clin Cancer Res* 1996; 2: in press.
28. Gasparini G, Barbareschi M, Boracchi P, Verderio P, Caffo O, Meli S, Dalla Palma P, Marubini E, Bevilacqua P. Tumor angiogenesis predicts clinical outcome of node positive breast cancer patients treated with adjuvant hormone therapy or chemotherapy. *Cancer J Sci Am* 1995; 1: 131-41.
29. Penault-Llorca F, Bertucci F, Adelaide J, Parc P, Coulier F, Jacquemier J, Dirnbaum D, Delapeyriere O. Expression of FGF and FGF receptor genes in human breast cancer. *Int J Cancer* 1995; 61: 170-6.
30. Toi M, Inada K, Hoshina S, Suzuki H, Kondo S and Tominaga T. Vascular endothelial growth factor and platelet-derived endothelial cell growth factor are frequently co-expressed in highly vascularized human breast cancer. *Clin Cancer Res* 1995; 1: 961-4.
31. Nguyen H, Watanabe H, Budson AE, Richie JP, Hayes DF and Folkman J. Elevated levels of an angiogenic peptide, basic fibroblast growth factor, in the urine of patients with a wide spectrum of cancers. *J Natl Cancer Inst* 1994; 86: 356-61.
32. Li V, Yu C, Rupnick M, Allred E, Sallan S, Hayes DF and Folkman J. Serum from breast cancer patients contains proliferative activity for capillary endothelial cells which correlates with risk of mortality. In: *Proc XXIX Meeting Amer Soc Clin Oncol* 1993; 12: 133 (abstr. n. 252).
33. Burrows FJ, Derbyshire EJ, Tazzari PL, Amlot P, Gazdar AF, King SW, Letarte M, Vitetta ES and Thorpe PE. Up-regulation of endoglin on vascular endothelial cells in human solid tumors: Implications for diagnosis and therapy. *Clin Cancer Res* 1995; 1: 1623-34.
34. Toi M. Endothelial growth factors: a target for antiangiogenesis. *Cancer J* 1995; 8: 315-9.
35. O'Reilly MS, Holmgren L, Shing Y, Chen C, Rosenthal RA, Moses M, Lane WS, Cao Y, Sage EH and Folkman J. Angiostatin: A novel angiogenesis inhibitor that mediates the suppression of metastases by a Lewis lung carcinoma. *Cell* 1994; 79: 315-28.
36. Fidler IJ and Ellis LM. The implications of angiogenesis for the biology and therapy of cancer metastasis. *Cell* 1994; 79: 185-8.
37. Ellis LM and Fidler IJ. Angiogenesis and breast cancer metastasis. *The Lancet* 1995; 3461: 388-90.

38. Karp JE and Broder S. Molecular foundations of cancer: New targets for intervention. *Nature Med* 1995; 1: 309-20.
39. Fidler IJ. Modulation of the organ microenvironment for treatment of cancer metastasis. *J Natl Cancer Inst* 1995; 87: 1588-92.
40. Folkman J. Tumor angiogenesis in women with node-positive breast cancer. *Cancer J Sci Am* 1995; 1: 106-8.

Breast Cancer. Advances in biology and therapeutics.
F. Calvo, M. Crépin, H. Magdelenat, eds. John Libbey Eurotext © 1996, pp. 175-181.

VEGF and breast cancer

Jean Plouet, Sylvie Sordello, Bernard Malavaud and Nathalie Ortega

Laboratoire de Biologie Moléculaire des Eucaryotes, CNRS UPR 9006, 118, route de Narbonne, 31062 Toulouse Cedex, France

Studies over the past 20 years have established that tumor progression requires a local enhancement of blood supply which is achieved by the sprouting of new capillaries from pre-existing vessels. Tumor angiogenesis also provides an essential exit route for metastasizing tumor cells from the tumor to the bloodstream. Extensive neovascularization has been reported to be a poor prognosis factor in prostate and breast cancer. This local hypervascularization is thought to result from release by the tumor of growth factors such as vascular endothelial growth factor (VEGF) or fibroblast growth factor 2 (FGF2). The cascade of events leading to angiogenesis consists of local degradation of the extracellular matrix followed by capillary endothelial cell proliferation, migration and differentiation into capillary tubes. In a recent study, Folkman [1] has listed the most potent angiogenic growth factors so far isolated. Some peptidic or non peptidic factors, such as Epidermal Growth Factor or Transforming Growth Factor α, angiogenin, Prostaglandin E2 and monobutyrin are angiogenic but not mitogenic *in vitro* for vascular endothelial cells. Other factors such as Transforming Growth Factor β, Tumor Necrosis Factor a inhibit endothelial cell proliferation and are supposed to act indirectly through stimulation of the local immune system which in turn releases direct angiogenic factors. We focused our study on FGF1, FGF2 and VEGF, which have in common a strong ability to bind to proteoheparansulfates, and present their potential implications for breast cancer.

Molecular characteristics of FGF1, FGF2, VEGF and their receptors

Up to ten different genes encode structurally related FGFs. FGF1 and FGF2, corresponding to acidic and basic FGF, are expressed in almost every tissue so far examined. Only one FGF2 gene and several FGF2 mRNA differing in the length of their untranslated 3' portion have been described in the human genome. Optional translation of a single FGF2 mRNA can be initiated by 3 unusual initiating CUG codons leading to the production of 3 different FGF2 forms of 210, 201, and 196 a.a. Four different tyrosine kinase gene products known as FGF-

R1-4 and ESL-1, the E selectin ligand, bind the different forms of FGF. A large number of variants of these FGF receptors are produced by optional splicing of their primary transcripts. FGF2 also binds to rich heparan sulfate proteoglycanes (HSPG) known as low affinity receptors. Several studies have shown that the presence of these low affinity receptors is necessary for binding of the ligand to the high affinity receptor [2].

An endothelial cell growth factor whose bioactivity seemed restricted to vascular endothelial cells was purified in 1989 and was then called Vascular Endothelial Growth Factor (VEGF) [3], Vascular Permeability Factor (VPF) [4] or Vasculotropin (VAS) [5]. Cloning of the VEGF gene has shown that the most abundant secreted form is a homodimer of 165 aminoacids. VEGF is synthesized as a profactor and secreted after the cleavage of a classical hydrophobic signal peptide. Alternative splicing of human VEGF pre-RNA messenger leads to the production of three VEGF isoforms of 121, 165 and 189 aminoacids [6]. The 121 and 165 a.a. forms are freely released but the 189 a.a. form remains cell associated. The role of the 189 a.a. form has not yet been established. It seems however that the proteolytic activity of plasmin or urokinase on this form of VEGF, produces truncated forms with activities similar to those of the 121 and 165 aminoacids forms. The loss of a single allele is lethal in the mouse embryo between day 11 and 12 [7]. Furthermore, VEGF-null embryonic stem cells exhibit a dramatically reduced ability to form tumors in nude mice. Two different genes encode type III tyrosine kinase receptors for VEGF: KDR [8] and flt-1 [9]. Recent results from our laboratory have shown that KDR mediates cell proliferation whereas flt-1 mediates vascular permeability and migration in vitro and in vivo. Knock out and physiopathological data suggest a schematic preferential expression in vivo of KDR/flk-1 in replicating endothelial cells [10] and Flt-1 in quiescent endothelial cells or during differentiation [11]. VEGF related genes, such as placenta growth factor (PlGF) which binds only to flt-1 [12], VEGF-C which binds to flt-4 and KDR [13] and VEGF-B [14] have also been described (*see Figure 1*).

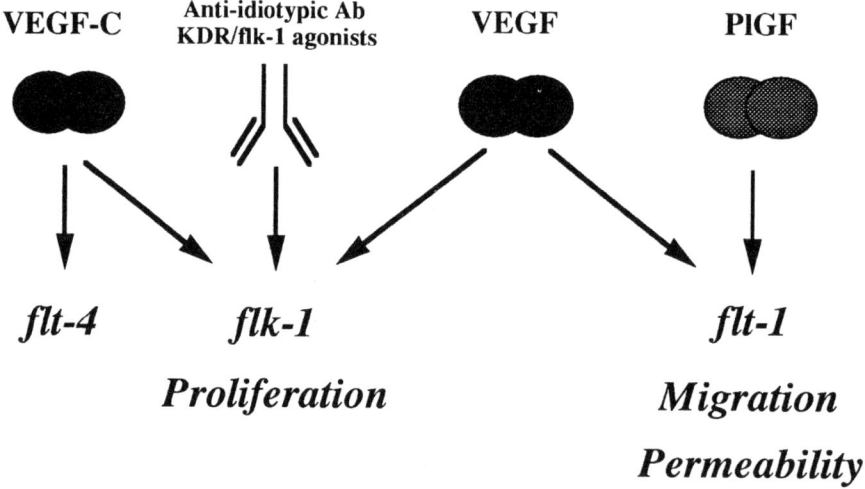

Figure 1. Schematic representation of the VEGF system.

VEGF has been found in adult tissues mainly in proliferating endometrium and ovarian corpus luteum, organs undergoing a physiological angiogenesis. The apparent capital role played by VEGF in the cyclic development of ovarian corpus lutei and uterine endometrium suggests an effect of sexual steroids on VEGF production. *In vitro* VEGF is expressed by transformed cell lines. Although VEGF has been reported as an elective mitogen for vascular endothelial cells [3-5], other cells such as IL-2 dependent lymphocytes, retinal pigment epithelial cells or dermal papilla cells express KDR and respond to the mitogenic effect of VEGF. The flt-1 receptor is also expressed *in vitro* in several non endothelial cell populations such as, corneal endothelium, lens epithelium, osteoblasts or monocytes in which its activation leads to differentiating functions (migration or permeability increase) rather than proliferation. *In vivo* VEGF binding sites have been primarily found expressed only in vascular endothelial cells. In situ hybridization have evidenced the expression of flt-1 and KDR in avascularized tissues, in accordance with the suggested roles of VEGF in survival and regulation of vascular permeability.

Expression of FGF1, FGF2, VEGF and their receptors in the normal and tumoral breast

The potential roles of FGF1 and FGF2 in breast cancer remain uncertain. FGF2 and FGF1 mRNAs are expressed at a significantly higher level in normal tissues and benign tumors than in malignant tumors [15]. Conversely VEGF and its receptors flt-1 and KDR are hardly detected in the normal breast or in epithelial cells of invasive lobular breast cancers but are dramatically up-regulated in invasive primary and metastatic comedo-type ductal breast cancers [16]. The endothelial cells of small vessels immediately adjacent to infiltrating malignant epithelial cells became strongly labeled for mRNAs of KDR and flt-1 whereas their expression was low in normal breast or infiltrating lobular carcinoma. VEGF is also present in tumor-associated macrophages of breast cancers [17].

Pathophysiological role of FGF and VEGF in breast cancer progression

The intensity of neovascularization [18] and the expression of tissue factor [19] have been correlated with prognosis in patients with carcinoma of the breast. It is tempting to correlate these independent prognosis factors with an increase in VEGF bioavailability which induces both the expression of tissue factor and neovascularization. Elucidation of the molecular mechanisms leading to the angiogenic switch of tumoral cells, *i.e.* increase of synthesis and/or bioavailability of angiogenic factors which would in turn confer an angiogenic phenotype to endothelial cells, is a multistep phenomenon. Several lines of evidence suggest that VEGF might represent a pivotal component of the angiogenic switch since its expression is up-regulated by (i) mutations of the tumor suppressor gene p53 or activation of the oncogenes ras or raf (ii) other growth factors such as FGF2 or TGFβ (iii) hormones and (iv) hypoxic fibroblasts surrounding the tumors [20]. Zhang *et al.* demonstrated that VEGF constitutive overexpression in MCF-7 cells confers a growth advantage *in vivo* [21]. However the demonstration in our laboratory that VEGF constitutive expression can lead to cell transformation, by up-regulating FGF-R1, raises serious problems about the exquisite target of VEGF on endothelial cells.
The demonstration that VEGF triggers tumoral angiogenesis is still dependent on indirect proofs such as the observation that VEGF immunoneutralization reduces tumor progression

[22]. Since angiogenic growth factors can interact with low affinity proteoheparansulfates receptors, it is unlikely that systemic delivery would provide direct receptor activation. Moreover the large number of angiogenic factor receptors and the partial overlapping of their biological functions makes this direct demonstration a difficult task. To overcome this difficulty, we took advantage of the anti-idiotypic network to design internal images of VEGF, FGF1 and FGF2 binding domains. Rabbits were immunized with rabbit immunoglobulins neutralizing FGF2 or VEGF bioactivities. The subsets of anti-idiotypic Ig produced in each rabbit were screened for their abilities to compete with binding of the corresponding iodinated growth factor to cells transfected with expression vectors carrying the coding sequence of VEGF or FGF receptors. 25% of the rabbits elicited internal images of the binding domains to the VEGF receptor KDR or its murine homologue flk-1 (anti-Id VEGF) or to the FGF-R1 (anti-Id FGF2) or FGF-R1 and FGF-R2b (anti-Id FGF1). Cultured vascular endothelial cells proliferate under any anti-Id stimulation. In contrast transformed breast epithelial MCF-7 cells which do not express FGF1, FGF2 or VEGF mRNA remain unresponsive to these anti-Id IgG whatever their hormonal environment *(Figure 2)*.

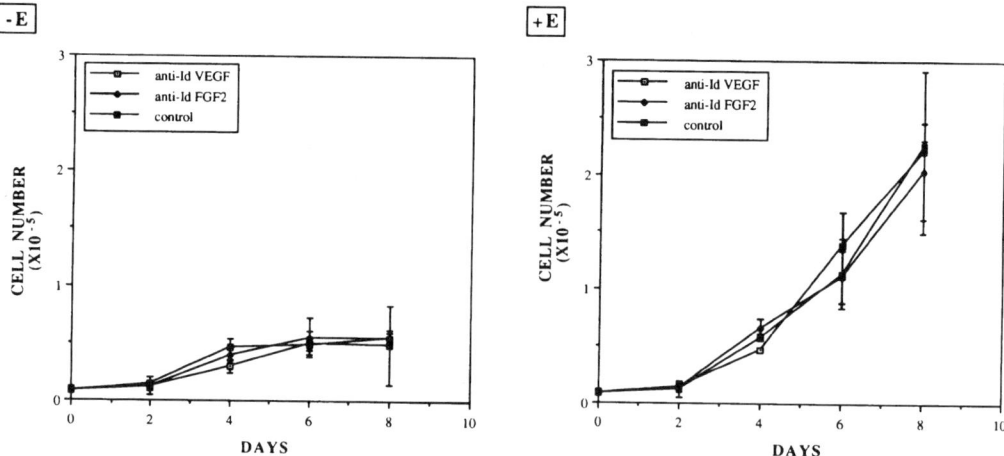

Figure 2. Anti-Id VEGF or FGF2 do not affect MCF-7 growth *in vitro*. MCF-7 cells were seeded at 5,000 cells per well in 12 multiwell plates and 10 ng/ml of anti-Id VEGF or FGF2 were added every other day in the presence (+E) or the absence (-E) of 10-9 M E1. The cells were trypsinized and counted every other day.

Ovariectomized nude mice received a slow-releasing pellet (25 days) of E and were grafted with 2×10^6 MCF-7 cells. Tumors grew as long as the hormone was efficiently released and reached a plateau after 30 days. Long lasting delivery of anti-Id VEGF or FGF2 induced a growth advantage to the tumor even in the absence of E. Histopathological analysis of the vascularization, as demonstrated by ulex-europeus, depicted an increase in staining, thus confirming the emergence of neovascularization. Mib-1 staining which only labels mitotic cells showed an increase of labelling in tumors treated with the anti-Id IgG compared with the untreated animals. Interestingly no Mib-1 staining could be detected in normal organs such as kidneys in either group. These results emphasize the ability of anti-idiotypic antibodies to demonstrate the functional roles of angiogenic growth factors receptors in tumor progression as well as a possible clue as to the mechanism of hormonal escape *(Figure 3)*.

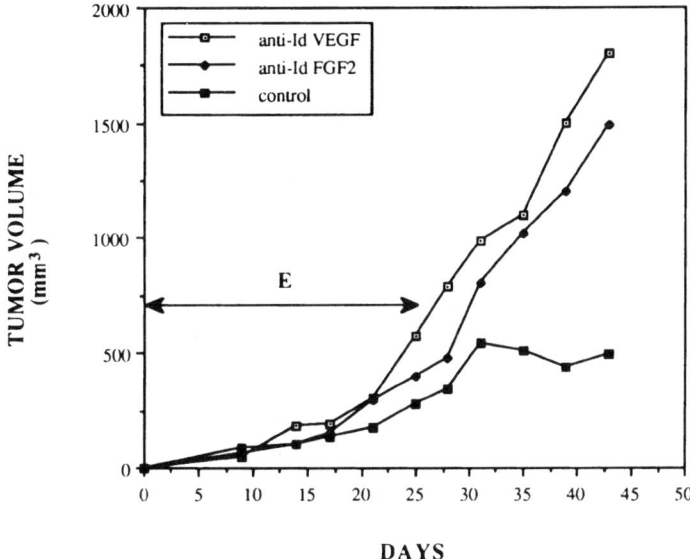

Figure 3. Systemic injections of Anti-Id VEGF or FGF2 increase the tumor volume of MCF-7 grafts. 2×10^6 MCF-7 cells were grafted in nude ovariectomized mice which had received a slow-releasing implant of E1. One week later the animals (n = 8-10 in each group) received 200 µg of anti-Id VEGF (open square), anti-Id FGF2 (diamond) or control IgG (closed square) twice weekly. The tumor burden was estimated twice weekly by measuring the largest and the lowest tumor dimensions with a caliper.

New anti-angiogenic treatments

The selective endothelial cell proliferation in tumors should make its selective blockade a useful tool for inhibiting breast tumor growth. Different therapeutic approaches, such as TNP 470 or heparinoid pentosanpolysulfates, have so far been proposed [23]. However these compounds might not be selective enough to avoid injurious side effects since most growth factors can act on various target cells. Several attempts to inhibit angiogenesis by reducing the bioavailability of VEGF have already been reported. Antisense mRNA or oligonucleotides targeted on the translation initiation codon or inhibition of VEGF bioavailability by antibodies or fusion proteins containing the extracellular domain of flt-1 or flk-1 and IgG reduce the retinal neovascularization by 50%. These treatments might lead to an inhibition of the survival effects of VEGF on the normal vasculature however. Other treatments such as lavenstudin inhibits the VEGF-dependent angiogenesis through the inhibition of tyrosine kinase activity. We developed an alternating strategy based on angiogenic growth factor receptors in our laboratory. Since such growth factors have half-lives in the minute range when injected by systemic route and can activate several distinct receptors, we relied on the anti-idiotypic method to construct specific circulating agonists for VEGF and FGF receptors. Systemic injections of these antibodies for two months trigger an increase in the proliferation of endothelial cells which have switched to the angiogenic phenotype but do not affect the resting endothelial cells of the adult vasculature. We are currently investigating the potential therapeutic interest of these anti-idiotypic antibodies conjugated to toxins as anti-angiogenic agents.

References

1. Folkman J. Angiogenesis in cancer, vascular, rheumatoid and other diseases. *Nature Med* 1995; 1: 27-30.
2. Schlessinger J, Lax I, Lemmon M. Regulation of growth factor by proteoglycans: what is the role of the low affinity receptors? *Cell* 1995; 83: 357-60.
3. Ferrara N, Henzel WJ. Pituitary follicular cells secrete a novel heparin binding growth factor specific for vascular endothelial cells. *Biochem Biophys Res Commun* 1989; 161: 851-6.
4. Connolly DT, Olander JV, Heuvelman D, Nelson R, Monsell R, Siegel N, Haymore BL, Leimgruber R, Feder J. Human Vascular Permeability Factor. *J Biol Chem* 1989; 264: 20017-24.
5. Plouët J, Schilling J, Gospodarowicz D. Isolation and characterization of a newly identified endothelial cell mitogen produced by ATt20. *EMBO J* 1989; 8: 3801-6.
6. Tischer E, Mitchell R, Hartman T, Silva M, Gospodarowicz D, Fiddes JC, Abraham JA. The human gene for vascular endothelial growth factor. *J Biol Chem* 1991; 266: 11947-54.
7. Ferrara N, Carver-Moore K, Chen L, Downd M, Lu L, Powell-Braxton L, Hilan KJ, Moore MW. Heterozygous embryonic lethality induced by targeted inactivation of VEGF gene. *Nature* 1996; 380: 439-42.
8. Terman BI, Vermazen MD, Carrion ME, Dimitrov D, Armellino DC, Gospodarowicz D, Bohlen P. Identification of the KDR tyrosine kinase as a receptor for vascular endothelial growth factor. *Biochem Biophys Res Commun* 1992; 34: 1578-86.
9. De Vries C, Escobedo J, Ueno H, Houck K, Ferrara N, Lewis LT. The fms-like tyrosine kinase, a receptor for vascular endothelial growth factor. *Science* 1992; 255: 989-91.
10. Shalaby F, Rossant J, Yamaguchi TP, Gertsenstein M, Wu XF, Breitman ML, Schuh AC. Failure of blood island formation and vasculogenesis in flk-1 deficient mice. *Nature* 1995; 376: 62-6.
11. Fong GH, Rossant J, Gertsenstein M, Breitman ML. Role of the Flt-1 receptor in regulating the assembly of vascular endothelium. *Nature* 1995; 376: 65-70.
12. Park JE, Chen HH, Winer J, houck KA, Ferrara N. Placenta growth factor. Potentiation of vascular endothelial growth factor bioactivity, *in vitro* and *in vivo*, and high affinity binding to flt-1 but not to flk-1/KDR. *J Biol Chem* 1994; 269: 25646-54.
13. Olofsson B, Pajusola K, Kaipanen A, von Euler G, Joukov V, Saksela O, Orpana A, Petterson RF, Alitalo K, Eriksson U. Vascular endothelial growth factor B, a novel growth factor for endothelial cells. *Proc Natl Acad Sci* 1996; 93: 2576-81.
14. Joukov V, Pajusola K, Kaipanen A, Chilov D, Lahtinen I, Kukk E, Saksela O, Kakkinen N, Alitalo K. A novel vascular endothelial growth factor, VEGF C, is a ligand for the flt-4 (VEGFR-3) and KDR (VEGFR-2) receptor tyrosine kinase. *EMBO J* 1996; 15: 290-8.
15. Bansal GS, Yiangou C, Coope RC, Gomm JJ, Luqmani YA, Coombes RC, Johnston CL. Expression of fibroblast growth factor 1 is lower in breast cancer than in normal human breast. *Br J Cancer* 1995; 72: 1420-6.
16. Brown LF, Berse B, Jackman RW, Tognazzi K, Guidi AJ, Dvorak HF, Senger DR, Connolly JL, Schnitt SJ. Expression of vacular permeability factor (vascular endothelial growth factor) and its receptor in breast cancer. *Hum Pathol* 1995; 26: 86-91.
17. Lewis CE, Leek R, Harris A, McGee JO'D. Cytokine regulation of angiogenesis in breast cancer: the role of tumor-associated macrophages. *J Leukoc Biol* 1995; 57: 747-51
18. Weidner N, Folkman J, Possa F. Tumor angiogenesis: a new significant and independent prognostic indicator in early-stage breast carcinoma. *J Natl Cancer Instit* 1992; 84: 1875-87.
19. Contrino J, Hair G, Kreutzer DL, Rickles FR. *In situ* detection of tissue factor in vascular endothelial cells: correlation with malignant phenotype of human breast cancer. *Nature Med* 1996; 2: 209-15.
20. Hlatky L, Tsionou C, Hahnfeldt P, Coleman CN. Mammary fibroblasts may influence breast tumor angiogenesis *via* hypoxia-induced vascular endothelial growth factor up-regulation and protein expression. *Cancer Research* 1994; 54: 6083-6.

21. Zhang HT, Craft P, Scott PAE, Ziche M, Weich HA, Harris AL, Bicknell R. Enhancement of tumor growth and vascular density by transfection of vascular endothelial cell growth factor into MCF-7 human breast carcinoma cells. *J Natl Cancer Inst* 1995; 87: 213-9.
22. Kim KJ, Li B, Winer J, Armanini M, Gillett N, Phillips HS, Ferrara N. Inhibition of vascular endothelial growth factor-induced angiogenesis suppresses tumor growth *in vivo*. *Nature* 1993; 362: 841-4.
23. Wellstein A. Growth factor targeted and conventional therapy of breast cancer. *Breast Cancer Res Treat* 1994; 31: 141-52.

Breast Cancer. Advances in biology and therapeutics.
F. Calvo, M. Crépin, H. Magdelenat, eds. John Libbey Eurotext © 1996, pp. 183-189.

Why is cathepsin D involved in breast cancer? A 1996 overview

Henri Rochefort, Valérie Laurent, Emmanuelle Liaudet, Nadine Platet, Danièle Derocq, Christian Rougeot, Jean-Paul Brouillet and Marcel Garcia

Université de Montpellier I and Unité Hormones et Cancer (U 148) INSERM 60, rue de Navacelles, 34090 Montpellier, France

Following the initial studies during the last decade on the overexpression of cathepsin D (cath-D) in breast cancer cell lines and primary tumours, and its association with experimental and clinical metastasis, there has been many criticisms and debate concerning the prognostic value of cath-D and its mechanism of action in tumors [1]. Some of the clinical studies did not show any prognostic value and people working on proteinases which are able to degrade extracellular matrix at neutral pH, pointed out that cath-D requires a too low pH to be active extracellularly to facilitate basement membrane effraction.

In this short review, we will clarify some of these questions and try to review the results indicating that this protease plays a role in breast cancer metastasis and possibly in other solid tumour metastasis.

Cath-D gene expression is stimulated by estrogen and growth factors

Estrogen responsive elements have been defined in the proximal promoter region of the gene which are responsible for the stimulation of cath-D gene expression in ER positive breast cancer [2]. Growth factors also stimulate cath-D mRNA accumulation [3]. Since estrogen and growth factors stimulate the growth of ER positive tumors, the induction of this protease appears to be associated with this growth stimulation. However, unlike other estrogen-regulated proteins having a good prognostic value, such as pS2 [4] and the progesterone receptor [5], cath-D is also overexpressed in ER negative breast cancer [6]. The mechanism responsible for this overexpression in ER negative breast cancer is important to specify.

Overexpression of cath-D is associated with increasing risk of breast cancer metastasis

Cath-D in breast cancer is overexpressed by 2- to 50-fold compared with its concentration in other cells such as fibroblasts or normal mammary glands [7]. Both mRNA and protein levels are increased, as shown by immunohistochemistry, *in situ* hybridization, cytosolic immunoassay and Northern and Western blot analyses. Overexpressed cath-D is mostly located in breast cancer cells and macrophages but not in tumor fibroblasts in contrast to other proteases, as shown by immunohistochemistry [8] and RNA *in situ* hybridization [9]. In contrast to some oncogenes such as c-er*B2*, this overexpression mechanism does not seem to involve any gene amplification or any major chromosomal rearrangements [10]. Clearly, most of the clinical studies from different and independent clinical centers using a standardized and validated cytosolic immunoassay, based on two monoclonal antibodies, indicate that the cath-D level in primary breast cancer cytosol is an independent prognostic parameter associated with the occurence of clinical metastases and shorter survival [reviewed in 11 and 12]. Quantification of the cath-D proteolytic activity in the cytosol after activation at an acidic pH gave similar results [13]. In contrast, studies performed by not yet standardized *in situ* immunohistochemistry assays or Western blot analysis are mostly discordant. These discrepancies could be due to the use of different tissue fixations and antibodies, absence of quantification or loss of the secreted form of cath-D during fixation [14]. Immunohistochemical assay of cath-D is also complicated by the fact that the relative contribution of infiltrating macrophages and cancer cells is not clear. We found that the cytosolic level was correlated with staining in cancer cells rather than with the number of macrophages [9] but other groups using different antibodies pointed out the importance of production by stromal cells [12].

Another reservation concerns node-negative breast cancer where the prognostic value of cath-D has not always been found unlike its value in the general population. However it might be important to measure this protease in order to complement the axillary lymph node status staging whose reliability depends on the pathologist's skill and experience and which always give inesthetic scars and sometimes *sequela* to the patient.

Moreover, in most studies, this prognostic parameter sometimes associated to lymph node status is independent of the other parameters, including the estrogen receptor (ER), Urokinase and its inhibitor (PAI-1), as shown in a recent study on 2,000 patients from Rotterdam [15]. As other strong prognostic markers, its determination will be indispensable as soon as its significance in term of response to the adjuvant therapy will be specified by further large scale prospective studies.

Experimental cath-D overexpression increases metastasis through its proteolytic activity

The role of cath-D in cancer metastasis was studied after stable transfection of an expression vector of human cath-D into a rat tumorigenic cell line (3Y1-Ad12) which does not secrete cath-D. Four cath-D clones displayed a higher metastatic potential than four corresponding control clones [16]. The incidence and size of gross liver metastases were significantly increased in mice injected with cath-D clones while these clones expressed moderate human cath-D concentrations (two-fold lower than the median concentration detected in human primary breast cancers). This was the first direct evidence that cath-D overexpression accelerates, and is not only associated with, the appearance of clinically detectable metastases.

The mechanism of cath-D action on metastasis could involve either its interaction with the plasma membrane M6P/IGFII receptor or its catalytic activity. To assess this question, the endoplasmic reticulum retention signal, KDEL, was inserted by mutagenesis at the C-terminal end of the cath-D coding sequence [17]. The consequence of pro-cath-D retention in the endoplasmic reticulum was to prevent its maturation *in vitro* and *in vivo* and to abolish its effects on metastases. We checked that a control peptide KDAS inserted in the same position did not prevent cath-D maturation and stimulated the metastatic potency. Moreover, the metastatic potential was unaffected in some KDEL clones secreting high concentrations of pro-cath-D-KDEL which displayed the same *in vitro* affinity to the M6P/IGFII receptor as the wild-type cath-D. This indicated that in this model system, pro-cath-D interaction with the plasma membrane M6P/IGFII receptor was not sufficient to stimulate metastasis and that maturation of cath-D into an active protease was a major requirement for its action on metastasis. Maturation also seems to occur *in vivo* in primary breast cancers since by assaying separately pro-cath-D and total cath-D, we found that the tumor contained only 4 to 6% of pro-cath-D, while the metastatic breast cancer cell lines secrete *in vitro* up to 50% of the precursor [18].

Pro-cath-D activation site: intracellular or extracellular or both?

While cath-D maturation is required to stimulate metastasis, where does maturation occur in the human tumor?

Extracellular activation of pro-cath-D at the contact of basement membrane

Most proteases are believed to play a role in degrading basement membrane following their secretion and extracellular activation [19]. Cancer cells can then cross the basement membrane border to invade the stroma and extravasate in blood. This mechanism was initially believed to be unlikely since a very acidic pH (at least 5,5) is required to activate pro-cath-D and this acidic pH is generally found in intracellular compartments. However, one major characteristic of cath-D and other cathepsins (B, L...) in cancer cells is their increased secretion. The mechanism of this secretion is not clear. It is unlikely to be due to an alteration of the protease structure but could be due to a alteration of the routing mechanism of pro-cathepsins general involving either the Man-6-P/IGF2 receptor [20], or an alternative pathway [21] or both. After secretion, pro-cath-D could potentially be activated extracellularly. Extracellular pH in tumor is generally more acidic than in the corresponding normal tissue [22]. We recently found that breast cancer cells as macrophages have a high potential to secrete proton in the extracellular milieu through lactic acid production and a functional H^+/ATPase pump at plasma membrane level. They are able to lower the pH down to 5.5 when measured under MCF7 cell monolayers and the acidifying potential of the invasive MDA-MB231 breast cancer cells is more important than in the estrogen responsive MCF7 cells (Montcourrier P., Silver I.A., Rochefort H., submitted for publication).

Intracellular activation of pro-cath-D and phagocytosis

Breast cancer cells display a high endocytotic activity (our unpublished observations) and our laboratory described large intracellular acidic vesicles (or LAVs) of ≥ 5μm in diameter [23]. These LAVs are more frequently found *in vitro* in breast cancer cells than in normal mammary cells and contain high levels of cath-D but no pro-cath-D. LAVs are also present *in vivo*, since they were found in primary cultures of pleural effusions from breast cancers, and large vesicles with the same diameter and highly concentrated in cath-D are found in parraffin sections of breast cancer biopsies [9]. We then showed that these acidic intracellular compartments (LAVs) contained phagocytosed extracellular material such as latex beads or pieces of extracellular matrix indicating that they were large heterophagosomes. In MDA-MB231 breast cancer cells, we found more LAV positive cells after migration through Matrigel than before migration [24]. Therefore breast cancer cells, as the professional phagocytotic cells macrophages, are able to phagocytose extracellular material, including extracellular matrix, and to digest this material within heterophagosomes. This heterophagocytosis associated with high proton secretion may facilitate the development of cancer cell colonies in distal parenchyma. In phagosomes, the large amount of engulfed extracellular material needs to be digested by cathepsins. This may explain why cancer cells overexpressing cath-D have a higher capability in developing metastasis.

In search of specific cath-D substrates involved in cancer metastasis

Cath-D in these vesicles is able to intracellularly digest many types of proteins, including proteins of the engulfed extracellular matrix, and thus to provide food, amino-acid supply and space for invasive breast cancer cells.

Most of our studies point out the role of cath-D in facilitating distant metastasis *via* an indirect mitogenic activity of this protease rather than stimulating local invasion and extravasation [19]. The mitogenic activity of cath-D, initially shown in MCF7 cells cultured in monolayer using purified pro-cath-D [25], was debated *in vitro* [26] but confirmed by cDNA transfection [16]. The cath-D gene inactivation by homologous recombination (knock out mice) shows that cath-D is not required for a normal prenatal development but that the 25 days-old mice rapidly died after weaning [27]. The lack of cath-D induces necrosis in epithelial small intestin and apoptosis in thymocytes. This strongly supports the idea that cath-D facilitates epithelial cell growth during tissue remodeling. Also, the original approach of Ann Chambers' group based on a direct *in vivo* video-microscopy observation of fluorescent cancer cells indicated that the limiting step for metastasis was not intravasation of cancer cells, their survival in the circulating or their extravasation, but was the ability of cancer cells to form colonies at distant sites in a foreign environment [29]. Cancer cells must find and utilize food and growth factors when they are transported in distant sites, and must therefore produce the enzyme(s) allowing them to multiply and form colonies in these sites.

In addition to the ability of cath-D to produce nutrients such as amino acids from the extracellular matrix, and to trigger a proteolytic cascade by activating pro-cathepsin B, and/or degrading cystatins [29], both knock out mice experiments and our data pointed out a specific modulation of growth factors and growth inhibitors by this overexpressed protease.

Increased liberation of growth factors from extracellular matrix

Several growth factors and cytokines are entrapped in an inactive form in the extracellular matrix, including pro-TGFb which may facilitate tumor cell invasion, and factors of the FGFs family which display a high angiogenic activity. The other neutral proteases can also liberate these factors, however, they are generally not produced by cancer cells but by stromal cells, unlike cath-D [9-30].
We previously showed that MCF7 breast cancer cells, cultured on an extracellular matrix secreted by bovine endothelial cells, could digest this matrix and liberate biologically active ^{125}I bFGF which had been preincorporated into the matrix. This bFGF could be incorporated into MCF7 cells, but not in presence of pepstatin A, indicating that in more biological culture conditions, an aspartyl protease, most likely cath-D, was activated to degrade ECM and liberate bFGF [31]. Consequently, the liberated bFGF could both stimulate the growth of cancer cells and increase angiogenesis by stimulating the growth of the surrounding endothelial cells.

Inactivation of density dependent growth inhibitor(s)

It has been proposed that in several hormone-dependent cancers, IGF-BP$_3$ can be specifically destroyed by cath-D, thus liberating IGF$_1$ to stimulate its receptor and the growth of cancer cells [32]. We recently showed, in 3YA1 rat tumor cells transfected with human cath-D-cDNA, that cath-D could also inactivate growth inhibitors. Stable cath-D transfected clones grew in vitro more rapidly in low serum conditions and more importantly reached 2-to 4.5-fold higher density at confluence than control clones [16]. Control cells reaching saturation density release an inhibitory activity that can prevent the growth of both control and cath-D clones. The production of this growth inhibitory activity was markedly reduced in cath-D clones [33]. Therefore, cath-D overexpression increases cell density by inhibiting the activity or secretion of growth inhibitors released by confluent cells. Cath-D probably acts intracellularly since the addition of the secreted proenzyme had no effect on the saturation density and no mature cath-D was detectable in the culture medium. Moreover, maturation of the intracellular proenzyme seems necessary since neutralization of acidic compartments by chloroquine or ammonium chloride prevented both cath-D maturation and its mitogenic effect. Further studies are in progress in order to identify and characterize the secreted growth inhibitor(s).

Conclusions

About ten years after the initial and unexpected findings that the estrogen-induced 52K protein secreted by cancer cells [34] was in fact the precursor of a protease associated with a shorter metastasis free survival, in breast cancers, data from our and other laboratories appear to confirm a major role of cath-D in breast cancer. This should not exclude the possible involvement of other proteases such as cathepsins (B, L...), plasminogen activators and metallo-proteinases [35]. It is likely that the nature of the proteases which are overexpressed to facilitate cancer cell growth and invasion vary considerably according to the type of cancer, the type of signal regulating their gene expression and the extracellular pH which should considerably vary according to several factors, such as the degree of tumor vascularization, the degree of macrophages invasion and the nature of the parenchyma in which the tumor cells will colonize.

Acknowledgements

This work was supported by the « Institut National de la Santé et de la Recherche Médicale », the University of Montpellier I, the « Ligue Nationale Contre le Cancer », and the « Association pour la Recherche sur le Cancer ». We thank Edith Moreno for secretarial assistance.

References

1. Cardiff RD. Cathepsin D and breast cancer: Useful? *Hum Pathol* 1994; 25: 847-8.
2. Augereau P, Mirallès F, Cavaillès V, Gaudelet C, Parker M, Rochefort H. Characterization of the proximal estrogen responsive element of human cathepsin D gene. *Mol Endocrinol* 1994; 8: 693-703.
3. Cavaillès V, Garcia M, Rochefort H. Regulation of cathepsin D and pS2 gene expression by growth factors in MCF7 human breast cancer cells. *Mol Endocrinol* 1989; 3: 552-8.
4. Rio MC, Bellocq JP, Daniel JY *et al*. Breast cancer-associated pS2 protein: synthesis and secretion by normal stomach mucosa. *Science* 1988; 241: 705-8.
5. Horwitz KB, McGuire WL. Estrogen control of progesterone receptor in human breast cancer. *J Biol Chem* 1978; 248: 6351-3.
6. Rochefort H, Capony F, Garcia M, Cavaillès V, Freiss G, Chambon M, Morisset M, Vignon F. Estrogen-induced lysosomal proteases secreted by breast cancer cells. A role in carcinogenesis? *J Cell Biochem* 1987; 35: 17-29.
7. Capony F, Rougeot C, Montcourrier P, Cavaillès V, Salazar G, Rochefort H. Increased secretion, altered processing, and glycosylation of pro-cathepsin D in human mammary cancer cells. *Cancer Res* 1989; 49: 3904-9.
8. Roger P, Montcourrier P, Maudelonde T, Brouillet JP, Pagès A, Laffargue F, Rochefort H. Cathepsin D immunostaining in paraffin-embedded breast cancer cells and macrophages. Correlation with cytosolic assay. *Human Path* 1994; 25: 863-71.
9. Escot C, Zhao Y, Puech C, Rochefort H. Cellular localisation by *in situ* hybridization of cathepsin D, stromelysin 3 and urokinase plasminogen activator RNAs in breast cancer. *Breast Cancer Res Treat* 1996; 38: 217-26.
10. Augereau P, Garcia M, Mattei MG, Cavaillès V, Depadova F, Derocq D, Capony F, Ferrara P, Rochefort H. Cloning and sequencing of the 52K cathepsin D cDNA of MCF7 breast cancer cells and mapping on chromosome 11. *Mol Endocrinol* 1988; 2: 186-92.
11. Rochefort H. Cathepsin D in breast cancer: a tissue marker associated with metastasis. *Eur J Cancer* 1992; 28A: 1780-3.
12. Westley BR, May FEB. Cathepsin D and breast cancer. *Eur J Cancer* 1996; 32A: 15-24.
13. Kute TE, Shao ZM, Sugg NK, Long RT, Russell GB, Case LD. Cathepsin D as a prognostic indicator for node-negative breast cancer patients using both immunoassays and enzymatic assays. *Cancer Res* 1992; 52: 5198-203.
14. Rochefort H. The prognostic value of cathepsin D in breast cancer. A long road to the clinic. *Eur J Cancer* 1996; 32A: 7-8.
15. Foekens JA, Peters HA, Look MP, Portengen H, Meijer-van Gelder ME, van Putten WLJ, Klijn JMG. The prognostic value of the urokinase system (uPA/uPAR/PAI-1/PAI-2) and cathepsin D in primary and recurrent breast cancer. *AACR Special Conference on « Proteases and Protease Inhibitors »*, Panama City Beach (Fl. USA), March 1-5, 1996.
16. Garcia D, Derocq D, Pujol P, Rochefort H. Overexpression of transfected cathepsin D in transformed cells increases their malignant phenotype and metastatic potency. *Oncogene* 1990; 5: 1809-14.
17. Liaudet E, Garcia M, Rochefort H. Cathepsin D maturation and its stimulatory effect on metastasis are prevented by addition of KDEL retention signal. *Oncogene* 1994; 9: 1145-54.
18. Brouillet JP, Spyratos F, Hacene K, Fauque J, Freiss G, Dupont F, Maudelonde T, Rochefort H. Immunoradiometric assay of pro-cathepsin D in breast cancer cytosol: Relative prognostic value versus total cathepsin D. *Eur J Cancer* 1993; 29A: 1248-51.
19. Liotta LA, Steeg PS, Stetler-Stevenson WG. Cancer metastasis and angiogenesis: an imbalance of positive and negative regulation. *Cell* 1991; 64: 327-36.

20. Mathieu M, Vignon F, Capony F, Rochefort H. Estradiol down regulates the mannose-6-phosphate/ IGFII receptor gene and induces cathepsin D in breast cancer cells: A receptor saturation mechanism to increase the secretion of lysosomal pro-enzymes. *Mol Endocrinol* 1991; 5: 815-22.
21. Diment S, Leech MS, Stahl PD. Cathepsin D is membrane-associated in macrophage endosomes. *J Biol Chem* 1988; 263: 6901-7.
22. Griffiths JR. Are cancer cells acidic? *Br J Cancer* 1991; 64: 425-7.
23. Montcourrier P, Mangeat P, Salazar G, Morisset M, Sahuquet A, Rochefort H. Cathepsin D in breast cancer cells can digest extracellular matrix in large acidic vesicles. *Cancer Res* 1990; 50: 6045-54.
24. Montcourrier P, Mangeat P, Valembois C, Salazar G, Sahuquet A, Duperray C, Rochefort H. Characterization of very acidic phagosomes in breast cancer cells and their association with invasion. *J Cell Science* 1994; 107: 2381-91.
25. Vignon F, Capony F, Chambon M, Freiss G, Garcia M, Rochefort H. Autocrine growth stimulation of the MCF7 breast cancer cells by the estrogen-regulated 52k protein. *Endocrinology* 1986; 118: 1537-45.
26. Stewart AJ, Piggott NH, May FEB, Westley BR. Mitogenic activity of procathepsin D purified for conditioned medium of breast cancer cells by affinity chromatography on pepstatinyl agarose. *Int J Cancer* 1994; 57: 715-8.
27. Saftig P, Hetman M, Schmahl W, Weber K, Heine L, Mossmann H, Köster A, Hess B, Evers M, Von Figura K, Peters C. Mice deficient for the lysosomal proteinase cathepsin D exhibit progressive atrophy of the intestinal mucosa and profound destruction of lymphoid cells. *EMBO J* 1995; 14: 3599-608.
28. Chambers AF, MacDonald IC, Schmidt EE, Koop S, Morris VL, Khokha R, Groom AC. Steps in tumor metastasis: New concepts from intravital videomicroscopy. *Cancer Met Review* 1995; 14: 279-301.
29. Lenarcic B, Kos J, Dolens I, Locovnik P, Krizaj I, Turk V. Cathepsin D inactivates cysteine proteinase inhibitors cystatins. *Biochem Biophys Res Commun* 1988; 154: 765-72.
30. Folkman J, Klagsbrun M, Sasse J, Wadjinski M, Ingber D, Vlodavsky I. A heparin-binding angiogenic protein-basic fibroblast growth factor- is stored within basement membrane. *Am J Pathol* 1988; 130: 393-400.
31. Briozzo P, Badet J, Capony F, Pieri I, Montcourrier P, Barritault D, Rochefort H. MCF7 mammary cancer cells respond to bFGF and internalize it following its release from extracellular matrix: a permissive role of cathepsin D. *Exp Cell Res* 1991; 194: 252-9.
32. Conover CA, Perry JE, Tindall DJ. Endogenous cathepsin D-mediated hydrolysis of insulin-like growth factor-binding proteins in cultured human prostatic carcinoma cells. *J Clin Endocrinol Met* 1995; 80: 987-92.
33. Liaudet E, Derocq D, Rochefort H, Garcia M. Transfected cathepsin D stimulates high density cancer cell growth by inactivating secreted growth inhibitors. *Cell Growth Diff* 1995; 6: 1045-52.
34. Rochefort H, Capony F, Cavalié-Barthez G, Chambon M, Garcia M, Massot O, Morisset M, Touitou I, Vignon F, Westley B. Estrogen-regulated proteins and autocrine control of cell growth in breast cancer. In: Rich MA, Hager JC, Taylor-Papadimitriou J, eds. *Breast Cancer: Origins, Detection, and Treatment*. Boston, Dordrecht, Lancaster: Martinus Nijhoff Publishing, 1985: 57-68.
35. Gottesman MM, ed. *Seminars in Cancer Biology. The Role of Proteases in Cancer* 1990; 1.

Clinical significance of the serine protease uPA (urokinase) and its inhibitor PAI-1 as well as the cysteine proteases cathepsin B and L in breast cancer

Manfred Schmitt, Christoph Thomssen, Fritz Jänicke, Heinz Höfler*, Kurt Ulm**, Viktor Magdolen, Ute Reuning, Olaf Wilhelm and Henner Graeff

*Frauenklinik, * Institut für Allgemeine Pathologie und Pathologische Anatomie; ** Institut für Medizinische Statistik und Epidemiologie, Technische Universität München, Germany*

Abstract

Proteases and their inhibitors have been implicated in tumor spread and metastasis. In breast cancer, several independent investigations have demonstrated that the serine protease uPA (urokinase-type plasminogen activator), and its inhibitor PAI-1 (plasminogen activator inhibitor type-1) and receptor (uPA-R), the aspartyl protease cathepsin D, as well as the cysteine proteases cathepsin B and L, are strong prognostic factors to predict disease recurrence and death. Based on the strong correlation between elevated proteolytic factors and cancer spread new tumor biology-oriented concepts involving proteolytic factors as targets for therapy were explored, especially factors of the plasminogen activation system (uPA, PAI-1, uPA-R). Suppression of uPA or uPA-R expression by antisense oligodeoxy-nucleotides or interruption of the uPA/uPA-R interaction by antibodies directed to uPA or uPA-R, naturally occurring and synthetic uPA inhibitors, as well as recombinant and synthetic uPA and uPA-R analogues were successfully tested. In addition to the plasminogen activation system, inactivation of different proteolysis systems, e.g. matrix metalloproteases and cysteine proteases, also in addition to conventional therapy protocols, may help to reduce tumor invasion and metastasis in humans even further.

Introduction

The capacity of breast cancer cells to invade tissues and to form distant metastases is closely related to their ability to disintegrate components of the surrounding extracellular matrix (tumor stroma). Proteases, e.g. plasmin, the urokinase-type plasminogen activator (uPA), the cathepsins B, D, L, and the matrix metalloproteases (MMP) have been shown to be related to these events [1-3]. By proteolytic action, tumor cells may intravasate lymph and blood vessels and disseminate. Extravasation and intravasation of tumor cells in solid malignant tumors are controlled by three steps: **1)** attachment to and interaction of tumor cells with components of the basement membrane and the extracellular matrix, **2)** local proteolysis, **3)** tumor cell migration. Proteases as well as their inhibitors and receptors are involved in these processes [1, 4].

There is substantial evidence that elevated concentrations of proteolytic factors in primary cancer tissues are conductive to tumor cell spread and metastasis [1-4]. Elevated antigen levels of the proteases cathepsin B/D/L, uPA, and the uPA-inhibitor PAI-1 are correlated with an increase in disease recurrence and early death of breast cancer patients [5-19]. In addition to the cathepsins [17-19], a strong, statistically independent prognostic value (relapse-free and/or overall survival) has been demonstrated for uPA and PAI-1 thus predicting the course of the breast cancer disease. The strong correlation between elevated uPA and PAI-1 values on the one hand and cancer spread on the other has prompted clinicians and basic researchers to explore new tumor biology-oriented concepts in order to suppress uPA, PAI-1 or uPA receptor (uPA-R, CD87) expression and synthesis. Various, very different approaches to block the expression of uPA, PAI-1, or uPA-R at the gene level or to interfere with the ligand-receptor interaction of uPA with its receptor, uPA-R were successfully tested [4,20]. Agents employed encompass antisense oligonucleotides, antibodies to uPA or uPA-R, naturally occurring and synthetic uPA inhibitors, as well as recombinant and synthetic uPA and uPA-R analogues.

Tumor-associated proteases uPA and cathepsin B/L

Four different classes of proteases are known to be correlated with invasion and metastasis in breast cancer: **1)** serine proteases; including plasmin and urokinase-type plasminogen activator (uPA) **2)** cysteine proteases; including cathepsins B and L **3)** aspartyl protease cathepsin D **4)** matrix metalloproteases (MMP); including collagenases, gelatinases and stromelysins [1]. Tumor-associated proteases are involved in the degradation of components of the extracellular matrix and/or the basement membranes. The extend of proteolysis, however, is limited by the action of specific protease inhibitors such as 2-macroglobulin/antiplasmin (to plasmin), plasminogen activator inhibitors PAI-1/-2 (to uPA), stefins and cystatins (to cathepsins B/L), and TIMPs (to MMP) [1, 4].

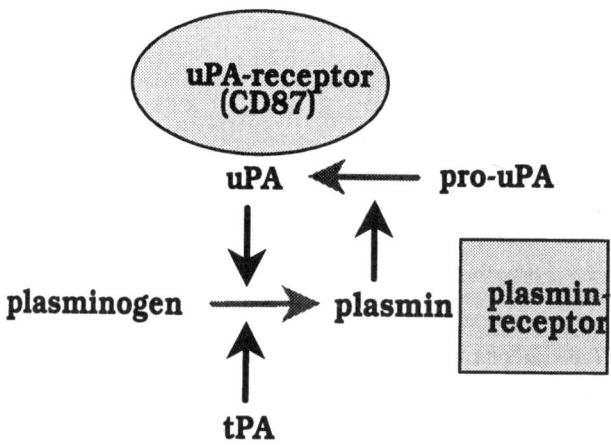

uPA is a central molecule in pericellular proteolysis. It converts enzymatically inactive plasminogen into the widely acting serine protease plasmin. Plasmin(ogen) and (pro)-uPA bind to receptors on the surface of tumor cells but also to receptors on normal cells (*e.g.* phagocytic cells, trophoblast cells, fibroblasts). tPA (tissue-type plasminogen activator), the second type of plasminogen activator of human origin, in contrast to uPA, is not involved in tumor spread. tPA does not bind to a tumor cell surface receptor and therefore does not promote tumor cell surface-focused pericellular proteolysis. uPA-mediated conversion of plasminogen into plasmin is controlled by two fast acting inhibitors, PAI-1 and PAI-2, which can inactivate enzymatically active uPA by binding to uPA in solution or when uPA is tightly bound to uPA-R [4]. uPA (M_r = 55,000) is produced by tumor cells but also by normal cells (*e.g.* kidney tubule cells, phagocytic cells, pneumocytes, keratinocytes, fibroblasts, trophoblasts) as a single-chain proenzyme (pro-uPA), with little or no intrinsic enzymatic activity. pro-uPA is activated into the enzymatically active high-molecular-weight two-chain form of uPA (HMW-uPA) by a variety of proteases including plasmin, cathepsins B/L, kallikrein, trypsin-like enzymes, thermolysin and nerve growth factor-γ [1, 4].

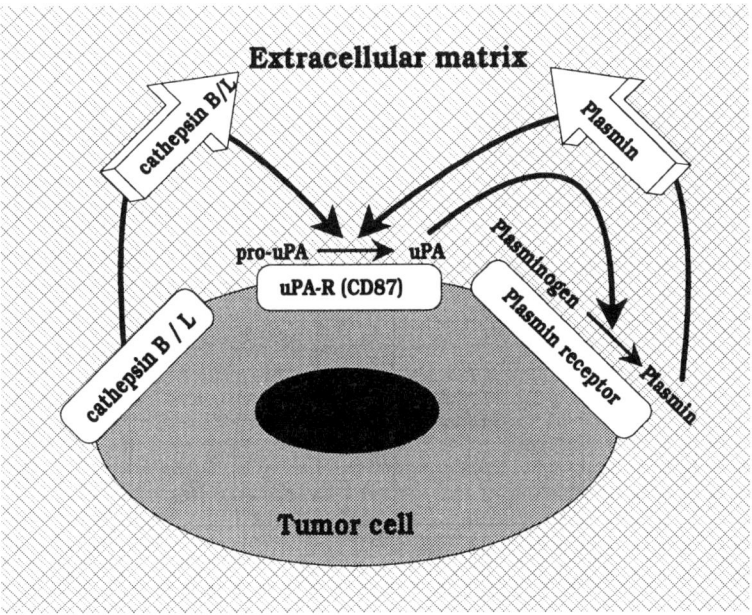

The interaction of uPA-R (CD87) with pro-uPA or HMW-uPA has been characterized in detail [21-24]. uPA binds to uPA-R in solution or to uPA-R present on the surface of tumor cells and normal cells via a defined peptide sequence (amino acids 13-30) of the N-terminus (aminoterminal fragment, ATF) of uPA. uPA-R is a cysteine-rich glycoprotein of M_r = 45 - 55,000 [25-27]. It is also present on tumor cells in malignant solid tumors [21, 28-31]. uPA-R is attached to the plasma membrane *via* a covalent linkage of the carboxyterminus of the protein to a glycosylated form of the phospholipid phosphatidyl inositol resulting in a glycolipid anchor termed glycosyl-phophatidylinositol (GPI) [23]. Binding of uPA to uPA-R is not sufficient to induce internalization (down regulation) of uPA-R by the cell. HMW-uPA-occupied uPA-R is internalized only after having reacted with PAI-1 or PAI-2. The uPA/PAI-mediated internalization of uPA-R is a complex pattern; besides uPA-R another cell surface receptor, LRP (low density lipoprotein-receptor-related protein, CD91), also known as α_2-macroglobulin receptor is involved in the internalization process [22]. Binding of uPA to uPA-R may elicit a mitogenic effect in tumor cells [31]. Previous work has also demonstrated that uPA stimulates the differentiation of leukemia cells, the migration of endothelial cells, chemotaxis of human neutrophils. Binding of uPA to uPA-R triggers tyrosine phosphorylation thereby establishing a link between the occupation of uPA-R and signal transduction [32].

Lysosomal cysteine proteases cathepsin B and L have also been shown to be associated with tumor invasion and metastasis in solid tumors [3, 33]. A direct and strong degrading action against components of the tumor stroma, e.g. laminin, collagen, and elastin has been described [34]. Cathepsin B and L are also strong activators of the proenzyme form of uPA (pro-uPA) [35, 36]. Overexpression and altered trafficking of cathepsins have been attributed to the malignant phenotype of tumor cells [37, 38]. The secreted precursors of cathepsin L have been assumed to be identical with MEP (major excreted protein), a protease which is involved in tumorigenesis as known by findings obtained with H-ras transformed mouse fibroblast cell lines [39]. Strong evidence has been presented that cathepsin B and regulation in tumor cells is different from that in normal cells, for instance decreased pH-dependent membrane association of pro-cathepsin L correlates with its increased secretion by tumor cells [40].

Clinical relevance of tumor-associated proteolytic factors uPA, PAI-1, and cathepsins B and L

Exploration of new tumor biological parameters that may identify breast cancer patients at risk is an important task in clinical cancer research. There is substantial evidence that high concentrations of the proteolytic factors uPA, PAI-1, and cathepsin B/L in primary breast cancer tissue are related to tumor cell invasion and metastasis [5-16, 19, 38]. uPA, PAI-1, and cathepsin B/L are strong and independent prognostic factors in breast cancer patients; elevated antigen levels of uPA or PAI-1 are correlated with short disease-free survival and early death [5-16]. A list of publications in which the prognostic relevance of factors of the tumor-associated plasminogen activator system (uPA, uPA-R, PAI-1, PAI-2) has been elucidated is shown in *Table I*. It should be noted that in all of these publications antigen contents were assessed by enzymometric techniques (ELISA) and not by immuno-histochemistry. Indeed, Jänicke *et al.* already in 1990 [6] and again in 1995 [41] have demonstrated that antigen determinations of these proteolytic factors by ELISA are superior to immunohistochemical assessment. In all of the investigations published so far on the prognostic value of factors of the plasminogen activator system in breast cancer *(Table I)* the same conclusion was reached: high levels of either uPA, uPA-R, or PAI-1 detected in primary cancer tissue extracts predict poor prognosis of the patient, both for disease-free and overall survival.

The lysosomal cysteine proteases cathepsin B and cathepsin L have also been implicated to be involved in tumor spread and metastasis. Thomssen *et al.* [19] and Lah *et al.* [38] evaluated the prognostic impact of these proteases in breast cancer patients. Thomssen *et al.* [19] applied commercially available ELISA to cathepsin B and L, Lah *et al.* used both ELISA and enzyme activity measurements to determine cathepsin B/L content in tumor tissue extracts. In the study of Thomssen *et al.*, patients with high cathepsin B (> 1.092 ng/mg protein) or cathepsin L content (> 376 ng/mg protein) in their primary tumors had a statistically significantly higher risk of recurrence than patients with low content of cathepsin B or cathepsin L. In multivariate analysis for disease-free survival, including cathepsin B and L as well as traditional histomor-

Table I. References in which the prognostic value of uPA, uPA-R, PAI-1 and/or PAI-2 in patients with breast cancer have been demonstrated by ELISA (tumor tissue extracts).

Factor	Author(s)	Year	Reference
uPA	Jänicke et al.	1989	Lancet 2 (8670): 1049
uPA	Jänicke et al.	1990	Fibrinolysis 4: 69
uPA	Duffy et al.		Lancet 335 (8681): 108
uPA	Duffy et al.		Cancer Research 50: 6827
uPA	Duffy et al.		Blood Coagul Fibrin 1: 681
uPA	Schmitt et al.		Blood Coagul Fibrin 1: 695
uPA	Bender and Schnurch	1991	Curr Opin Obstet Gynecol 3: 58
uPA	Duffy et al.		Clin Chem 37: 101
uPA, PAI-1, PAI-2	Foucre et al.		Br J Cancer 64: 926
uPA	Graeff et al.		Geburtsh Frauenheilk 51: 90
uPA, PAI-1	Jänicke et al.		Sem Thromb Hem 17: 303
uPA	Reilly et al.		Blood Coagul Fibrin 2: 47
uPA	Schmitt et al.		Biomed Biochim Acta 50: 731
uPA	Duffy	1992	Clin Exp Metastasis 10: 145
uPA	Duffy et al.		Fibrinolysis 6, suppl. 4: 55
uPA	Foekens et al.		Cancer Research 52: 6101
uPA, PAI-1	Reilly et al.		Int J Cancer 50: 208
uPA, PAI-1	Schmitt et al.		Biol Chem Hoppe-Seyler 373: 611
uPA	Spyratos et al.		J Natl Cancer Inst 84: 1266
uPA, PAI-1	Grondahl-Hansen et al.	1993	Cancer Res 53: 2513
uPA, PAI-1	Harbeck et al.		Gynäkol Geb Rundsch 33 suppl 1: 303
uPA, PAI-1	Jänicke et al.		Breast Cancer Res Treat 24: 195
uPA	Ferrer et al.		ECCO 7, Abstract 316, S63
uPA	Klijn et al.		Cancer Treat Rev suppl B: 45
uPA	Klijn et al.		Cancer Surv 18: 165
uPA	Rosenquist et al.		Breast Cancer Res Treat 28: 223
uPA, PAI-1, PAI-2	Bouchet et al.	1994	Br J Cancer 69: 398
uPA	Duffy et al.		Cancer 74: 2276
uPA, PAI-1	Foekens et al.		Excerpta Medica 1050: 197
uPA, PAI-1	Foekens et al.		J Clin Oncology 12: 1648
uPA, PAI-1	Jänicke et al.		Excerpta Medica 1050: 207
uPA, PAI-1	Jänicke et al.		Cancer Res 54: 2527
uPA	Romain et al.		Br J Cancer 70: 304
uPA-R	Duggan et al.	1995	Int J Cancer 61: 597
uPA, PAI-2	Foekens et al.		Cancer Res 55: 1423
uPA, PAI-1	Foekens et al.		J Natl Cancer Inst 87: 751
uPA, PAI-1	Foekens et al.		Int J Cancer 64: 130
uPA, PAI-1	Graeff		Geburtsh Frauenheilk 55: M17
uPA-R	Grondahl-Hansen et al.		Clin Cancer Res 1: 1079
uPA, PAI-1	Jänicke et al.		CRC Press. In: *Fibrinolysis in Disease*, p. 19
uPA, PAI-1	Schmitt et al.		J Obst Gynaecol 21: 151
uPA, PAI-1	Schmitt et al.		Karger Verlag: In: *Hormone-dependent tumors*, p. 73
uPA, PAI-1	Schmitt et al.		Springer Verlag, In: *Malignome und Hämostase*, p. 167
uPA	Yamashita et al.		Surgery 117: 601
uPA	Fernö et al.	1996	Eur J Cancer, in press
PAI-1	Fernö et al.		AACR-Meeting, Florida, USA

phological prognostic factors, cathepsin L turned out to be a strong and independent prognostic factor with a prognostic impact comparable to that of axillary lymph node status and grading. To evaluate the relationship between tumor biological factors and the metastatic potential of primary node-negative breast cancer, in a recent study, we assessed proteolytic factors uPA, PAI-1, and cathepsin L in comparison with traditional prognostic factors by multivariate analysis and CART (classification and regression trees). In extracts of primary tumors of node-negative breast cancer patients tumor-associated proteolytic factors (cathepsin L, uPA, PAI-1) were quantified by ELISA in comparison to traditional prognostic factors (tumor size, steroid hormone receptor status, grading, vessel invasion, menopausal status). The median follow-up was 53 months. In this analysis, PAI-1, cathepsin L, tumor size, grading, and steroid hormone receptor status were of prognostic relevance for disease-free survival (univariate analysis). Multivariate analysis of disease-free survival (Cox proportional hazards model) disclosed PAI-1 (relative risk = 8,6) to be the only strong and statistically independent prognostic factor. By CART-analysis, however, we found that the combination of PAI-1 ($\leq$ 14 ng/mg protein) and cathepsin L ($\leq$ 1,100 ng/mg protein) identifies a subgroup comprising 68% of the node-negative breast cancer patients having a low risk of disease recurrence (incidence of 0,8% per year). Thus, by the combined determination of PAI-1 and cathepsin L tumor levels, a maximum number of patients with low risk to experience disease recurrence may be identified. These patients most probably will not benefit from systemic adjuvant therapy.

The uPA/uPA receptor system as a target for tumor therapy

Inactivation of the genes (« knock-out ») for proteolytic factors of the uPA/uPA-R system in mice has been anticipated to result in a lethal phenotype. Surprisingly, mice in which the gene for uPA, uPA-R, PAI-1, tPA, or plasminogen had been eliminated were viable, fertile and appeared healthy or showed only minor pathophysiological symptoms [42, 43]. This very recent, surprising finding implies the non-essentiality of the plasminogen activator system for reproduction and survival in mammals under physiological conditions. On the other hand, substantial clinical and biochemical evidence has accumulated that uncontroled regulation and expression of the plasminogen activator system is an important aspect in tumor invasion and metastasis [4]. Interference of the uPA/uPA-R system at the gene and/or at the protein level may therefore be a feasible approach in inhibiting tumor spread of solid malignant tumors. Indeed, inhibition of proliferation, invasion, and/or metastasis by preventing the uPA/uPA-R interaction has been achieved [20]. At the gene level, antisense plasmids or antisense oligo-deoxynucleotides to uPA, uPA-R, or the transcription factor NF-κB have successfully been applied to block expression and synthesis of these factors *in vitro (Table II).*

At the protein level, two strategies have been shown to be successful: **1)** inhibition of the proteolytic activity of uPA by naturally occurring or synthetic inhibitors **2)** disturbance of the interaction of uPA with uPA-R. Various, very different reagents have been applied to interrupt the uPA/uPA-R interaction such as inactive uPA or fractions thereof, recombinant uPA-R, antibodies to uPA or uPA-R, and synthetic uPA-derived peptides. Key references describing the *in vitro* or *in vivo* effects of these agents on cell proliferation, tumor invasion and/or metastasis are listed in *Table II*. The results obtained so far are sufficiently encouraging to continue the search for substances interfering with the plasminogen activator system. Some of these agents even may be candidates for therapeutic intervention in humans. Based on the phenotypes of the plasminogen-activator-system-deficient « knock-out »-mice, one may speculate that if the uPA-R/uPA system is blocked in man other proteases such as cathepsins or metalloproteases might function as an *in vivo* back-up system by substituting for uPA/plasmin action in order to maintain the capability of cells to degrade cellular proteins or components of the extracellular matrix. It is worth mentioning, however, that also very potent synthetic inhibitors directed to the metalloproteases and cysteine proteases have been developed recently which efficiently inhibit tumor spread [44, 45]. In view of this, combined inactivation of different proteolytic factors, also in addition to conventional therapy protocols, may help to reduce tumor invasion and metastasis in humans even further.

Table II. Agents directed to factors of the plasminogen activation system which have been employed to block tumor cell proliferation, invasion and/or metastasis.

Factor	Reagent applied	Reference
uPA	uPA antisense oligonucleotide	Wilhelm *et al.* (1995), *Clin Exp Met* 13: 296
uPA-R	Antisense plasmid to uPA-R	Kook *et al.* (1994), *EMBO J* 13: 3983
uPA-R	uPA-R antisense oligonucleotide	Quattrone *et al.* (1995), *Antic Drug Des* 10: 97
uPA-R	uPA-R antisense oligonucleotide	Quattrone *et al.* (1995), *Cancer Res* 55: 90
uPA, PAI-1	NFκ-B antisense oligonucleotide	Reuning (1995), *Nucl Acids Res* 23: 3887
uPA	Antibody to uPA	Ossowski *et al.* (1983), *Cell* 35: 611
uPA	Antibody to uPA	Hearing *et al.* (1988), *Cancer Res* 48: 1270
uPA	Antibody to uPA	Kobayashi *et al.* (1994), *Thr Haemost* 71: 474
uPA	Antibody to uPA	Jarrad *et al.* (1995), *Invasion Metastasis* 15: 34
uPA-R	Antibody to uPA-R	Mohanam *et al.* (1993), *Cancer Res* 53: 4143
PAI-1	Antibody to PAI-1	Tsuchiya *et al.* (1995), *Gen Diagn Path* 141: 41
uPA-R	uPA	Howell *et al.* (1994), *Blood Coag Fibrin* 5: 445
uPA, uPA-R	Inactive uPA	Cohen *et al.* (1991), *Blood* 78: 479
uPA, uPA-R	Inactive uPA	Crowley *et al.* (1993), *PNAS* 90: 5021
uPA, uPA-R	ATF	Kirchheimer *et al.* (1989), *PNAS* 86: 5424
uPA-R	ATF-albumin	Lu *et al.* (1994), *FEBS Lett* 356: 56
uPA, uPA-R	ATF, uPA peptides	Rabbani *et al.* (1992), *J Biol Chem* 267: 14151
uPA, uPA-R	uPA peptides	Schlechte *et al.* (1989), *Cancer Res* 49: 6064
uPA, uPA-R	uPA peptides	Kobayashi *et al.* (1993), *Br J Cancer* 67: 537
uPA-R	uPA-peptide	Kobayashi *et al.* (1994), *Int J Cancer* 57: 727
uPA	uPA-R	Wilhelm *et al.* (1994), *FEBS Lett* 337: 131
uPA	PAI-2	Baker *et al.* (1990), *Cancer Res* 50: 4676
uPA	PAI-2	Laug *et al.* (1993), *Cancer Res* 53: 6051
uPA	PAI-2	Evans *et al.* (1995), *Am Surg* 61: 692
uPA	PAI-2	Mueller *et al.* (1995), *PNAS* 92: 205
Plasmin	Urinary trypsin inhibitor (UTI)	Kobayashi *et al.* (1994), *Clin Exp Met* 12: 117
Plasmin	Urinary trypsin inhibitor (UTI)	Kobayashi *et al.* (1994), *Cancer Res* 54: 844
Plasmin	UTI, UTI-peptide 3	Kobayashi *et al.* (1995), *Int J Cancer* 63: 455
uPA-R, plasmin	uPA-UTI	Kobayashi *et al.* (1995), *J B Chem* 270: 8361
uPA, PAI-1	Dexamethasone	Reeder *et al.* (1993), *Terat Carc Mutag* 13: 75
uPA	Benzo[b]thiophene derivative	Towle *et al.* (1993), *Cancer Res* 53: 2553
uPA	Phenylacetate	Samid *et al.* (1993), *J Clin Invest* 91: 2288
uPA	Estramustine, taxol	Santibanez *et al.* (1995), *Cell Bio Funct* 13: 217
uPA, PAI-1	N-(4-hydroxylphenyl)-retinamide	Kim *et al.* (1995), *Anticancer Res* 15: 1429
uPA	p-aminobenzamidine	Billstrom *et al.* (1995), *Int J Cancer* 61: 542
uPA	Pyroglutamyl-Leu-Arg-CHO	Kawada and Umezawa (1995), *BBRC* 209: 25

References

1. Schmitt M, Jänicke F, Graeff H. Tumor-associated proteases. *Fibrinolysis* 1992; 6, Suppl. 4: 3-26.
2. Stetler-Stevenson WG, Liotta LA, Kleiner DE. Extracellular matrix 6: Role of matrix metalloproteinases in tumor invasion and metastasis. *Faseb J* 1993; 7: 1434-41.
3. Sloane BF. Cathepsin B and cystatins: evidence for a role in cancer progression. *Sem Cancer Biol* 1990; 1: 137-52.
4. Schmitt M, Wilhelm O, Jänicke F, Magdolen V, Reuning U, Ohi H, Moniwa N, Kobayashi H, Weidle U, Henner Graeff. Urokinase-type plasminogen activator (uPA) and its receptor (CD87). A new target in tumor invasion and metastasis. *J Obstet Gynaecol* 1995; 21: 151-65.
5. Jänicke F, Schmitt M, Ulm K, Gössner W, Graeff H. Urokinase-type plasminogen activator antigen and early relapse in breast cancer. *Lancet* 1989; 334: 1049.
6. Jänicke F, Schmitt M, Hafter R, Hollrieder A, Babic R, Ulm K, Gössner W, Graeff H. Urokinase-type plasminogen activator (u-PA) antigen is a predictor of early relapse in breast cancer. *Fibrinolysis* 1990; 4: 69-78.
7. Jänicke F, Schmitt M, Graeff H. Clinical relevance of the urokinase-type and the tissue-type plasminogen activators and of their inhibitor PAI-1 in breast cancer. *Sem Thromb Hemost* 1991; 17: 303-12.
8. Jänicke F, Schmitt M, Pache L. Urokinase (uPA) and its inhibitor PAI-1 are strong and independent prognostic factors in node-negative breast cancer. *Breast Cancer Res Treatm* 1993; 24: 195-208.
9. Jänicke F, Pache L, Schmitt M, Ulm K, Thomssen C, Prechtl A, Graeff H. Both the cytosols and detergent extracts of breast cancer tissues are suited to evaluate the prognostic impact of the urokinase-type plasminogen activator and its inhibitor plasminogen activator inhibitor type 1. *Cancer Res* 1994; 54: 2527-30.
10. Duffy M, O'Grady P, Devaney D, O'Siorain L, Fennelly JJ, Lijnen HJ. Urokinase-plasminogen activator, a marker for aggressive breast carcinomas. *Cancer* 1988; 62: 531-3.
11. Duffy MJ, Reilly D, O'Sullivan C, O'Higgins N, Fenelly JJ, Andreasen P. Urokinase-plasminogen activator, a new and independent prognostic marker in breast cancer. *Cancer Res* 1990; 50: 6827-9.
12. Duffy MJ, Reilly D, O'Sullivan C, O'Higgins N, Fennelly JJ. Urokinase plasminogen activator and prognosis in breast cancer. *Lancet* 1990; 335: 108.
13. Foekens JA, Schmitt M, van Putten WLJ, Peters HA, Brontenbal M, Jänicke F, Klijn JGM. Prognostic value of urokinase-type plasminogen activator in 671 primary breast cancer patients. *Cancer Res* 1992; 52: 6101-5.
14. Foekens JA, Schmitt M, van Putten WLJ. Plasminogen activator inhibitor-1 and prognosis in primary breast cancer. *J Clin Oncol* 1994; 12: 1648-58.
15. Grøndahl-Hansen J, Christensen IJ, Rosenquist C, Brünner N, Mouridsen HT, Danø K, Blichert-Toft M. High levels of urokinase-type plasminogen activator (uPA) and its inhibitor PAI-1 in cytosolic extracts of breast carcinomas are associated with poor prognosis. *Cancer Res* 1993; 53: 2513-21.
16. Fernö M, Bendahl P, Borg A, Brundell J, Hirschberg L, Olsson H, Killander D. Urokinase plasminogen activator, a strong independent prognostic factor in breast cancer, analysed in steroid receptor cytosols with a luminometric immunoassay. *Eur J Cancer* 1996; in press.
17. Spyratos F, Martin PM, Hacene K, Romain S, Andrieu C, Ferrero-Poüs M, Deytieux S, Le Doussal V, Tubiana-Hulin M, Brunet M. Multiparametric prognostic evaluation of biological factors in primary breast cancer. *J Natl Cancer Inst* 1992; 84: 1266-72.
18. Spyratos F, Maudelonde T, Brouillet J.-P, Brunet M, Defrenne A, Andrieu C, Hacene K, Desplaces A, Rouesse J, Rochefort H. Cathepsin D: An independent prognostic factor for metastasis of breast cancer. *The Lancet* 1989; November 11, 8672: 1115-8.
19. Thomssen C, Schmitt M, Goretzki L, Oppelt P, Pache L, Dettmar P, Jänicke F, Graeff H. Prognostic value of the cysteine proteases cathepsin B and cathepsin L in human breast cancer. *Clin Cancer Res*, 1995; 1: 741-6.
20. Wilhelm O, Schmitt M, Senekowitch R, Höhl S, Wilhelm S, Will C, Rettenberger P, Reuning U, Weidle U, Magdolen V, Graeff H. The urokinase / urokinase receptor system - A new target for cancer therapy? Elsevier Excerpta Medica International Congress Series 1050. 1994; 145-56.
21. Chucholowski N, Schmitt M, Rettenberger P, Schüren E, Moniwa N, Goretzki L, Wilhelm O, Weidle U, Jänicke F, Graeff H. Flow cytofluorometric analysis of the urokinase receptor (uPA-R) on

tumor cells by fluorescent uPA-ligand or monoclonal antibody #3936. *Fibrinolysis* 1992; 6, Suppl. 4: 95-102.
22. Andreasen PA, Sottrup-Jensen L, Kloller L, Nykjaer A, Moestrup SK, Munch-Petersen C, Gliemann J. Receptor-mediated endocytosis of plasminogen activators and activator/inhibitor complexes. *FEBS Lett* 1994; 338: 239-45.
23. Ploug M, Behrendt N, Lober D, Dano K. Protein structure and membrane anchorage of the cellular receptor for urokinase-type plasminogen activator. *Sem Thromb Hemost* 1991; 17: 183-93.
24. Nykjaer A, Petersen CM, Moller B, Jensen PH, Moestrup SK, Holtet TL, Etzerod M, Thorgersen HC, Munch M, Andreasen PA, Gliemann J. Purified alpha-2 macroglobulin receptor / LDL receptor-related protein binds urokinase plasminogen activator inhibitor type-1 complex. Evidence that the alpha 2-macroglobulin receptor mediates cellular degradation of urokinase receptor-bound complexes. *J Biol Chem* 1992; 267: 14543-6.
25. Nielsen LS, Kellermann GM, Behrendt N, Picone R, Dano K, Blasi F. A 55,000-60,000 Mr receptor protein for urokinase-type plasminogen activator. Identification in human tumor cell lines and partial purification. *J Biol Chem* 1988; 263: 2358-63.
26. Ploug M, Ronne E, Behrendt N, Jensen AL, Blasi F, Dano K. Cellular receptor for urokinase plasminogen activator: Carboxyl-terminal processing and membrane anchoring by glycosyl-phosphatidylinositol. *J Biol Chem* 1991; 266: 1926-33.
27. Vassalli JD, Baccino D, Belin D. A cellular binding site for the Mr 55,000 form of the human plasminogen activator, urokinase. *J Cell Biol* 1985; 100: 86-92.
28. Casslén B, Gustavsson B. Expression of cell membrane receptors for urokinase plasminogen activator (uPA) in the human endometrium increases during the ovarian cycle. *Fibrinolysis* 1991; 5: 243-8.
29. Ronne E, Behrendt N, Ellis V, Ploug M, Dano K, Hoyer-Hansen G. Cell-induced potentiation of the plasminogen activation system is abolished by a monoclonal antibody that recognizes the NH2-terminal domain of the urokinase receptor. *FEBS Lett* 1991; 288: 233-6.
30. Pedersen N, Schmitt M, Ronne E, Nicoletti MI, Hoyer-Hansen G, Conese M, Giavazzi R, Dano K, Kuhn W, Jänicke F, Blasi F. A ligand-free, soluble urokinase-receptor is present in the ascitic fluid from patients with ovarian cancer. *J Clin Invest* 1993; 92: 2160-7.
31. Berdel WE, Wilhelm O, Schmitt M, Maurer J, Reufi B, von Marschall Z, Oberberg D, Graeff H, Thiel E. Urokinase-type plasminogen activator (uPA), a protease with cytokine-like activity in human HL-60 leukemic cell line. *Int J Oncol* 1993; 3: 607-13.
32. Dumler I, Petri T, Schleuning WD. Tyrosine phosphorylation of a 38 kDa protein upon interaction of urokinase-type plasminogen activator (u-PA) with its cellular receptor. Excerpta Medica International Congress Series 1993; 1041: 163-169.
33. Kane SE, Gottesmann MM. The role of cathepsin L in malignant transformation. *Semin Cancer Biol* 1990; 1: 127-36.
34. Yee C, Shiu RPC. Degradation of endothelial basement membrane by human breast cancer cell lines. *Cancer Res* 1986; 46: 1835-9.
35. Kobayashi H, Schmitt M, Goretzki L, Chucholowski N, Calvete J, Kramer M, Günzler WA, Jänicke F, Graeff, H. Cathepsin B efficiently activates the soluble and the tumor cell receptor-bound form of the proenzyme urokinase-type plasminogen activator (pro-uPA). *J Biol Chem* 1990; 266: 5147-52.
36. Goretzki L, Schmitt M, Mann KH, Calvete J, Chucholowski N, Kramer M, Günzler WA, Jänicke F, Graeff, H. Effective activation of the proenzyme form of the urokinase-type plasminogen activator (pro-uPA) by the cysteine protease cathepsin L. *FEBS Lett* 1992; 297: 112-8.
37. Sloane BF, Cao L, Sameni M. Trafficking of cathepsin B in tumor cells. *Proc Am Assoc Cancer Res* 1993; 34: 603.
38. Lah TT, Kokali-Kunovar M, Strukelj B, Pungercar J, Barlic-Maganja D, Drobnic-Kosorok M, Kastelic L, Babnik J, Golouh R, Turk V. Stefins and lysosomal cathepsins B, L and D in human breast carcinoma. *Int J Cancer* 1992; 50: 36-44.
39. Denhardt DT, Greenberg AH, Egan SE, Hamilton RT, Wright JA. Cysteine proteinase cathepsin L expression correlates closely with the metastatic potential of H-ras transformed murine fibroblasts. *Oncogene* 1987; 2: 55-9.
40. Godbold GD, Chapman RL, Yeyeodu S, Erickson A. Binding of procathepsin L to the lysosomal proenzyme receptor is altered in tumor cells. Abstract at the AACR-Meeting: Proteases and protease inhibitors. *Panama City*, Fl, USA. 1996.

41. Jänicke F, Schmitt M, Graeff H. Both uPA and PAI-1 are independent prognosticators of relapse and death in breast cancer. In: *Fibrinolysis in Disease*. Glas-Greenwalt, P ed. CRC Press, Boca Raton, New York, London, Tokyo, 1995; 19-25.
42. Carmeliet P, Schoonjans L, Kieckens L, Ream B, Degen J, Bronson R, de Vos R, van den Oord JJ, Collen D, Mulligan RC. Physiological consequences of loss of plasminogen activator gene function in mice. *Nature* 1994; 368: 419-24.
43. Bugge T, Flick MJ, Daugherty CC, Degen JJ. Plasminogen deficiency causes severe thrombosis but is compatible with development and reproduction. *Genes & Develop* 1995; 9: 794-807.
44. Kohn EC, Liotta LA. Molecular insights into cancer invasion: Strategies for prevention and intervention. *Cancer Res* 1995; 55: 1856-62.
45. Calkins CC, Sloane BF. Mammalian cysteine protease inhibitors: Biochemical properties and possible roles in tumor progression. *Biol Chem Hoppe Seyler* 1995; 376: 71-80.

Urokinase plasminogen activator receptor in breast cancer

Nils Brünner, Claus Holst-Hansen[1], Anders N. Pedersen[1], Charles Pyke[2], Gunilla Hoyer-Hansen[1], John Foekens[3] and Ross W. Stephens[1]

[1] *Finsen Laboratory, Rigshospitalet, Strandboulevarden 49, DK-2100, Copenhagen, Denmark.*
[2] *Novo Nordisk, Copenhagen, Denmark.*
[3] *Dr. Daniel den Hoed Cancer Center, Rotterdam, The Netherlands*

Introduction

The invasive nature of malignant tumors is due to the co-ordinated expression of proteolytic enzymes, contributed by tumor cells and/or the stromal cells they recruit into the process [1]. The complex interactions between tumor cells and stromal cells also include a dynamic equilibrium between proteases and protease inhibitors, as well as modulation of cellular adhesion and migration by the effect of proteases on adhesion proteins and other components of the extracellular matrix. A central role in this invasive process can be ascribed to the urokinase plasminogen activator (uPA). The specific cleavage of plasminogen by uPA gives rise to plasmin, a less specific protease able to degrade many structural components of the extracellular matrix [2].

uPA is secreted as an inactive proenzyme (pro-uPA), and both uPA and pro-uPA bind with high affinity to a cell-surface receptor (uPAR). This cell surface binding enhances the rate of activation of pro-uPA and localizes newly-formed uPA activity at the cell-surface contacts with other cells and the matrix. uPAR is a glycolipid-anchored three-domain 55 kDa glycoprotein whose N-terminal domain 1 contains the binding site for the growth factor domain of uPA [3, 4]. In order to realise its full proteolytic potential, assembly of the uPA system requires cell-surface display of uPAR, occupancy of the receptor by pro-uPA, and the proximity of bound plasmin/plasminogen in order to activate pro-uPA and continuously propagate uPA and plasmin activities [5]. Within this assembly, some of the essential components may be contributed by tumor cells, others by the stromal cells. The most aggressive tumors are now known to efficiently bring together a highly active uPA system, but the contributing cells may differ substantially between different types of cancer.

In this short review we summarize findings from studies of both the quantitation and cellular origin of uPAR in breast cancer, and their implications in prognosis and therapy.

Cellular uPAR localization

As already mentioned, several studies have indicated that extracellular tissue degradation in cancer is a result of an interaction between the epithelial tumor cells and the infiltrating stromal cells [1].
We have investigated by immunohistochemistry the cellular localization of uPAR in breast cancer samples derived from 60 patients with invasive ductal breast carcinomas [6]. We used two monoclonal antibodies, R2 and R4, which are directed against different epitopes on domains 2 and 3 [7]. These antibodies work both on frozen and paraffin sections. In the majority of the samples (49/60) uPAR immunoreactivity was observed in macrophages located in close vicinity to the infiltrating epithelial cancer tissue. Double-staining with a macrophage specific antibody (CD68) confirmed the macrophage identity of the uPAR stained cancer cells. In 8 out of 51 uPAR positive samples, uPAR immunoreactivity was found in the epithelial cancer cells. In most specimens, a subpopulation of tissue neutrophils was also positive. In contrast, normally appearing epithelium was negative, as were 10 samples of normal female breast tissue.
In a study by Bianchi *et al.* [8], the cellular localization of uPAR was studied in 59 invasive breast cancer samples, 12 normal breast tissue cases and 4 fibroadenomas. By using an anti uPAR polyclonal antibody, they found 49/59 invasive breast carcinomas to express uPAR immunoreactivity. Strong surface staining of tumor-associated macrophages was evident in most of the cases. Staining of tumor cells was observed in 21/59 cases while no staining was seen in normal breast tissue or in the fibroadenomas.
The expression of uPAR in tumor-infiltrating macrophages in breast cancer is consistent with the pattern of uPAR mRNA expression in human colon adenocarcinomas [9]. It has been a matter of dispute whether tumor-infiltrating macrophages inhibit or promote cancer progression. The immunohistochemical findings of uPAR localized predominantly to a population of periductal tissue macrophages in areas of infiltrating breast carcinomas point to macrophages playing a role in promoting tumor progression, probably by contributing to extracellular proteolysis required for invasion. This tumor promoting effect may, however, be exerted only by a subfraction of macrophages on which plasmin is generated.

uPAR quantitation

Methods for an objective quantitation of uPAR in tissues and bodily fluids are a prerequisite for studies on the diagnostic and/or prognostic impact of uPAR in human cancer. We have established a highly sensitive and specific uPAR ELISA, which consists of one polyclonal anti-uPAR antibody as catching antibody and three monoclonal anti-uPAR antibodies as detecting antibodies [10]. The three monoclonal antibodies were selected so that they detect different epitopes on uPAR (R2 is directed against an epitope on domain 2+3 while R3 and R5 are directed against different epitopes on domain 1). The detection limit of the assay is 1,6 pM. There is a linear dose-response over a 40-fold concentration range and the signal is completely dependent on the specific immune reaction. The intra- and interassay coefficients of variation are 7 and 13%, respectively.
We applied this assay on 20 different human breast tumors [10] each extracted with three different buffers: Buffer A (pH 7,5) is the one being routinely used for biochemical steroid

horrnone receptor assays, buffer B is a Triton X-100 containing buffer, pH 4,2 and buffer C is a Triton X-114 containing buffer, pH 8,1. All extracts contained measurable amounts of uPAR. Buffer C was the most efficient for extraction of uPAR while buffer B extracted 51% and buffer A 28% of the amount extracted by buffer C.

We also studied uPAR in a set of 94 breast tumor extracts made with buffer A and B [10]. uPAR was found in all tumor extracts and the regression coefficient between the uPAR values obtained using the two buffers was 0,45.

Prognostic significance of uPAR

Several studies have described the prognostic impact of uPA and PAI-1 in extracts from breast cancers [11-15]. In all of these studies high tumor levels of uPA or PAI-1 were found to predict a shorter survival. In order to study the prognostic role of tumor uPAR content in breast cancer, we applied the uPAR ELISA on extracts from 505 breast tumors [16]. uPAR was extracted by two different buffers, one being the EORTC steroid hormone receptor buffer (buffer A), the other containing Triton X-114. In all but 12 cases the level of uPAR was above the detection limit. In a Cox univariate analysis using the median uPAR value to divide patients into two groups, one with uPAR values below the median and one with values above, it was found that high levels of uPAR in the cytosol buffer (buffer A) were significantly associated with a shorter overall survival, while only a non-significant trend was found towards a similar association between uPAR and overall survival in the Triton X-114 containing buffer.

It was found in both univariate and multivariate analysis that cytosolic uPAR was a significant prognostic factor in postmenopausal node-positive patients. In contrast, triton-extracted uPAR was not related to prognosis in this group of patients *(Figure 1)*.

In a study by Duffy *et al.* [17], including 141 primary breast carcinomas, uPAR was measured in cytosolic extracts using a different uPAR ELISA than we used. They showed that high cytosolic uPAR significantly predicted shorter disease-free interval and shorter overall survival when compared to patients with low uPAR levels.

It is interesting that the uPAR level in cytosolic tumor extracts is a much stronger prognostic marker than is the uPAR level in detergent extracts. The uPAR found in cytosols may represent a water-soluble degradation product of native uPAR which has lost its lipid anchor due to the action of either proteases or lipases. Such a water-soluble form of uPAR has been described in ascites fluid from ovarian cancer patients [18]. Water-soluble uPAR could also be formed as a result of uPA mediated uPAR cleavage, resulting in liberation of domain 1 of uPAR [19]. On the cell surfaces plasmin formation happens in close vicinity to uPAR, and the amount of water-soluble domain 1 of uPAR may therefore be a good indirect measure of the level of uPA mediated plasmin formation in a tissue.

We have studied uPAR in the human MDA-MB-231 breast cancer cell line. In cell culture, uPAR is cleaved between domain 1 and 2 [20], and this cleavage can be inhibited by anticatalytic antibodies against uPA [20], indicating that the cleavage is mediated by either uPA or plasmin generated by uPA. Significant amounts of uPAR can be detected in conditioned medium from MDA-MB-231 cells [21]. Also, when grown as xenografts in nude mice, uPAR in MDA-AIB-231 is cleaved [21] and human uPAR can be detected in plasma from tumor bearing mice (unpublished data). We have recently found that also in patient breast cancers, uPAR can be detected both as a full length protein and in a cleaved form (unpublished data). By comparing uPAR in plasma from healthy controls and from stage IV breast cancer patients, it

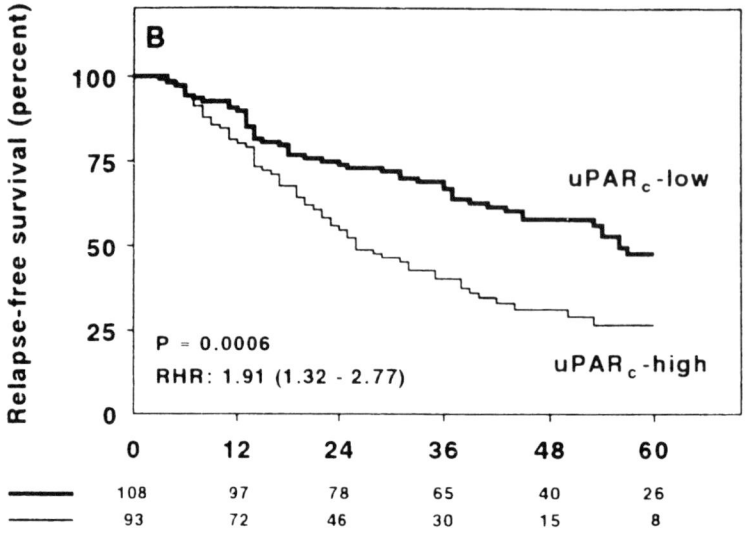
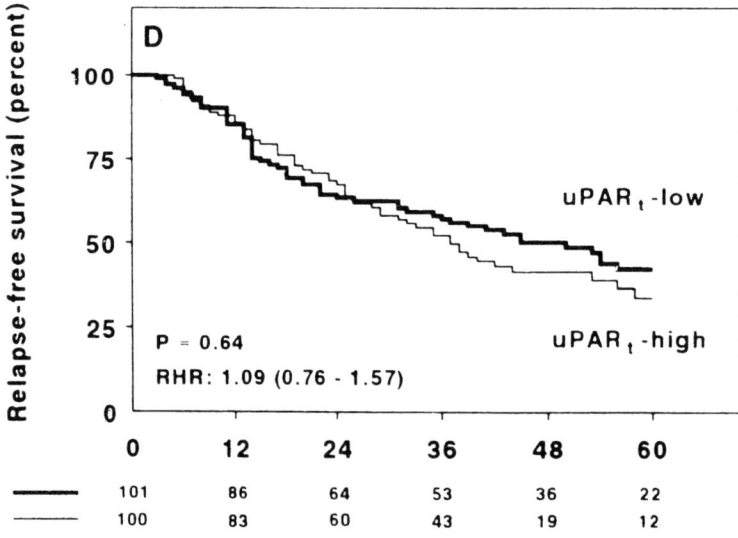

Figure 1. Actuarial relapse-free survival curves for 201 postmenopausal, node-positive breast cancer patients divided according to the level of uPAR in cytosols (uPARc, B) and Triton extracts (uPARt, D) of tumor tissue. Patients were divided into groups with uPAR levels below (low) and above (high) the median value. P values were calculated using the likelihood ratio test, relative hazard risks (RHR) with 95% confidence intervals were calculated using the Cox regression model and the number of patients at risk are indicated. Reproduced with permission from [16].

was found that the cancer patients had significantly elevated uPAR plasma levels (unpublished data), indicating that a water-soluble form of uPAR is released from the cancer cells and entering the blood stream. We are currently characterizing plasma uPAR.

Therapeutic applications

It is well established that cancer invasion and metastasis require extracellular proteolysis, and molecules mediating tissue degradation may hence be attractive targets for anti-invasive therapy. Indeed, preclinical experiments have shown that interference with the proteolytic pathways in cancer cells may inhibit their invasive activity in *in vitro* assays [22, 23], and significantly decrease their invasion and metastatic spread in animals [24].

uPAR plays a critical role in uPA mediated plasminogen activation which preceeds cancer cell invasion. Inhibition of uPA binding to uPAR leads to diminished plasmin formation *in vitro*, and since plasmin activates various growth factors as well as latent forms of some metalloproteinases, interference with uPA: uPAR interaction might have severe impact on tumor progression. Indeed, a number of preclinical *in vitro* [22, 23] and *in vivo* [24, 25] tumor studies now support this assumption.

We have studied the effect of inhibiting uPA binding to uPAR in an *in vitro* model system of human breast cancer cells [21]. By inhibiting uPA:uPAR interaction with a monoclonal antibody (R3) directed against the ligand binding domain of uPAR (domain 1), we have shown that *in vitro* plasmin formation as well as *in vitro* invasion through Matrigel can be significantly impaired. *Figure 2* shows an example from an *in vitro* invasion assay employing the inhibitory anti-uPAR antibody (R3) and as control an uPAR antibody (R4) directed against domain 2+3. We have also developed *in vivo* assays to study the role of uPAR in tumor invasion and metastasis [26]. One important observation is that, in the xenotransplantation model, the host

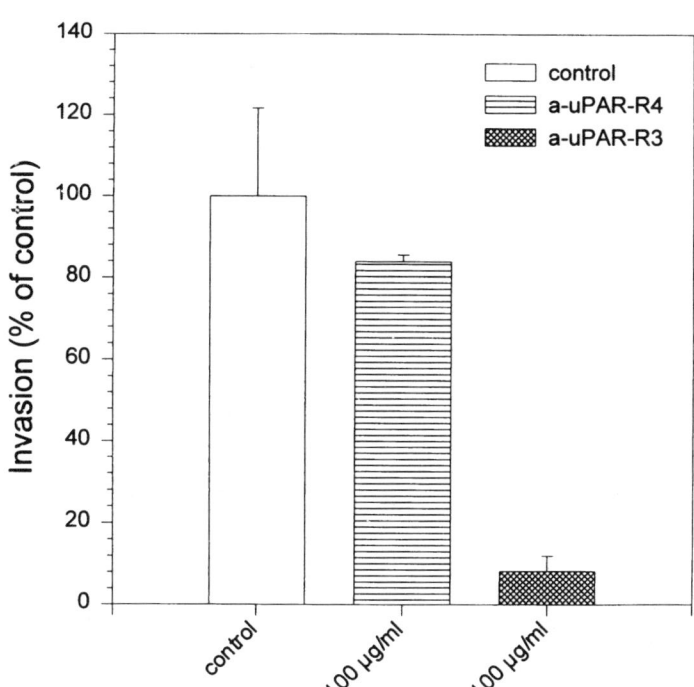

Figure 2. Matrigel invasion by MDA-MB-231 BAG human breast cancer cells. Transwell filters were coated with 100 μg Matrigel supplemented with human plasminogen. 2×10^5 cells were resuspended in 0,5 ml media ± antibodies (anti-uPAR clone R4, or anti-uPAR clone R3), and the cells were added to the upper chambers. Lower chambers received the same media as the upper chambers. Transwells were incubated for 24 hours and invasion was defined as the accumulation of cells on the lower aspect of the membrane and in the outer well, as a function of the total number of cells. Cell number was determined by the vital stain MTT. Means of triplicate assay points are shown.

stromal cells also participate in generation of extracellular proteolysis, *e.g.* mouse uPA and mouse uPAR are expressed in the tumor-infiltrating stromal cells [27]. One implication of this finding is that, when testing potential uPAR antagonists in this *in vivo* model, the presence of mouse uPA and uPAR has to be taken into consideration.

References

1. Danø K, Grøndahl-Hansen J, Eriksen J, Nielsen BS, Rcmer J, Pyke C. The receptor for urokinase plasminogen activator. Stromal cell involvement in extracellular proteolysis during cancer invasion. Proteolysis and protein turnover. In: AJ Barrett and J Bond (eds), *Portland Press*, London 1992.
2. Danø K, Andreasen PA, Grøndahl-Hansen J, Kristensen P, Nielsen LS, Skriver L. Plasminogen activators, tissue degradation and cancer. *Adv Cancer Res* 1985; 44: 139-266.
3. Behrendt N, Rønne E, Ploug M, *et al*. The human receptor for urokinase plasminogen activator. *J Biol Chem* 1990; 265: 6453-60.
4. Behrendt N, Ploug M, Patthy L, Houen G, Blasi F, Danø K. The ligand-binding domain of the cell surface receptor for urokinase-type plasminogen Activator. *J Biol Chem* 1991; 266: 7842-7.
5. Ellis V, Behrendt N, Danø K. Plasminogen activation by receptor-bound urokinase. *J Biol Chem* 1991; 266: 12752-8.
6. Pyke C, Græm N, Ralfkiær E, *et al*. Receptor for urokinase is present in tumor-associated macrophages in ductal breast carcinoma. *Cancer Research* 1993; 53: 1911-5.
7. Ronne E, Behrendt N, Ellis V, Ploug M, Danø K, Høyer-Hansen G. Cell-induced Potentiation of the Plasminogen Activation System is Abolished by a Monoclonal Antibody that Recognizes the NH-terminal Domain of the Urokinase Receptor. *FEBS Letters* 1991; 288: 233-6.
8. Bianchi E, Cohen RL, Thor AT, *et al*. The urokinase receptor is expressed in invasive breast cancer but not in normal breast tissue. *Cancer Res* 1994; 54: 861-6.
9. Pyke C, Kristensen P, Ralfkiær E, *et al*. Urokinase-type plasminogen activator is expressed in stromal cells and its receptor in cancer cells at invasive foci in human colon adenocarcinomas. *Amer J Pathol* 1991; 138: 1059-67.
10. Rønne E, Høyer-Hansen G, Brunner N, *et al*. Urokinase receptor in breast cancer tissue extracts. Enzyme-linked immunosorbent assay with a combination of mono-and polyclonal antibodies. *Breast Cancer Res Treat* 1995; 199-207.
11. Duffy MJ, Reilly D, O'Sullivan C, O'Higgins N, Fennelly JJ, Andreasen P. Urokinase-plasminogen activator, a new and independent prognostic marker in breast cancer. *Cancer Research* 1990; 50: 6827-9.
12. Jänicke F, Schmitt M, Hafter R, *et al*. Urokinase-type plasminogen activator (u-PA) antigen is a predictor of early relapse in breast cancer. *Fibrinolysis* 1990; 4: 69-78.
13. Foekens JA, Schmitt M, van Putten WLJ, *et al*. Prognostic value of urokinase-type plasminogen activator in 671 primary breast cancer patients. *Cancer Research* 1992; 52: 6101-5.
14. Foekens JA, Schmitt M, van Putten WL, *et al*. Plasminogen activator inhibitor-1 and prognosis in primary breast cancer. *J Clin Oncol* 1994; 12: 1648-58.
15. Grøndahl-Hansen J, Christensen IJ, Rosenquist C, *et al*. High levels of urokinase-type plasminogen activator and its inhibitor PAI-1 in cytosolic extracts of breast carcinomas are associated with poor prognosis. *Cancer Research* 1993; 53: 2513-21.
16. Grøndahl-Hansen J, Peters HA, van Putten LJ, *et al*. Prognostic significance of the receptor for urokinase plasminogen activator in breast cancer. *Clinical Cancer Res* 1995; 1: 1079-87.
17. Duggan C, Maguire T, McDermott E, O'Higgins N, Fennelly JJ, Duffy MJ. Urokinase plasminogen activator and urokinase plasminogen activator receptor in breast cancer. *Int J Cancer* 1995; 61: 597-600.
18. Pedersen N, Schmitt M, Rønne E, *et al*. A Ligand-Free, Soluble Urokinase-Receptor is Present in the Ascitic Fluid from Patients with Ovarian Cancer. *J Clin Invest* 1993; Submitted.
19. Høyer-Hansen G, Rønne E, Solberg H, *et al*. Urokinase plasminogen activator cleaves its cell surface receptor releasing the ligand-binding domain. *J Biol Chem* 1992; 267: 18224-9.

20. Solberg H, Rømer J, Brunner N, *et al*. A cleaved form of the receptor for urokinase-type plasminogen activator in invasive transplanted human and murine tumors. *Int J Cancer* 1994; 58: 877-81.
21. Holst-Hansen C, Johannesen B, Høyer-Hansen G, Rømer J, Ellis V, Brunner N. Urokinase-type plasminogen activation in three human breast cancer cell lines correlates with their *in vitro* invasiveness. *Clin Exp Metastasis* 1996; in press.
22. Quax PHA, Pedersen N, Masucci MT, *et al*. Complementation between urokinase-producing and receptor-producing cells in extracellular matrix degradation. *Cell Regulation* 1991; 2: 793-803.
23. Hollas W, Blasi F, Boyd D. Role of the urokinase receptor in facilitating extracellular matrix invasion by cultured colon cancer. *Cancer Res* I 991; 51: 3690-5.
24. Crowley CW, Cohen RL, Lucas BK, Liu G, Shuman MA, Levinson AD. Prevention of metastasis by inhibition of the urokinase receptor. *Proc Natl Acad Sci USA* 1993; 90: 5021-5.
25. Ossowski L, Russo-Payne H, Wilson EL. Inhibition of urokinase-type plasminogen activator by antibodies: The effect on dissemination of a human tumor in the nude mouse. *Cancer Research* 1991; 51: 274-81.
26. Brünner N, Thompson EW, Spang-Thomsen M, Rygaard J, Danø K, Zwiebel JA. lacZ transduced human breast cancer xenografts as an in vivo model for the study of invasion and metastasis. *Eur J Cancer* 1992; 28A: 1989-95.
27. Rømer J, Pyke C, Lund LR, *et al*. Urokinase-Type Plasminogen Activator and its Receptor are Expressed by Both Neoplastic and Stromal Cells During Invasion of Human Breast Carcinoma Xenografts in Nude Mice. *Int J Cancer* 1994; 57: 553-60.

Multiparameter analysis of prognostic factors in breast cancer

Wim L.J. van Putten, Jan G.M. Klijn, Marion E. Meijer-van Gelder, Maxime P. Look and John A. Foekens

Department of Biostatistics and Division of Endocrine Oncology, Department of Medical Oncology, Rotterdam Cancer Institute (Daniel den Hoed Kliniek)/Academic Hospital, Groene Hilledijk 301, 3075 EA Rotterdam, The Netherlands

Breast cancer is a heterogeneous disease with widely variable outcomes between patients. A partial explanation for this variation by prognostic factors may help in a better understanding of the disease. This will be most fruitful if this is supported by a biological model for the impact of a potential prognostic factor. Identification of prognostic factors may also help in the selection of subgroups of patients for which special forms of treatment are required. However, this depends on the extent of separation into patients with a very good and those with a very poor prognosis that may be achieved. In addition, it depends on the firm establishment of the benefit of alternative treatments in subgroups of patients with poor prognosis. For that purpose large randomized clinical trials are required. Unfortunately, most cell biological factors are not studied within the framework of such trials. Therefore it is not possible to determine whether the generally modest benefits of adjuvant therapy are different in subgroups defined by these cell biological factors. As a consequence, the immediate impact of the study of prognostic factors on choice of therapy is limited. Yet, the identification of prognostic factors may be of use in the design of clinical trials, the understanding of the biology of the disease, and for the design of new treatments based on a specific cell biological phenotype of a tumor. In the Daniel den Hoed Cancer Center (DDHCC) we have been studying prognostic factors in breast cancer for almost a decade, both in primary and in advanced disease. Our initial study involved 205 patients [1]. The examples of analysis in the present paper are based on the current database with 2,204 patients with a median follow up of 5.4 years, and a maximum follow up of 17 years. Of these patients 1,004 have relapsed, with actuarial 5 and 10 years disease free survival probabilities 57.6 and 43.8%. The main aim of the project is to study the relation between cell biological characteristics and the course of disease. Here we describe the statistical methods we use and the approaches we follow in our studies in primary breast cancer.

Patient selection

The DDHCC is a referral cancer center. The majority of the patients with breast cancer are referred from regional hospitals for adjuvant radiotherapy after primary surgery, especially after lumpectomy and/or in case of positive axillary nodes, or later for treatment for advanced disease. During the eighties most hospitals in the area sent tumor tissue to the laboratory of Biochemistry/Tumor Endocrinology for determination of cytosolic ER and PgR, which were performed according to methods recommended by the European Organization for Research and Treatment of Cancer (EORTC) [2]. Rest tissue and cytosol were stored in a tumor bank kept in liquid nitrogen.

The study population of primary patients is defined as patients with:
- primary diagnosis of breast cancer between 1978 and 1990 (at least 5 years of potential follow up);
- cytosol and/or rest tissue of the primary breast tumor, untreated, in the tumor bank;
- no metastatic disease at diagnosis;
- no previous diagnosis of carcinoma, except basal cell carcinoma of the skin and cervical cancer stage I;
- diagnosis and primary surgery for breast cancer at the DDHCC, or
- adjuvant primary treatment in the DDHCC within 3 months of surgery elsewhere;
- no evidence of disease within one month of primary surgery;
- data available in the DDHCC hospital charts.

In case of mastectomy after an initial lumpectomy because of residual disease, the mastectomy is considered as (part of) the primary treatment. Patients without primary surgery, *i.e.* inoperable T4 tumors, are excluded. Identification of patients is a two-step process. Potentially eligible patients are identified from the tumor bank database, in which for each sample is recorded: the amount of rest tissue and cytosol, the date of surgery, the hospital in which the primary surgery was performed, the type of tissue, and the DDHCC hospital registration number for patients referred to the DDHCC.

For all patients a limited amount of data is collected to describe the patient (date of birth, length, weight, menopausal status), the tumor and primary treatment (date of diagnosis; date and type of primary surgery; pTNM; number of positive nodes and number of nodes examined; which breast(s); multifocality; histology; differentiation grade; radiotherapy of breast, axilla and other regions; adjuvant chemotherapy and/or hormonal therapy), and follow up (first local, regional and distant relapse with date, location and treatment; incidence of secondary malignancy; survival status, date of last contact or death and cause of death).

Statistical methods

The analysis of the prognostic value of cell biological factors may be subdivided into three parts: description of the distribution of each of the factors separately, the analysis of associations between factors and the study of the relation between the factors and outcome. Many biological factors are measured on a continuous scale, expressed as amount per mg protein. The distribution of such factors is summarized by the median, quartiles, mean and standard deviation. Often a log transformation is applied in order to create more symmetrically distributed factors for regression analysis later on. For that purpose we also generate ordered categorical variables by subdivision in a limited number of classes of equal size, *e.g.* below and above the median, or quartiles. The number of classes depends on the number of patients in the study population. To prevent undue influence of outliers in a regression analysis we also generate shrinked copies of continuous covariates with long tails, by replacing values above the 95th- and below the 5th-percentile by these percentile values.

The second step is the analysis of the relation between factors. This analysis is important for a better understanding of the biological meaning of a factor, and also for an explanation of possible differences in outcomes of univariate and multivariate regression analyses. Associations are examined by the calculation of means and medians in subgroups, non-parametric tests, scatterplots and Spearman rank correlations. The size of an association is more important than its statistical significance. With large numbers (n>1,000) small correlations (*e.g.* $r_s \approx .10$) may be formally statistically significant (*i.e.* $P < 0.05$), while the size of the association and the scatterplot do not point into the direction of a meaningful association.

The third step is the analysis of the relation with outcome. The major endpoint in the primary breast cancer series is disease free survival (DFS) where patients with relapse count as failures. Patients who died without documented previous relapse, but with cause of death unknown are also counted as failures. The associations between factors and DFS are visualized in univariate analyses by actuarial survival curves, using a natural classification as for tumor size (T1-T4), or the ordered categorical subdivisions mentioned above. Cox regression analysis is used for univariate tests for trend or differences in DFS between groups. Such an analysis is in general purely exploratory, unless it tries to confirm the association between a factor and DFS described by others. Thus, inevitably, the exploration of the data requires different ways of assessment of the relation of a factor with outcome, *e.g.* subdivision in classes, and tests for trend using the original covariate, a log transform or shrinked versions of covariates. All these analyses produce different P-values, and it may be tempting to choose the smallest and regard this as statistical evidence for an association. There is no universally accepted solution for this multiplicity problem. We follow the approach that only when a statistically significant association is found in a robust test for trend based on a shrinked and symmetrically transformed covariate, further exploration of a cutpoint or a transformation is warranted. For this purpose we have used isotonic regression analysis [3]. An Example will be given in the next section. Factors that have shown an association in univariate analysis are included in multivariate analysis to see whether a factor adds prognostic information to well established prognostic factors as tumor size and nodal status, and to determine which factor retains statistical significance in the presence of others. Such an analysis may lead to a more refined prognostic index. Not only the factors that remain statistically significant are of biological relevance. Also loss of statistical significance in a multivariate analysis is useful information. This is generally due to an association of a factor with others, and this may help in a biological explanation of the association between the factors and the risk of relapse. In the past with smaller sample sizes our analyses often stopped at this point. Further analysis of variable transformations, interactions between covariates, analysis in subgroups and an analysis of the basic assumption of the proportional hazards model of Cox, *i.e.* the constant proportionality of the hazard rate over time, was generally not feasible due to the limited statistical power of such analyses, lack of the required software tools and the time consuming nature of these analyses. In recent years many papers have been published about model-fitting and model-checking applied to Cox regression analysis, *e.g.* [4-6]. Moreover, these types of advanced analyses can currently be performed with the statistical package Stata, which is the primary tool for our analyses. Stata contains modules for fractional polynomials analysis, for spline regression, for the calculation of residuals and for smoothing, all of which are useful for regression diagnostic purposes. In the next section we will give some examples of the application of the methods mentioned here.

Results - Examples

The classical prognostic factors tumor size and number of positive nodes show a strong association with DFS, comparable to other series, e.g. [7]. Adjusted for other prognostic factors the number of positive nodes is the strongest prognostic factor *(Figure 1)*. With one single positive node the hazard rate increases only slightly (RHR = 1.12), but with more positive nodes the relative hazard rate increases steadily up to 4.4 for patients with 10 or more nodes. The smooth curve with 95% confidence interval in *Figure 1*, generated by restricted cubic spline regression, follows the point estimates closely. Also tumor size is an important factor with a RHR for T2 of 1.4 and for T3/4 of 2.0, as compared to T1. The effect of age is more complicated. Cox regression with age as a linear covariate shows a statistically significant decreasing hazard rate with increasing age (P = .004). In this case spline regression is useful to check the linearity of the effect of age. The result in *Figure 2* shows that the risk does not further decrease above the age of 45-50 years. An analysis of the RHR in the four age-quartiles shows almost identical RHR's around 0.79 in the three higher quartiles compared to the first quartile with patients below the age of 47. However, the graph is still slightly misleading, while it suggests that the risk for relapse is the highest for the youngest patients, and decreases steadily up till the age of 45-50. Further analysis revealed that for patients younger than 40 years the risk of relapse is higher than for older patients, but within this young age group the risk seems constant. This is not picked up by the spline regression analysis, which may be sensitive to the choice of the knots. Although young age generally implies premenopausal status, the premenopausal status of the patient does not seem to be the explanation for this age effect. The unfavourable effect of young age (taken here as below 47) remains if the analysis is restricted to premenopausal patients, similar to what has been reported by de la Rochefordiere *et al.* [8]. Adjusted for T, number of nodes and age, also ER/PR status shows a prognostic effect with a RHR = 0.79 (P = 0.004) for ER or PR positive patients (*i.e.* ≥ 10 fmol/mg protein). A spline regression analysis of a log transformed ER (details not shown)

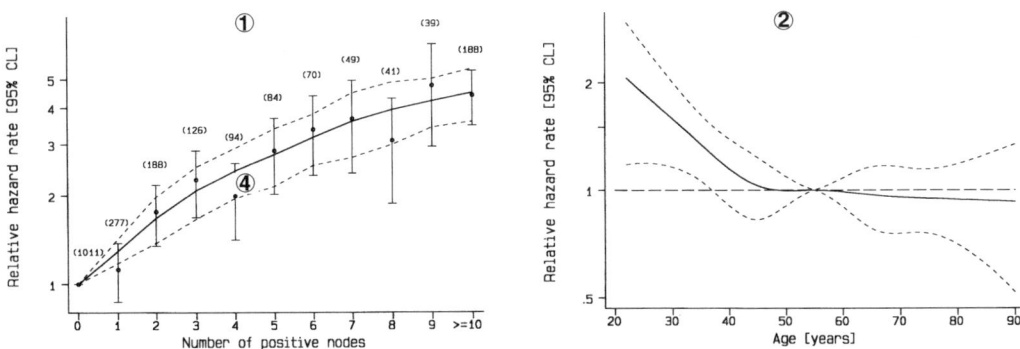

Figure 1. Relative hazard rates for numbers of positive nodes compared to node negative patients, adjusted for T stage, young age and ER/PR status. Cox regression analysis with endpoint relapse. Point estimates and spline regression analysis with 95% confidence region. Within brackets (number of patients).

Figure 2. Relative hazard rates for age with 55 years as reference age, adjusted for T stage, number of positive nodes and ER/PR status. Cox regression analysis with endpoint relapse. Spline regression analysis with 95% confidence region.

Table I. Multivariate Cox regression analysis.

		Relative hazard rates		
		Cathepsin-D	uPA	PAI-1
RHR[1,2]				
	Q2	1.20±0.12	1.36±0.14	1.30±0.13
	Q3	1.48±0.15	1.33±0.14	1.73±0.18
	Q4	1.40±0.14	2.17±0.21	2.13±0.21
Chisquare values 3				
	A[4]	38.84	62.70	79.76
	B[2]	21.79	64.05	74.97
	C[5]	0.53	15.86	25.08

[1] Relative hazard rates with respect to first quartile.
[2] Adjusted for T, number of nodes, young age and ER/PR status.
[3] Chisquare values for tests of trend for CD, uPA and log(PAI-1). All covariates shrinked and values of CD above 50 replace by 50.
[4] Univariate analysis not adjusted.
[5] In addition adjusted for the other two biochemical factors.

suggested a more complicated picture, with a decreasing hazard rate up till ER ≈ 75 fmol/mg protein, followed by an increase for higher values of ER, similar to a pattern found by Knorr et al. with logistic regression analysis [5]. However, the variation in the hazard rate among the ER positive patients was not statistically significant, and the main difference is between receptor negative and positive patients.

Adjusted for these classical prognostic factors the impact of three biochemical factors was analysed: Cathepsin-D (CD), uPA and PAI-1. *Table I* shows the estimated RHR for the quartiles and chisquare values of tests for trend in univariate and multivariate analyses. All three factors are highly statistically significant in univariate analysis, and they remain so after adjustment for the classical prognostic factors. The reduction in the chisquare value of CD from 38.8 to 21.8 could be due to the (weak) positive associations between CD and tumor size and number of positive nodes, while the further reduction and loss of prognostic impact after adjustment for uPA and PAI-1 is to be attributed to the correlation of CD with uPA ($r_s = 0.45$) and PAI-1 ($r_s = 0.39$). In contrast, the size of the chisquare values for uPA and PAI-1 hardly change after adjustment for tumor size, nodes and receptor status. This fits with the lack of an association of uPA and PAI-1 with these factors. The chisquare values for both uPA and PAI-1 are considerably lower after adjustment for the effect of one another. This can be explained by the strong correlation between these two factors ($r_s = 0.59$). However, both factors remain statistically highly significant, after adjustment for the other, despite this rather high correlation, higher than the correlation with CD. An explanation for this phenomenon should be found in a biological model.

The RHR's for the quartiles, adjusted for tumor size, nodes and ER/PR status, are easily calculated and useful for an assessment and comparison of the sizes of the effect and to give a first impression of the shape of the relation. For example: the RHR's for the fourth quartile compared with the first immediately show that the effects of uPA and PAI-1 are much larger than the effect of CD, which is also reflected in the chisquare values. The continuous increase of the RHR's for PAI-1 quartiles already suggests that the search for a cutpoint is useless. PAI-1 must be considered as a continuous covariate. The same, to a lesser degree, applies to uPA. This suggestion was supported by an analysis of residuals and by spline regression (details not shown). The values of the RHR's for CD suggest an increase in the hazard rate with increasing values of CD up to about the median, but no further increase with higher values of CD. This is also found by spline regression analysis and isotonic regression analysis *(Figure 3)*, both adjusted for tumor size, nodes and ER/PR status. It is clear from *Figure 3* that the association between CD and relapse rate is nonlinear with a steady increase for values of CD up to about 50, and no evidence of further increase with higher values. The choice of a cutpoint for CD to discriminate between negative and positive values would be rather arbitrary. It is better to consider CD as a continuous covariate, adjusting for the plateau by transforming or shrinking all values above 50 to 50.

The results of the analyses presented above only give an impression of the average strength of an association of a covariate with the hazard rate over time. There are several techniques to study the variation of the relative hazard rates over time. Here we follow the approach used by Gore [9]. About half of all relapses occurred within the first two years of follow up. Therefore we have performed a Cox regression analysis restricted to the first two years of follow up and another analysis restricted to the patients with a disease free survival longer than two years. The estimated RHR's for the covariates of both analyses are compared in *Figure 4*. A point below (above) the line y = x implies that the RHR after two years is less (higher) than corresponding RHR in the first two years. The unfavourable effect of positive nodes is slightly reduced after two years, but still very large. The reduction in the effect of tumor size is larger, but the effect remains statistically significant. The unfavourable effect of young age slightly increases, but this is not statistically significant. Positive ER/PR status shows a remarkable effect: during the first two years it is a favourable factor with a lower relapse rate RHR = 0.59 (P < 0.0001), while in the period after two years it is an unfavourable factor with a higher relapse rate RHR = 1.6 (P = 0.002). The effect of uPA remains the same in both periods, while the effect of PAI-1 is strongest during the first two years, and no longer significant after two years.

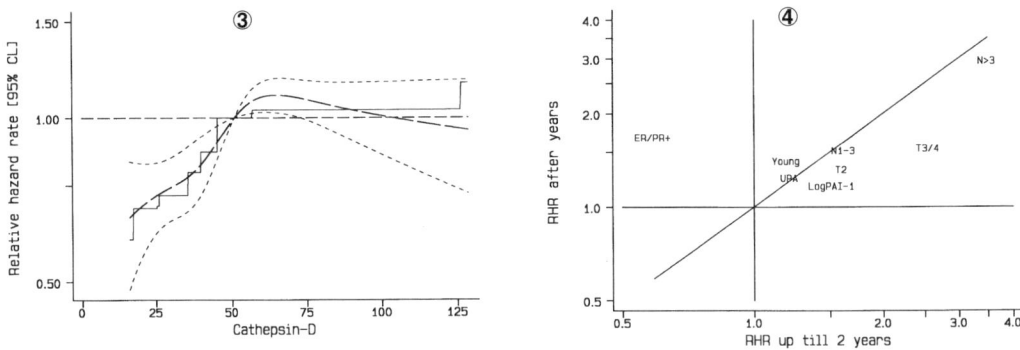

Figure 3. Relative hazard rates for Cathepsin-D with 50 as reference value, adjusted for T stage, number of positive nodes, young age and ER/PR status. Cox regression analysis with endpoint relapse. Spline regression analysis (smooth curve) with 95% confidence region and isotonic regression analysis (stepfunction).

Figure 4. Comparison of the relative hazard rates estimated by Cox regression analyses restricted to the relapses in the first two years (X-axis) and the relapses after two years (Y-axis). Abbreviations: N1-3, N > 3: 1-3 or more than 3 positive nodes compared to node negative; T2 and T3/4 compared to T1; Young: patients younger than 47 years compared to older patients; ER/PR+: receptor positive compared to receptor negative; uPA: continuous covariate in fmol/mg protein with 5% shrinkage of the tails; LogPAI-1: continuous covariate log(PAI-1) with 5% shrinkage of the tails.

Conclusion

The scope of this paper does not allow an extensive discussion of these results. Its main purpose is to show the methods that we use in our project. Until some years ago our life seemed simple: the analysis of a new potential prognostic factor was done with multivariate Cox regression analysis, supplemented in some cases by analyses in subgroups. We did not go into details about goodness of fit and validation of the model assumptions. We just have entered the era of model fitting, tests for interactions and regression diagnostics. Now we have to face a high dimensional world of complex interactions, violations of model assumptions, nonlinear relationships, a mixture of structure and random variation. The challenge for the future will be to retain simplicity for the prognostic classification of patients, while at the same time link the often complex interactions between covariates and the risk of relapse with underlying biological models.

References

1. Foekens JA, Portengen H, van Putten WLJ, Peters HA, Krijnen HLJM, Alexieva-Figusch J, Klijn JGM. Prognostic value of estrogen and progesterone receptors measured by enzyme immunoassays in human breast cancer cytosols. *Cancer Res* 1989; 49: 5823-8.
2. EORTC Breast Cancer Cooperative Group. Revision of the standards for the assessment of hormone receptors in human breast cancer. *Eur J Cancer* 1980; 16: 1513-5.
3. Barlow RE, Bartholomew DJ, Bremner JM, Brunk HD. *Statistical inference under order restrictions*. London: Wiley, 1972.
4. Gray RJ. Flexible methods for analyzing survival data using splines, with applications to breast cancer prognosis. *JASA* 1992; 87: 942-52.
5. Knorr KL, Hilsenbeck G, Wenger CR, Pounds G, Oldaker T, Vendely P, Pandian MR, Harrington D, Clark GM. Making the most of your prognostic factors: presenting a more accurate survival model for breast cancer patients. *Breast Cancer Res Treat* 1992; 22: 251-62.
6. Grambsch PM, Therneau TM. Proportional hazard tests and diagnostics based on weighted residuals. *Biometrika* 1994; 81: 515-26.
7. Nemoto T, Vana J, Bedwani RN, Baker HW, McGregor FW, Murphy GP. Management and survival of female breast cancer: Results of a National Survey by the American College of Surgeons. *Cancer* 1980; 45: 2917-24.
8. De la Rochefordiere A, Asselain B, Campana F, Scholl SM, Fenton J, Vilcoq JR, Durand JC, Pouillart P, Magdelenat H, Fourquet A. Age as prognostic factor in premenopausal breast carcinoma. *Lancet* 1993; 341: 1039-43.
9. Gore SMG, Pocock SJ, Kerr GR. Regression models and non-proportional hazards in the analysis of breast cancer survival. *Appl Stat* 1984; 33: 176-95.

Interpretation of data in prognostic studies

Gary M. Clark

Division of Medical Oncology, University of Texas Health Science Center, San Antonio 7703 Floyd Curl Drive, San Antonio, Texas 78284-7884, USA

The diagnosis of breast cancer presents several dilemmas for the patient and her physician. Among these is whether or not to use systemic adjuvant therapy following surgery. If so, which therapy is best for a particular patient? In order to address these questions, one must first determine the likelihood that the patient will have a recurrence of her disease in the future if no additional therapy is administered. Then, the efficacy of the available therapies must be estimated and weighed against the potential side effects to determine the probable benefit for this patient. Unfortunately, the clinical course of primary breast cancer varies considerably from patient to patient. Some patients have very long disease-free survival, while others experience a rapid deterioration with early recurrence of their breast cancer, followed shortly by death. Some of this variability is undoubtedly explained by differences in tumor growth rates, invasiveness, metastatic potential, and other mechanisms that we do not yet fully understand. It would obviously be useful to have biomarkers that measure these characteristics, either directly or indirectly, so that individual patients could be classified into subsets with varying risks of disease recurrence.

The role of prognostic factors in optimizing treatment for breast cancer patients has clearly changed with the trend toward general use of systemic adjuvant therapy. Several years ago, patients with axillary node-negative breast cancer were considered to have a relatively good prognosis and few received adjuvant therapy after local surgery. In 1985, an NCI Consensus Development Conference concluded that there was no standard therapy for patients with node-negative breast cancer [1]. It was recognized that some of these patients were destined to have early recurrences of their disease, but despite attempts by several groups to identify subsets of patients with an increased risk of disease recurrence and death using prognostic factors, a consensus could not be reached concerning the identity of such high-risk patients. However, with the publication of early results from several randomized clinical trials showing a benefit from adjuvant therapy for patients with node-negative breast cancer, and the publication of overview analyses by the Early Breast Cancer Trialists' Collaborative Group [2] many clinicians began to adopt the treatment strategy of administering systemic adjuvant therapy to all breast cancer patients regardless of their prognostic factors. A subsequent NCI Consensus Development Conference in 1991 [3] recognized that clinical outcomes varied among patients with primary breast cancer, but generally concluded that aside from the standard factors of nodal status, tumor size, and histopathologic subtype, none of the newer prognostic factors had been proven to have clinical utility. Thus, currently, the clinical role of prognostic factors for primary breast cancer remains unclear.

Clinical utility of prognostic factors

We have previously described three clinical situations where prognostic factors would be useful [4]. The first is to identify patients whose prognosis is so good following local surgery that the benefits of additional systemic adjuvant therapy would not out-weigh the toxicities. Since approximately 70% of node-negative patients and 25% of node-positive patients who receive only local surgery remain alive after 10 years, the strategy of administering adjuvant therapy to all breast cancer patients must surely result in needless toxicities and, in some cases, decreased quality of life. The issue is whether we can identify subsets of patients with extremely low risks of disease recurrence.

The second situation is to identify patients whose prognosis is so poor with conventional treatment that other forms of more aggressive therapy might be warranted. Despite improvements in adjuvant therapies, there are some patients who recur rapidly after diagnosis despite conventional adjuvant therapy who might be candidates for more aggressive regimens such as investigational, high-dose therapy followed by bone marrow or peripheral stem cell rescue.

But, the third, and perhaps the most useful types of prognostic markers are predictive factors that could indicate which patients are or are not likely to benefit from specific therapies. While it is useful to accurately predict the likely clinical outcome of a patient's breast cancer, we would also like to alter the natural history of the disease and prevent its recurrence. Therefore, biomarkers that are predictive of resistance or sensitivity to specific therapies would be extremely useful in the clinic.

Prognostic factor models

We have previously described models that identify patients with a *very high risk* of early death using only standard prognostic factors (number of positive lymph nodes, tumor size, ER, PgR, S-phase by flow cytometry) [4, 5]. These models have been validated in two different sets of patients. We first identified significant predictors of overall survival and created a prognostic index, and then we defined a cutpoint for the resulting index such that patients with a high index had the same survival as patients with 10 or more positive lymph nodes. The presence of 10 or more positive lymph nodes indicates a very poor prognosis and is a standard eligibility criterion for clinical trials of high dose therapy followed by bone marrow transplantation or peripheral blood stem cells. The number of patients in the validation sets with a high index was two-fold higher than the number of patients with 10 or more positive lymph nodes. In addition to identifying high risk patients with less than 10 positive nodes, the model also identified patients with many positive nodes whose survival with conventional adjuvant therapy was significantly better than that of the high index patients. Similar models identified high risk subsets comprising more than 40% of patients with 4 to 9 positive nodes whose survival was equivalent to that of patients with 10 or more positive nodes. Such patients would also be good candidates for trials of aggressive adjuvant therapy.

One criticism of these models is that S-phase fraction is an important component that is not universally available for patients with primary breast cancer. We have been leaders in the application of flow cytometry for measuring S-phase fractions in primary breast tumors, but we recognize that there are many technical issues with reproducibility between laboratories that have limited its clinical use. Therefore, we have begun to evaluate new markers of proliferation to see if S-phase fraction by flow cytometry can be replaced by more reliable factors which are easier to measure. One such marker, Ki67, is a monoclonal antibody that is specific for a resulting nuclear protein that is expressed only in proliferating cells (late G_1, S, M, and G_2 phases of the cell cycle). The Ki67 antibody developed by Gerdes and associates [6] can be used with fresh or frozen sections of breast tissue and can be detected by a rapid IHC assay. Newer antibodies, polyclonal Ki67 and monoclonal MIB1, have been raised against peptides from recombinant fragments of the gene for the Ki67 antigen and are effective in fixed, archival sections. In 674 tumors from our node-negative bank, Ki67 provided significant prognostic information in addition to that contained in tumor size and S-phase fraction [7].

Based on the results of ongoing studies, we may be able to replace S-phase fraction in these models with Ki67/MIB1 or other markers of proliferation that should be more easily and reliably measured, and expand our models to include particularly promising new markers to see if we can further improve the predictive accuracy of our prognostic indices.

Predicting response to adjuvant endocrine therapy

The ability of ER and PgR, determined by biochemical ligand binding assays, to predict response to endocrine therapies of patients with metastatic breast cancer, and to predict longer disease-free survival of patients with primary breast cancer who are treated with hormonal therapies has been validated in several studies, including our own [8, 9]. Because of the decreasing size of newly diagnosed breast cancer and the inability of biochemical assays to assess intratumoral heterogeneity, histochemical techniques have been proposed for determining steroid receptor levels. Indeed, these techniques are being adopted with increasing frequency. However, very few comparative studies with clinical follow-up have been performed, and appropriate cutpoints for predicting response to tamoxifen have not been established. It is likely, as a result, that many patients are being mistreated because optimal cutoffs for IHC have not been determined. Some patients are not receiving tamoxifen when they should, and others are receiving it when the benefit will be nil.

It has been hypothesized that the p53 tumor suppressor gene could alter a breast tumor's responsiveness to hormonal therapy and result in estrogen-independent growth. One possible mechanism might be through its role in apoptosis induced by anticancer agents. If p53 is mutated, it is possible that tamoxifen-induced apoptosis might be inhibited. Also, p53 mutations can alter growth factor interactions potentially important in the therapeutic response to tamoxifen. Finally, p53 negatively regulates cell proliferation and entry of cells into the S-phase. Since ER also influences cell proliferation and transit through the cell cycle, it is possible that mutated p53 might alter the ability of ER to control the cell cycle so that the cell would no longer be responsive to tamoxifen. To address these issues, we determined p53 status by IHC in 205 paraffin-embedded blocks of tumors from patients entered onto a prospective trial. All patients had metastatic, ER-positive breast cancer, and were treated with tamoxifen. Although response to tamoxifen and time to treatment failure in this small pilot study were not associated with p53 status, patients with higher p53 did have worse survival. Thus, p53 and its related family members are attractive candidates for predictive markers for tamoxifen resistance.

The bcl-2 gene can block apoptosis induced by a wide range of insults and stimuli [10]. It is trans-regulated by p53 and by estrogen and has been shown in preclinical experimental systems to be involved in resistance to a variety of cytotoxic agents. It is possible that it may also interfere with response to tamoxifen. We evaluated the prognostic significance of bcl-2 expression determined by IHC in node-positive breast tumors, and surprisingly, found that high levels of expression were correlated with several good prognostic factors, and with *prolonged disease-free survival* in univariate analyses [11]. We also examined bcl-2 expression in specimens from a clinical trial of metastatic breast cancer. Higher levels of bcl-2 were associated with higher levels of ER, *better* response to tamoxifen, *longer* time to treatment failure, and *better* survival. In multivariate analyses that included other factors such as p53, ER and PgR levels, bcl-2 remained significantly associated with longer time to treatment failure and survival. These results are consistent with other studies that have found strong associations between high levels of bcl-2 and favorable clinical outcome, but not with apoptosis [12]. This paradox is an excellent example of how hypotheses developed from *in vitro* data may need to be revised when studied in clinical specimens.

Bax is a homologue of bcl-2 that functions as a *promoter* of apoptosis rather than a *blocker*, and it may be upregulated by p53 [13]. Analysis of several types of tumors, including breast and ovarian cancers, revealed marked reductions in bax protein levels in a significant proportion of cases, sometimes in association with p53 mutations and/or development of drug resistance [10]. Therefore, by studying p53, bcl-2, and bax by IHC in the same tumors, it might be possible to identify patients who might be particularly resistant or sensitive to adjuvant tamoxifen. It may well be that the ratio of these markers will determine whether a cell undergoes treatment-induced apoptosis.

Direct preclinical and clinical evidence indicates that HER-2/neu and EGFR may also be predictors of resistance to hormonal therapies. In animal models, transfection of breast tumor cells with HER-2/neu resulted in resistance to tamoxifen [14], and the effect of HER-2/neu overexpression on resistance to tamoxifen has been demonstrated in patients with metastatic breast cancer [15]. Several groups have shown that metastatic tumors expressing EGFR are more likely to be resistant to endocrine therapy. Conversely, EGFR-negative tumors, especially if they are also ER-positive, tend to have high response rates.

Predicting response to adjuvant chemotherapy

Several factors, including p53, bcl-2, and bax are involved in regulating apoptosis, and all have been linked, at least in experimental systems, to resistance to a variety of cytotoxic agents. We have studied p53 by IHC using 564 paraffin-embedded blocks from an ECOG-coordinated Intergroup trial to determine if abnormal p53 was associated with response or lack of response to adjuvant CMFP chemotherapy [16]. Although p53 status was not a significant prognostic factor for either the untreated control group or the treated group, there was a trend for patients with normal p53 to receive greater benefit from chemotherapy. Reduced expression of bax has been associated with poor response rates to combination chemotherapy and shorter survival in women with metastatic breast cancer [13], and overexpression of bcl-2 was reported to be predictive of efficacy of adjuvant chemotherapy [17]. However, there is *in vitro* evidence that overexpression of bcl-2 results in resistance to chemotherapy, and that overexpression of bcl-x_s, the short form of bcl-x, sensitizes cells to apoptosis induced by chemotherapy [18]. Recently, additional proteins that inhibit apoptosis (bcl-x_L, Bag-1, Mcl-1) or promote apoptosis (Bad, myc) have been described [13, 18]. If antibodies suitable for IHC studies become available, these proteins will be candidates for additional predictive factor studies.

There may be a relationship between HER-2/neu overexpression and resistance to adjuvant CMF-based chemotherapy. Using IHC on paraffin blocks from an ECOG-coordinated Intergroup trial, patients whose tumors expressed normal levels of HER-2/neu had improved disease-free and overall survival when treated with adjuvant CMFP chemotherapy compared to controls [19]. However, patients whose tumors overexpressed HER-2/neu did not respond to CMFP. Subsequently, other groups have reported similar findings [20, 21], although the results may be different if Adriamycin-containing regimens are used [22]. If we can confirm that HER-2/neu overexpression predicts for resistance to CMF then the thousands of patients treated each year with this regimen can instead be treated with Adriamycin-based regimens which should be more effective, thereby sparing many recurrences and deaths.

Factor integration

The final objective of all of these analyses is to predict clinical outcomes for individual patients with breast cancer. These predictions should be accurate and reliable, and easy to interpret by physicians and patients. A major question is how to best present these results.

We have developed an interactive computer program that allows health care professionals to estimate outcomes for breast cancer patients in scenarios with and without adjuvant therapy [23]. Estimates of patient outcomes in terms of overall and breast cancer specific mortality are computed based on the patient's age, estimated risk of breast cancer related mortality at 5 years, a selected model of reduction in annual risk of mortality over time, and the proportional mortality risk reduction expected with a given adjuvant therapy. Help features provide data for breast cancer specific mortality estimates based on tumor size and number of involved nodes from the SEER data base and the Early Breast Cancer Trialists' Collaborative Group meta-analysis estimates of the efficacies of adjuvant chemotherapy and hormonal therapy in different groups of patients [2]. We now need to enhance this program by including more refined estimates of recurrence, mortality, and expected treatment benefits based on the patient's prognostic and predictive factors. This is now one of the primary focuses in our research laboratories.

References

1. Breast Cancer Chemotherapy - Consensus Conference. Adjuvant chemotherapy for breast cancer. *JAMA* 1985; 254: 3461-3.
2. Early Breast Cancer Trialists' Collaborative Group. Systemic treatment of early breast cancer by hormonal, cytotoxic, or immune therapy. *Lancet* 1992; 339: 1-15, 71-85.
3. National Institutes of Health Consensus Development Panel. Consensus statement: Treatment of early-stage breast cancer. *J Natl Cancer Inst Monographs* 1992; 11: 1-5.
4. Clark GM. Do we really need prognostic factors for breast cancer? *Breast Cancer Res Treat* 1994; 30: 117-26.

5. Clark G, Hilsenbeck S, Ravdin P, Osborne C. Validation of a model that identifies high risk breast cancer patients for clinical trials of intensive therapy. *Proc Am Soc Clin Oncol* 1995; 14: 92 (Abstract).
6. Gerdes J, Schwab U, Lemke H, Stein H. Production of mouse-monoclonal antibody reactive with a human nuclear antigen associated with cell proliferation. *Int J Cancer* 1983; 31: 13-20.
7. Brown RW, Allred DC, Clark GM, Osborne CK, Hilsenbeck SG. Prognostic value of Ki-67 compared to S-phase fraction in axillary node-negative breast cancer. *Clin Cancer Res* 1996; 2: 585-92.
8. Ravdin PM, Green S, Dorr TM, McGuire WL, Fabian C, Pugh RP, Carter RD, Rivkin SE, Borst JR, Belt RJ, Metch B, Osborne CK. Prognostic significance of progesterone receptor levels in estrogen receptor-positive patients with metastatic breast cancer treated with tamoxifen: results of a prospective Southwest Oncology Group study. *J Clin Oncol* 1992; 10: 1284-91.
9. Clark GM, McGuire WL, Hubay CA, Pearson OH, Marshall JS. Progesterone receptor as a prognostic factor in Stage II breast cancer. *N Engl J Med* 1983; 309: 1343-7.
10. Reed JC. Bcl-2 and chemoresistance in cancer. *ASCO Educational Book* 1995; 408-10.
11. Berardo M, de Moor CA, Clark GM, Osborne CK, Allred DC. Bcl-2 expression in node-positive breast cancer. *Breast Cancer Res Treat* 1995; 37 (Supplement): 37 (Abstract 17).
12. Joensuu H, Pylkkanen L, Toikkanen S. Bcl-2 protein expression and long-term survival in breast cancer. *Am J Pathol* 1994; 145: 1191-8.
13. Krajewski S, Blomqvist C, Franssila K, Krajewska M, Wasenius V-M, Niskanen E, Nordling S, Reed JC. Reduced expression of proapoptotic gene BAX is associated with poor response rates to combination chemotherapy and shorter survival in women with metastatic breast adenocarcinoma. *Cancer Res* 1995; 55: 4471-8.
14. Benz CC, Scott GK, Sarup JC, Johnson RM, Tripathy D, Coronado E, Shepard HM, Osborne CK. Estrogen-dependent, tamoxifen-resistant tumorigenic growth of MCF-7 cells transfected with HER2/neu. *Breast Cancer Res Treat* 1992; 24: 85-95.
15. Wright C, Nicholson S, Angus B, Sainsbury JRC, Farndon J, Cairns J, Harris AL, Horne CHW. Relationship between c-erbB-2 protein product expression and response to endocrine therapy in advanced breast cancer. *Br J Cancer* 1992; 65: 118-21.
16. Elledge RM, Gray R, Mansour E, Yu Y, Clark GM, Ravdin P, Osborne CK, Gilchrist K, Davidson NE, Robert N, Tormey DC, Allred DC. Accumulation of p53 protein as a possible predictor of response to adjuvant combination chemotherapy with cyclophosphamide, methotrexate, fluorouracil, and prednisone for breast cancer. *J Natl Cancer Inst* 1995; 87: 1254-6.
17. Gasparini G, Barbareschi M, Doglioni C, Palma PD, Mauri FA, Boracchi P, Bevilacqua P, Caffo O, Morelli L, Verderio P, Pezzella F, Harris AL. Expression of bcl-2 protein predicts efficacy of adjuvant treatments in operable node-positive breast cancer. *Clin Cancer Res* 1995; 1: 189-98.
18. Sumantran VN, Ealovega MW, Nuñez G, Clarke MG, Wicha MS. Overexpression of Bcl-x_s sensitizes MCF-7 cells to chemotherapy-induced apoptosis. *Cancer Res* 1995; 55: 2507-510.
19. Allred DC, Clark GM, Tandon AK, Molina R, Tormey DC, Osborne CK, Gilchrist KW, Mansour EG, Abeloff M, Eudey L, McGuire WL. HER-2/neu in node-negative breast cancer: prognostic significance of overexpression influenced by the presence of in situ carcinoma. *J Clin Oncol* 1992; 10: 599-605.
20. Gusterson BA, Gelber RD, Goldhirsch A, Price KN, Säve-Söderborgh J, Anbazhagan R, Styles J, Rudenstam CM, Golouh R, Reed R, Martinez-Tello F, Tiltman A, Torhorst J, Grigolato P, Bettelheim R, Neville AM, Bürki K, Castiglione M, Collins J, Lindtner J, Senn H-J. Prognostic importance of c-erbB-2 expression in breast cancer. International (Ludwig) Breast Cancer Study Group. *J Clin Oncol* 1992; 10: 1049-56.
21. Têtu B, Brisson J. Prognostic significance of HER-2/neu oncoprotein expression in node-positive breast cancer. The influence of the pattern of immunostaining and adjuvant therapy. *Cancer* 1994; 73: 2359-65.
22. Muss HB, Thor AD, Berry DA, Kute T, Liu ET, Koerner F, Cirrincione CT, Budman DR, Wood WC, Barcos M, Henderson IC. c-erbB-2 expression and response to adjuvant therapy in women with node-positive early breast cancer. *N Engl J Med* 1994; 330: 1260-6.
23. Ravdin PM, Clark GM, Hilsenbeck SG, Osborne CK. A personal computer based program for providing outcome estimates and cooperative group trial eligibility information for adjuvant therapy. *Proc Am Soc Clin Oncol* 1995; 14: 96 (Abstract 82).

3
Therapy

Clinical circumvention of antioestrogen resistance

Anthony Howell and Elizabeth Anderson

CRC Department of Medical Oncology, University of Manchester, and Department of Tumour Biochemistry, Christie Hospital, Manchester, UK M20 4BX

The importance of endocrine therapy for treatment of patients with advanced breast cancer has been known since Beatson published his classical paper reporting responses to oophorectomy one hundred years ago [1]. Since that time we have realised that responders to treatment have a median survival of approximately three years whereas the median survival for nonresponders is approximately fourteen months [2]. Some patients may have remissions lasting several years but eventually all become resistant to the series of endocrine therapies we have available currently. The response rates to endocrine therapy and durations of remission have not improved appreciably since Beatson's time.

Our understanding of the mechanisms of response to treatment and of resistance has been significantly increased by the discovery of the oestrogen receptor (ER) [3], by new insights into the mechanism of gene transcription by the oestrogen/ER complex [4] and, more recently, by the discovery of « cross talk », between steroid receptors and growth factor pathways within the breast tumour cells [5]. The purpose of this chapter is to outline our current understanding of the mechanisms of response and resistance to endocrine therapy and to discuss how this might lead to new approaches to the circumvention of the antioestrogen resistance that we see in the clinic every day.

We will argue that all endocrine therapies are essentially « antioestrogenic » and thus circumvention of resistance to all types of endocrine therapy in common use will have to be considered. First however, we will consider our current knowledge of the endocrine control of the normal and malignant breast proliferation since it is the understanding of these mechanisms together with clinical information that may give us new insights into methods of avoiding « antioestrogen » resistance.

Oestrogen control of normal and malignant breast growth

When the pituitary gland is intact, there is strong evidence to suggest that E2 is the major mitogenic steroid for both the normal breast and for breast tumours [6, 7]. The effects of E2 are mediated by the oestrogen receptor (ER) which we know is a ligand-dependant nuclear transcription factor. Binding of E2 to the ER induces formation of an ER dimer which in turn binds to a short palindromic DNA sequence (the oestrogen response element or ERE) situated in the vicinity of E2 regulated genes. The ER has two transcriptional activating functions (AF's). It is thought that the first AF (AF-1) is activated merely by the binding of the ER to the ERE and it is, therefore not ligand dependent. In contrast the second AF (AF-2) appears to be strictly ligand dependent as it can only interact with the proteins that mediate its action when the ER is occupied by its physiological ligand (E2 [4, 8]

All endocrine therapies are anti-oestrogenic

It may be argued that all endocrine therapies are essentially anti-oestrogenic. This supposition is undisputed in the case of treatment with ovarian ablation, aromatase inhibitors, the steroidal and non-steroidal antioestrogens. However, progestogens may also be regarded as anti-oestrogenic in that they down-regulate the ER and suppress serum E2 levels by up to 70%. Therefore the progestagens have not one but two mechanisms of opposing oestrogen action [9, 10].

Growth factors interact with oestrogen

Although oestrogen is apparently the major mitogenic steroid for the normal and malignant breast it is clear that it acts in concert with growth factors produced by epithelial cells or by local stromal cells. Synergistic and additive effects between E2 and growth factors in MCF-7 human mammary tumour cells was reported by Westley *et al.* [11]. In these studies there was a synergistic effect on growth between E2 and insulin - like growth factor-1 (IGF1) or basic fibroblast growth factor (bFGF) and an additive effect between E and transforming growth factor alpha (TGF alpha).
Later it became clear that the interaction between E2 and growth factors occured at the level of the ER since growth factor action could be inhibited by antioestrogens [12]. [Oestrogen initiates gene transcription by binding to the hormone binding domain of ER and inducing the activity of two activating factors (AF1 and AF2) *(Figure 1)*] In particular there is evidence that growth factors activate AF1 on the receptor. Knowledge of receptor function is important for our understanding of the mechanism of action of the two classes of antioestrogens. Tamoxifen inhibits ER activity at AF2 but stimulates at AF1 [4, 8]. Thus if a tumour becomes resistant to the inhibitory effect of tamoxifen on AF2 it might stimulate growth *via* AF1. Stimulation by tamoxifen may be synergistic with growth factors acting via AF1. The specific ('pure') antioestrogens are known to inhibit both AF1 and AF2 and is the likely reason that they are active against tamoxifen resistant tumours [13, 14].

Sensitivity of tumours to changes in oestradiol concentration

Endocrine therapy is standard therapy after surgery for breast cancer, for advanced disease and is in clinical trial for disease prevention in high risk groups. Approximately half of patients with advanced disease respond to treatment and a proportion will respond to a second, third or even fourth endocrine treatment *(Figure 2)*. A major paradox of endocrine therapy is how these multiple responses are obtained if, as we have argued, all treatments are basically « antioestrogenic ». The answer to this question is likely to provide important new insights into ways of circumventing endocrine resistance and into general breast tumour biology.

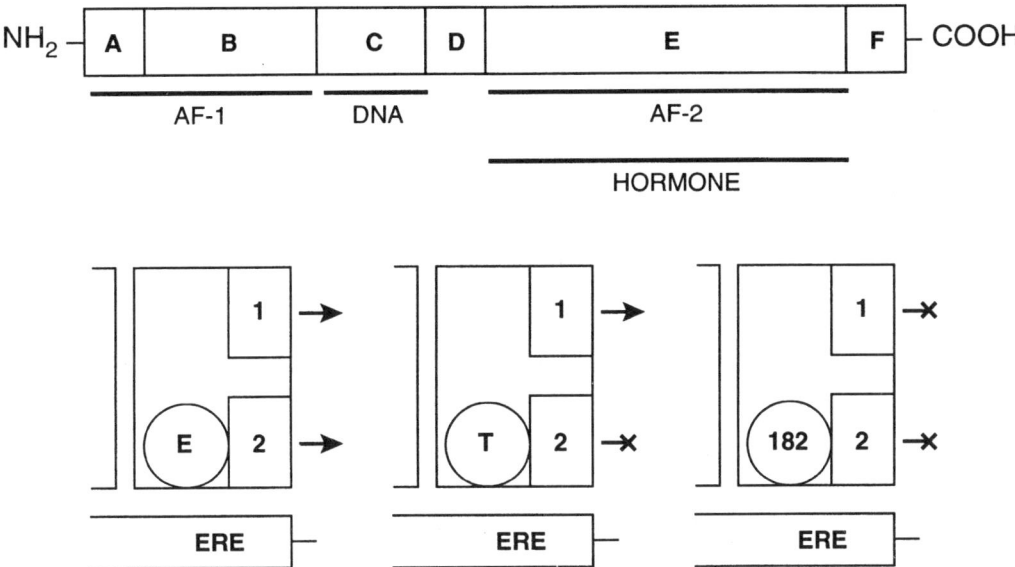

Figure 1. The domains of the oestrogen receptor (above) and the effect of oestrogen (E), tamoxifen (T) and the specific antioestrogen ICI 182780 (182) on gene transcription *via* the two activating factors AF1 and AF2. Oestradiol stimulates *via* AF1 and AF2, tamoxifen inhibits activity of AF2 only, and ICI 182780 inhibits both AF1 and AF2.

Why does a tumour respond to two sequential treatments both of which are anti-oestrogenic eg oophorectomy, followed by tamoxifen or an aromatase inhibitor? After oophorectomy there is little evidence that serum E2 levels rise with time, thus the tumour appears to become sensitive to the lower levels of E2 present after removal of the ovaries. In this case a tumour might be expected to respond to further lowering E2 levels with an aromatase inhibitor or to blocking the growth stimulatory effect of the low level of E2 with tamoxifen. The suggestion that tumour cells may 'adapt' to lowered oestradiol concentrations is supported by reported responses to the sequential use of increasingly more potent aromatase inhibitors [15, 16].

What is the evidence that a change in sensitivity of the tumour to E2 can occur? An elegant demonstration of the ability of the MCF-7 cell line to alter sensitivity to oestradiol was reported by Santen *et al.* [17]. Under standard serum containing culture conditions the MCF-7 cells were maximally stimulated by 10-8 M E2 whereas when the cells were retested for responsiveness after a period in oestrogen free conditions maximal stimulation was seen at an E2 concentration of 10-14 M. In addition, the sensitive cells produced more tumours when transplanted into oestrogen treated nude mice. The ER content of the oestrogen deprived cells was four times higher than that of the wild type cells which does not appear to account for the 10,000 fold difference in concentration of oestradiol required to maximally stimulate proliferation. Whatever the mechanism of increased sensitivity of tumour cells to E2 there is a major question which needs to be answered in order to design ways to circumvent this type of resistance. This question is whether it was an adaptive response in all tumour cells or whether there was a pre-existing clone of cells in the original tumour which were sensitive to low levels of oestradiol and which gradually grew out after those requiring higher concentrations were growth inhibited by low levels of E2. Such a clonal selection hypothesis would require that the highly sensitive clone was inhibited by standard oestrogen concentrations in postmenopausal women which is plausible given the bell-shaped dose response to oestradiol shown in the diagram taken from Santen's work.

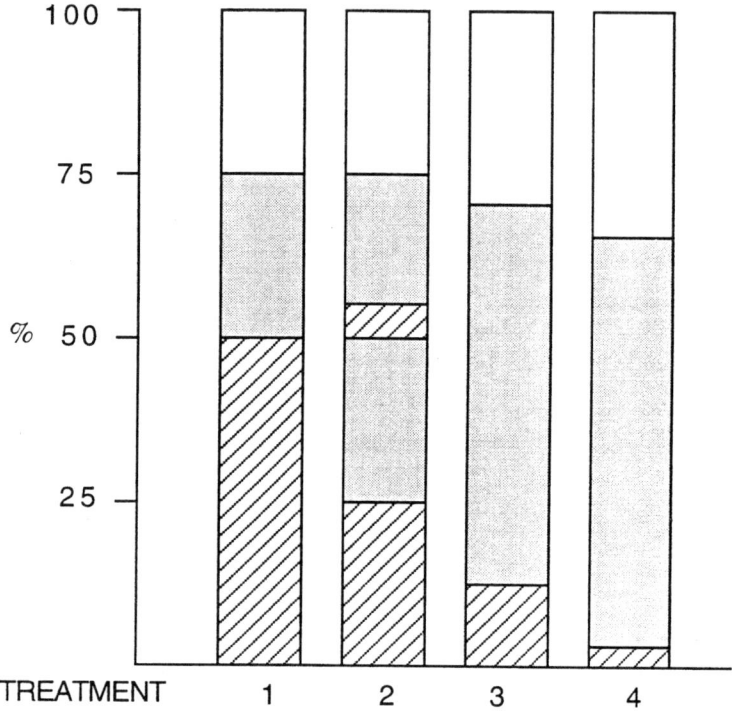

Figure 2. Effect of sequential endocrine therapy in relation to oestrogen receptor (ER) status of the tumour in advanced breast cancer. Although several responses may be obtained the proportion of responders diminishes with each treatment.

▨ ER+ responders   ▨ ER+ non-responders   ☐ ER-ve non-responders

A small proportion of ostensibly ER-ve tumours repond but are not represented here. They are probably ER+ve but below the sensitivity level of assays used. Note that secondary resistant tumours would usually be offered chemotherapy.

These considerations lead to the first suggestion for circumventing 'antioestrogen' resistance. We now have available in the clinic a series of aromatase inhibitors of differing potencies with respect to their ability to lower serum E2 levels. It should be possible to devise clinical experiments where E2 levels are sequentially reduced with the aim of comparing this approach to the maximal immediate suppression which we do at present by using the highly potent new imidazole compounds [18].

Tamoxifen resistance

Tamoxifen has become the treatment of first choice for adjuvant therapy and for advanced disease since it was first introduced into the clinic in 1969 [19]. In advanced disease approximately half of patients respond to therapy for a median duration of approximately eighteen months. After tamoxifen failure, approximately half of the responders and 10% of the non-responders will respond to a second form of endocrine therapy *(Figure 2)*. Thus tumours fall into two groups, those which are totally endocrine resistant after tamoxifen therapy and those that are resistant to tamoxifen but are still sensitive to alternative endocrine therapies. Two major types of mechanism have been postulated to account for tamoxifen resistance in tumours which are responsive to second therapies. Either tamoxifen itself or one of its metabolites may stimulate growth or tamoxifen may be sequestered away from the ER thus allowing endogenous E2 to restimulate growth.

Stimulation of tumour growth by tamoxifen

Direct evidence for stimulation of human mammary growth by tamoxifen is derived from studies on patients who progress whilst being treated with tamoxifen but respond when treatment is withdrawn [20 for review]. The demonstration of tumour agonism is particularly compelling in studies on nude mice, transplanted with MCF-7 tumours and treated with tamoxifen where growth is inhibited for a few months by the antioestrogen. If the tumours which grow out are retransplanted to other mice, tamoxifen can be shown to stimulate growth since growth is stopped by withdrawing tamoxifen or treating the mice with the specific 'pure' antioestrogen ICI164384 [21]. The latter result is particularly important since it suggests that tamoxifen is no longer acting by inhibiting growth *via* AF2 but only acting via AF1 where it is known to have an agonist effect [4,8]. The specific antioestrogens act by inhibiting both ER-activating functions.
Tamoxifen may also gain agonist properties by intracellular conversion to oestrogenic metabolites [22]. However this conversion is thought to be unlikely since fixed ring structures of tamoxifen, which are unable to be metabolised, are capable of stimulating MCF-7 cell-growth [23].

Tamoxifen « sequestration »

A second potential mechanism for tamoxifen failure is sequestration of the drug away from the ER. Tamoxifen may be bound to intracellular proteins [24] or be excreted from the tumour cell [25, 26]. This would result in there being insufficient intracellular tamoxifen to compete with circulating E2 which in turn could restimulate tumour growth *via* the 'vacated' rececptor. The relative importance of the two postulated mechanisms of tamoxifen failure, agonism and sequestration, is not known but the clinical data indicate that withdrawal responses occur in only 10-20% of patients [20] which suggests that sequestration may be the most common mechanism of treatment failure. However data from two trials where patients were treated with oophorectomy after tamoxifen failure suggest tamoxifen agonism certainly does occur. In one study there were responses to oophorectomy [27] whereas in a second study, rather surprisingly, none of the patients responded [28]. In the first study tamoxifen was stopped at treatment failure whereas, in the second, treatment with tamoxifen was continued after operation, suggesting that tamoxifen treatment abrogated the effect of oophorectomy, possibly *via* an agonist effect on tumour growth.

As argued in the previous section concerning changes in sensitivity to oestradiol, it is not known whether resistance to tamoxifen occurs as an adaptive response in all the tumour cells or whether a clone of resistant cells already present within the primary tumour is selected which grows when the tamoxifen sensitive cells are inhibited [29].

Complete resistance to endocrine therapy in ER+ve tumours

Oestrogen receptor positive tumours may fail to respond to endocrine therapy de-novo or become completely resistant after treatment with one or more types of endocrine therapy. Usually the ER is still present [30] indicating that receptor loss is not a common mechanism of this type of resistance. It is possible that tumour cells with defective receptors are selected out by treatment and it has been reported that some mutations in the ER result in tamoxifen agonism in *in vitro* experiments. [31]. However, to date, mutations of this type have rarely been detected in the ER of primary tumours although few have been assessed at the time of treatment failure [32]. It is also possible that splice variants of the ER might arise, for example, deletion of exon 5 which gives the ER the capacity to switch on gene transcription without binding hormone or anti-hormone (dominant positive effect) [33]. However a search for such ER splice variants has failed to establish this as a major mechanism for endocrine failure [34]. Since growth factor pathways are known to inter act with the ER, a major mechanism of endocrine failure may be stimulation of tumour growth through these pathways which would be unresponsive to the mediating effects of 'antioestrogen' treatment. This is an active and highly important area of current research [35, 36].

Clinical circumvention of 'antioestrogen' resistance

A variety of actual and potential mechanisms of resistance to oestrogen deprivation have been outlined above and there are probably others waiting to be discovered. However the insights that we already have can lead to design of strategies for circumventing resistance. Some of these are already being explored in clinical trials, others may be explored in the future.

Delaying resistance by alternating therapies

In advanced breast cancer the current endocrine therapies are not curative and any treatment which could delay the onset of resistance would have a therapeutic advantage. Such a strategy may extend the period advanced breast cancer patients spend in remission, alleviate symptoms, and possibly extend survival. The question is: how can we prevent the emergence of the mechanisms of endocrine resistance outlined above? How can we delay the onset of partial and complete resistance. If we assume that endocrine therapy selects for endocrine resistance almost as soon as a response has been obtained it may be logical to stop therapy at this time in order to prevent the emergence of resistant tumour cells. However the tumour may be then stimulated by endogenous oestradiol to the detriment of the patient and therefore one approach may be to alternate an agent such as tamoxifen with no treatment at, say, three monthly intervals. If the tumour consists of tamoxifen stimulated and tamoxifen inhibited clones the proportions of these types of cell might reciprocally rise and fall but stability of tumour size would be maintained. [29]. We prefer to obtain 'responses' to treatment (partial or complete remissions) but it is quite possible that we should accept a situation where the tumour remains stable. This would test the hypothesis and may result in longer periods of effectiveness of endocrine therapy for the benefit of the patient. We and others have shown that stablisation of disease (or 'no change'), is associated with equivalent durations of response and overall survival compared with patients who show objective partial remissions [37]. Do we have any data to support the alternating on or off treatment approach? A trial is currently in progress under the auspices of the EORTC comparing continuous tamoxifen with a three month on three month off strategy; the results of this study are soon to be reported and will be of great mportance to our approaches to therapy.

We have reported two patients who responded to tamoxifen, who both had a withdrawal response when treatment was stopped at progression and who both then had a further, albeit brief, response to the reintroduction of tamoxifen when they progressed after their response to withdrawal [20]. This is not alternating therapy as in the scheme outlined above but it does perhaps give an indication that this approach may be effective in endocrine responsive tumours. Alternating on/off approaches may now be able to be tested with relative ease with the new potent aromatase inhibitors that have no action on the adrenal gland, low toxicity and a relatively short half life such as the recently introduced imidazole derivative, anastrazole. Both adaptive or clonal mechanisms for intermediate endocrine resistance, should be delayed if treament is changed before they become « fixed » by prolonged continuous therapy.

An alternative approach to intermittent therapy is to use two drugs and various methods of alternating tamoxifen and progestagens (megestrol acetate or medroxyprogesterone acetate) have been attempted with mixed results [38]. Interpretation of these studies is difficult because of the difficulty of obtaining true alternation of therapy because of the long serum half lives of the agents used to date. Now the alternating therapy hypothesis can be truly tested because these are effective triphenylethylene antioestrogens, draloxifene [39], and potent aromatase inhibitors which are quickly eliminated [18].

Delaying resistance by stepwise reduction of oestradiol levels

The responses to sequential aromatase inhibitors reported by several groups suggest another approach to delaying resistance to oestrogen suppression. It is rather surprising that the recently introduced highly potent imidazole aromatase inhibitors introduced recently do not appear to give superior response rates compared to less oestradiol suppressive inhibitors such as aminoglutethimide [39]. A working hypothessis to explain these observations is that tumours respond to small changes in serum oestradiol but large changes produce no additional affect.

Stepwise reduction of oestradiol levels using progressively more potent aromatase inhibitors in sequence may give the tumour an oppportunity to respond two or three times [15, 16].

Delaying resistance by using inhibitors of both AF1 and AF2 of the ER

Tamoxifen is thought to inhibit growth by inhibiting AF2 of the oestrogen receptor. As indicated above one mechanism of resistance to tamoxifen is presumed to be the development of ER with AF2 unresponsive to tamoxifen leaving its agonist effect on AF1 resulting in promotion of tumour growth. The specific or 'pure' antioestrogens such as ICI 182780 are known to block both AF1 and AF2. Of interest is the demonstration of prolonged remissions with ICI 182780 treatment after failure of treatment with tamoxifen [14]. Prolonged remissions of MCF-7 tumours in nude mice have been reported with first line ICI 182780 treatment [40] and we await the initiation of trials of this agent as first line therapy in patients with advanced breast cancer.

Restablishment of crosstalk *via* ER

One general probable mechanism for the total loss of endocrine sensitivity in receptor positive tumours, as we have argued above, is loss of control by steroids of the crosstalk between steroids and growth factors via the ER which appears to be the major mechanism for the control of growth in the breast. It is impossible to intervene in this area at present since we do not have a detailed enough knowledge about the mechanism of loss of control. However it is important for clinicians to be aware of the rapid developments in this area in order to respond to any new insights as to how the breakdown in crosstalk may be prevented or if it has occurred how it may be reestablished. Pharmacological inhibition of growth factor pathways with agents such as tyrosine kinase inhibitors is already being explored [41]. It may be possible, for example, to delay the onset of loss of crosstalk using such agents or they may be effective after it has occurred.

References

1. Beatson GT. On the treatment of inoperable cases of carcinoma of the mamma. Suggestions for a new method of treatment with illustrative cases. *Lancet* ii 1896; 104-7.
2. Howell A, DeFriend D, Anderson E. Mechanisms of response and resistance to endocrine therapy for breast cancer and the development of new treatments. *Rev End Rel Cancer* 1993; 43: 5-21.
3. Jensen EU, Desombre ER. Mechanism od action of the female sex hormones. *Ann Rev Biochem* 1972; 41: 203-8.
4. Tora L, White J, Brou C, Tasset D, Webster N, Scheer E and Chambon P. The human estrogen receptor has two independent nonacid transcriptional activation functions. *Cell* 1989; 59: 477-7.
5. Ignar-Trowbridge DM, Nelson KG, Bidwell MC, Curtis SW, Washburn TF, McLachlan JA and Korach KS. Coupling of duel signalling pathways: epidermal growth factor action involves the oestrogen receptor. *Proc Natl Acad Sci USA* 1992; 89: 4658-62.

6. Pearson O and Bronson SR. Results of hypophysectomy in the treatment of metastatic mammary carcinoma. *Cancer* 1959; 12: 85-92.
7. Laidlaw I, Anderson E, Clarke R, Potten CS and Howell A. The proliferation of normal human breast tissue implanted into athymic nude mice is stimulated by oestrogen but not progesterone. *Endocrinology* 1995; 136: 164-71.
8. McDonnell DP, Dana SL, Hoener PA, Lieberman BA, Imhof MO, Stein RB. Cellular mechanisms which distinguish between hormone and antihormone activated estrogen receptor. *Ann N Y Acad Sci* 1995; 761: 121-37.
9. Horwitz KB, Tung L and Takimoto GS. Why are there two progesterone receptors? *The Breast* 1996; 5: In press.
10. Lundgren S, Helle SI, Lonning PF. Profound suppression of plasma estrogens by megestrol acetate in postmenopausal breast cancer patients. *Clin Cancer Res* 1996; In press.
11. Stewart AJ, Westley BR & May FEB. Modulation of the proliferative response of breast cancer cells to growth factors by oestrogen. *Br J Cancer* 1992; 66: 640-8.
12. Vignon F, Bouton MM, Rochefort H. Antioestrogens inhibit the mitogenic effect of growth factors on breast cancer cells in the total absence of estrogens. *Biochem Biophys Res Commun* 1987; 146: 1202-508.
13. DeFriend DJ, Anderson E, Bell J, Wilks DP, West CML, Howell A. Effects of 4-hydroxytamoxifen and a pure antioestrogen (ICI 182780) on the clonogenic growth of human breast cancer cells *in vitro*. *Br J Cancer* 1994; 70: 2043-211.
14. Howell A, DeFriend D, Robertson J, Blamey R, Walton P. Response to a specific antioestrogen (ICI 182780) in tamoxifen-resistant breast cancer. *Lancet* 1995; 345: 29-30.
15. Murray R, Pitt P. Aromatase inhibition with 4-OH androstenedione after prior aromatase inhibition with aminoglutethimide in women with advanced breast cancer. *Breast Ca Res Treat* 1995; 35: 249-53.
16. Lonning PE, Dowsett M, Jones A *et al*. Influence of aminoglutethimide on plasma oestrogen levels in breast cancer patients on 4-hydroxyandrostenedione treatment. *Breast Ca Res Treat* 1992; 23: 57-92.
17. Masamura S, Santner SJ, Heitjan DF, Santen RJ. Estrogen deprivation causes estradiol hypersensitivity in human breast cancer cells. *J Clin End Metab* 1995; 80: 2918-25.
18. Jonat W, Howell A, Blomqvist C *et al*. A randomised trial comparing two doses of the new selective aromatase inhibitor anastrozole (Arimidex) with megestrol acetate in postmenopausal patients with advanced breast cancer. *Eu J Cancer* 1996; 32A: 404-12.
19. Cole MP, Jones CTA and Todd IDJ. A new antioestrogenic agent in late breast cancer. An early clinical appraisal of ICI 46, 474. *Br J Cancer* 1971; 25: 270-5.
20. Howell A, Dodwell DJ, Anderson H, Redford J. Response after withdrawal of tamoxifen and progestogens in advanced breast cancer. *Ann Oncol* 1992; 3: 611-7.
21. Gottardis MM, Jiang SY, Yeng MH, Jordan VC (1989). Inhibition of tamoxifen-stimulated growth of an MCF-7 variant in athymic mice by novel steroidal antioestrogens. *Cancer Res* 49, 4090-3.
22. Osborne CK, Coronado E, Allred DC *et al*. Acquired tamoxifen resistance: correlation with reduced breast tumour levels of tamoxifen and isomerisation of trans-4-hydroxytamoxifen. *J Natl Cancer Inst* 1991; 83: 1477-82.
23. Wolf DM, Langan-Fahey SM, Parker CJ, McCague R, Jordan VC. Investigation of the mechanism of tamoxifen stimulated breast tumour growth with nonisomerizable analogues of tamoxifen and metbolites. *J Natl Cancer Inst* 1993; 85: 806-12.
24. Pavlik EJ, Nelson K, Srinivasan S *et al*. Resistance to tamoxifen with persisting sensitivity to estrogen: possible mediation by excessive antiosrtogen binding site activity. *Cancer Res* 1992; 52: 4106-12.
25. Osborne CK, Coronado-Heinsohn EB, Allred DC. Acquired tamoxifen resistance: correlation with reduced breast tumor levels of tamoxifen and isomerization of trans-4-hydroxytamoxifen. *J Natl Cancer Inst* 1991; 83: 1477-82.
26. Johnston SRD, Haynes BP, Smith IE, Jarman M, Sacks NPM, Dowsett M. Acquired tamoxifen resistance in human breast cancer and reduced intra-tumoral drug concentration. *Lancet* 1993; 342: 1521-2.

27. Pritchard KI, Thomson DB, Myers RE, Sutherland JA, Mobbs BG, Meaken JW Tamoxifen therapy in premenopausal patients with metastic breast cancer. *Cancer Treat Reports* 1980; 64: 787-96.
28. Hoogstraten B, Gad-el-Mawla N, Maloney TR, Fletcher WS, Vaughan CB, Tranum BL, Athens JW, Costanzi JJ, Foulkes M. Combined modality therapy for first recurrence of breast cancer. A Southwest Oncology Group Study. *Cancer* 1984; 54: 2248-56.
29. Howell A, Dodwell D, Laidlaw I, Anderson H and Anderson E (1990). Tamoxifen as an agonist for metastatic breast cancer. In: *'Endocrine Therapy of Breast Cancer IV'*, Ed. A Goldhirsch: 49-58, Springer Verlag, Berlin.
30. Robertson JFR. Oestrogen receptor: a stable phenotype in breast cancer. *Br J Cancer* 1996; 73: 5-12.
31. Wrenn CK, Katzenellenbogen BS. Structure function analysis of the hormone binding domain of the human estrogen receptor by region-specific mutagenesis and phenotypic screening in yeast. *J Biol Chem* 1993; 268: 24089-98.
32. Roodi N, Bailey LR, Kao WY, Verrier CS, Yee CJ, Dupont WD, Parl FF. Estrogen receptor gene analysis in estrogen receptor-positivs and receptor negative primary breast cancer. *J Natl Cancer Inst* 1995; 87: 446-51.
33. Fuqua SAW, Fitzgerald SD, Chamness GC, Tandon AK, McDonnell DP, Nawaz Z, O'Malley BW, McGuire WL. Variant human breast tumour estrogen receptors with constituitive transcriptional activity. *Cancer Res* 1991; 51: 105-9.
34. Leygue ER, Watson PH, Murphy LC. Estrogen receptor variants in normal human mammary tissue. *J Natl Cancer Inst* 1996; 88: 284-90.
35. Ignar-Trowbridge DM, Pimentel M, Parker M, McLachlan JA, Korach KS. Peptide growth factor cross-yalk with the estrogen receptor requires the A/B domain and occurs independently of protien kinase C or estradiol. *Endocrinology* 1996; 137: 1735-42.
36. Nicholson RI, Gee JMW. Growth factors and modulation of endocrine response in breast cancer. Wayne V Vedeckis, Ed. *Hormones and Cancer* 1996; Birkhäuser, Boston.
37. Howell A, Mackintosh J, Jones M, Redford J, Wagstaff J and Sellwood R.A. (1988). The definition of the 'No Change' category in patients treated with endocrine therapy and chemotherapy for advanced carcinoma of the breast. *Eur J Cancer Clin Oncol* 1988; 24: 1567.
38. Crawford DJ, George WD, Smith DC, Stewart M Paul J, Leake RE. Comparison of cyclical tamoxifen versus megestrol acetate with tamoxifen alone in advanced breast cancer. *Breast* 1992; 1: 35-40.
39. Howell A, Downey S and Anderson E. New endocrine therapies in breast cancer. *Eur J Cancer* 1996; 4: 576-89.
40. Osborne CK, Coronado-Heinsohn EB, Hilsenbeck SG, McCue BL, Wakeling AE, McLelland RA, Manning DL, Nicholson RI. Pure steroidal antioestrogens are superior to tamoxifen in a model of human breast cancer. *J Natl Cancer Inst* 1995; 87: 746-50.
41. Katzenellenbogen BS. Estrogen receptors: bioactivities and interactions with cell signalling pathways. *Biology of Reproduction* 1996; 54: 287-93.

Breast cancer: should we control rather than kill tumor cells?

H. Schipper[1], M. Baum[2] and E.A. Turley[3]

[1] University of Manitoba, Winnipeg, Canada; [2] University College, London, England; [3] Manitoba Institute of Cell Biology, Winnipeg, Canada

The treatment of breast cancer is now the commonest indication for bone marrow transplant in the United States, our maximal dose-intensive therapy. More experience and improved technologies have decreased the procedure-related morbidity and mortality to the point where the procedure is no longer experimental, though the indication remains so [1]. Peripheral stem cell utilization, the use of colony stimulating factors, and better management of transient marrow suppression are at the point of making our most intensive chemotherapy an out-patient procedure [2, 3]. Transplants in this setting are safer, less disabling and cheaper than they were even months ago. The double-barreled question is, are transplants better, and does the exercise take us toward a biologic breakthrough in the management of epithelial cancers, and breast cancer in particular?

The argument we wish to advance is that while these higher dose technologies may provide incremental improvement in disease-free survival and possibly overall survival, there is little evidence to suggest that the biology of the disease will be beneficially altered. To the contrary, killing strategies may exacerbate the malignant process producing more refractory recurrence. In essence we have produced a therapeutic blind alley. In contrast to the treatment of leukemia, in which the ablated organ is the defective one, transplant in breast cancer is intended to rescue an innocent bystander organ, the marrow. The hope is that by further escalating marginally effective drugs we will reach a point on the dose response curve where complete response is a commonplace, and more important, it is sustained. There is little evidence that this is likely to be so.

Drawing this conclusion comes from a « rethinking » of the malignant process. The argument has been elaborated earlier, but can be summarized as follows. [4-6]. To date we have viewed the malignant cell as autonomous, avaricious and irretrievably deranged. The result is a kill or be killed strategy, somewhat akin to microbiology. (It bears noting that even here, where the metabolic process of microbe and host are so different as to allow an effective therapeutic margin, we now recognize a concept of balance restoration between environmental pathogens and host response). More recent evidence suggests a subtler, step-wise process which offers opportunities for regulation, and a different model, which has five principles:

1. Cancer is a process, not a morphologic entity. Individual cancers, while likely originating

from single cells, are constantly adapting to the local environment in a process of clonal evolution.
2. The cancer cell is largely normal, both genetically and functionally. The malignant properties are the result of a small number of genetic and/or environmental changes which have a profound effect on certain aspects of its behaviour.
3. The process is unstable, characterized by regulatory imbalance, rather than autonomy.
4. The imbalance is potentially reversible.
5. Killing strategies may be counterproductive, because they impair host response, and drive the already defective regulatory process toward further aberrance.
Three corollaries follow:
1. Host response is critical, and determines long term outcome.
2. Cancer growth rates are variable, depending on the regulatory balance.
3. Functional cure does not require a complete response. Conversely, complete response may not be the best predictor of long term survival.
What evidence is there to support such a paradigm shift?

Cancer is a process

To date no single substance or metabolic process has been uniquely identified with cancer. The disease is characterized by growth, invasion and metastasis, all of which have their equivalents in normal tissues. Clonality, previously considered a hallmark of cancer, is neither always present in malignancy nor restricted to it [7, 8]. It has been demonstrated in a few malignancies, mostly of lymphoid origin. Some such as Hodgkin's Disease may be overtly polymorphous. The HIV related lymphomas may be polyclonal [9,10]. Conversely, there are non-malignant clonal expansions, as seen in Epstein-Barr viral infection [11]. However, the natural history of most malignancies - characterized by progressive expression of gene products which serve to facilitate growth, invasion and metastasis - serves to emphasize a dynamic process. Further, there is evidence that this process can be induced or accelerated by therapy, as in the example of the multiple drug resistance (*mdr*) gene coding for P-glycoprotein [12, 13].

Cancer cells are largely normal

By definition cancer originates from host normal tissues, with the exception of trophoblastic neoplasia and rare tumours inadvertently transplanted into the host. Most cancers are diagnosed by virtue of their morphologic or histochemical similarity to their tissue of origin. The metabolic machinery is intact to the point where the tumour has a growth advantage over the host. In addition, there are no truly specific « tumour specific » markers [14].
At the genetic level, with the exception of deletions, all necessary information is preserved, and the defective portion of DNA is very tiny. Most oncogenes code for normal proteins, the abnormality being in expression control. Data continues to emerge suggesting that the key processes which characterize malignancy are genetically controlled through the expression, or lack thereof, of proteins which also serve normal and essential cellular functions in ontogeny and homeostasis. [15-21].

Regulatory imbalance and instability

At one time tumours were considered to be completely autonomous, but that view has changed. There has long been clinical evidence to the contrary. Spontaneous remissions, though rare, do occur. Lymphomas, hormone-sensitive malignancies (particularly breast cancers), and chronic myelogenous leukemia are examples of tumours in which spontaneous cycling to the point of near complete remission is common. Surgical and autopsy studies have shown the incidence of occult tumours of breast and prostate to be much higher than the observed clinical rate [22, 23]. The growth rate of residual tumour frequently increases after chemotherapy [24]. Many tumours relapse after long disease-free intervals, often in association with demonstrable changes in the known regulatory environment.

In the laboratory, resection of primary tumour transiently increases cell cycling in distant metastases [25-27]. This old observation forms the basis of adjuvant chemotherapy. It also clearly implies that malignant tumours are still functionally part of a regulatory/communications network. There is both morphologic and functional evidence of reversible cell-to-cell communications defects in epithelial tumours, whose extent correlates with malignant behaviour in cell culture [28, 29].

Cells in a malignant tumour are no longer viewed as groups of like individuals, limited in their growth by anatomic and nutritional factors. As described by the autocrine model, the tumour mass, as an aggregate of cells, genes and milieu, serves as a biologic information storage system, the data being used to shape responses to subsequent stimuli. Polypeptides such as growth factors serve as communications couplers, converting individual cells into a network. The same polypeptide may up - or down - regulate depending on the local milieu [30]. Specific lesions in receptors for growth factor, or in the ligand itself, have malignant correlates. These considerations begin to explain the enigmatic function of hormones, wherein estrogens, androgens and anti-estrogens all appear to work in similar circumstances. The dynamic relationship between cells and milieu may hold important clues to the aetiology of overtly polymorphic tumours such as Hodgkin's Disease.

Reversibility

Following closely on the concept of regulatory imbalance is potential reversibility. Any regulatory pathway is essentially a cascade whose direction is dependent on the relative concentrations and specific affinities of the substrates. Few are intrinsically irreversible. The hormones and peptides governing growth, invasion and metastasis, have normal functions. Their malignant gene correlates, such as *c-myc*, can be pharmacologically regulated [31]. Defective regulatory receptors can be bypassed, as seen in the therapeutic success of all-trans retinoic acid in overwhelming a defective vitamin A receptor in acute promyelocytic leukemia [32-34]. Cell-to-cell communication disorders can be corrected [28,35]. Apoptosis is inhibited by specific genetic alteration, and may be reversible, leading to resumption of programmed cell death [36, 37]. Disorders of p53, which has an effect on apoptosis, cell cycling and drug resistance gene amplification, may also be subject to modulation [38-41].

There is clinical and morphologic evidence as well. Some years ago Mintz demonstrated that malignant teratoma cells developed into normal mice when transplanted into mouse blastocysts [42]. The clinical correlate is the frequent finding of mature teratoma following *cis*-platinum chemotherapy for embryonal carcinoma. Similar evidence of post-treatment differentiation has been reported by Brambilla in small cell lung cancer [43]. Functional reversibility must be possible if we are to explain the induction of complete remissions in Mediterranean and MALT lymphomas by antibiotics, and the earlier described spontaneous remissions and natural cycling of tumours [44-46].

Killing

The central premise of the classical model is that it is both necessary and possible to kill the last tumour cell, and that achieving complete clinical and laboratory remission leads to cure. Yet there are some disturbing inconsistencies in our experience over the past two decades.

There is clinical evidence to suggest that the killing model achieves remission but does not directly cure. Despite increasing intensity, cytotoxic therapies beyond remission have not flattened survival curves except in germ cell tumours, and lymphomas. Particularly disappointing is the recent evidence that dose intensive regimens do not provide a therapeutic advantage in a range of responsive lymphoid malignancies [47-49]. Epithelial tumours continue to relapse after intensive treatment, both in the adjuvant setting, and despite induction of rigorously assessed complete remission in advanced disease [50, 51]. Even though we frequently achieve complete clinical remission when treating small cell lung cancer, further treatment intensification only infrequently prevents relapse [52, 53].

Where we have achieved apparent cure, it seems processes other than cell kill are of critical importance. In marrow transplantation for acute leukemia, survival correlates with low grade graft-versus-host disease rather than marrow remission [54, 55]. The platinum-based drugs seem capable of inducing differentiation in those diseases where their role seems curative [43]. Interferons and interleukins seem to exert regulatory actions on susceptible cell lines, an excellent example being hairy cell leukemia [56, 57]. Metaphase and polymerase chain reaction studies in CML show that persistence of *bcr-abl* containing cells does not always mean inevitable relapse [58-61].

How specifically does this model relate to breast cancer? The contemporary breast cancer paradigm holds that breast cancer is a systemic disease from the time of clinical diagnosis, and that the outcome is pre-determined by the extent of micrometastases prior to diagnosis. Further, nodal metastasis is a hallmark of an intrinsic tumour property, namely its metastatic potential. Fisher's major conceptual evolution from the days of Halstead is not simply from that of nodal spread as a time dependent, stepwise process to a systemic illness, but also that an individual tumour has a mix of genetically governed growth, invasion and metastatic potential that is determined early on. What the instability model further contributes is the notion of a continuum of evolution in an unstable environment which can be perturbed. Malignancy is a partnership between the cancer cell and the local and systemic microenvironment. The model operates across the cancer spectrum, from prevention through the treatment of advanced disease.

With respect to prevention, the early data relating to BRCA1, among other sites supports the instability model. Rearrangements and defects are seen in the tumour gene locus in a substantial proportion of patients who do not have family histories or evidence of the gene in normal tissues. The facilitative defect is not as profound as that consequent on the *ras* mutation in the Li-Fraumeni syndrome, but would appear to make breast and ovarian epithelial tissues (and perhaps colon in the case of BRCA2) more susceptible to the consequences of hormonal flux.

Early diagnosis, most particularly using mammography is intended to bring forward the time of diagnosis to a sub-clinical phase before metastasis takes place. The modest improvements seen in post-menopausal women may reflect the time-shift part of the model. The continued recurrence, and possible adverse effect of early surgical intervention as suggested by the Canadian study might be the result of critically timed adverse perturbation of a particularly unstable form of breast cancer.

We now accept that conservative surgery is of equal value to more radical approaches. That follows logically from Fisher's systemic model of the disease. The paradox is that the same model predicts a benefit for « adjuvant » therapy because the surgery perturbs the tumour host interaction, leading to a period of proliferation at occult metastatic sites. The 5-10% added to the probability of fifteen year survival by current cytotoxic therapies may be due to killing, but it comes at a price. Disease-free survival is prolonged more than survival, suggesting the remaining tumour is adversely perturbed by the intervention. There is ample evidence that sub-lethal killing is destabilizing, and drives the malignant process forward.

There are further inconsistencies in the conventional paradigm. Adjuvant chemotherapy has been assumed to work through the simple mechanism of killing off cancer cells according to the classic teachings of Skipper et. However, the recent observations that a number of classic cytotoxic drugs both restore apoptosis by down-regulation of gene product, and up-regulate resistance pathways suggests there is a limit to the extent to which the classic cytotoxic mechanism can be driven. Moreover, there is a growing body of opinion that the benefits of chemotherapy in premenopausal women could be in part related to ovarian suppression and additional benefits of chemotherapy could be related to immunomodulation by the disproportionate reduction in suppresser T cells which appear to be more sensitive to alkylating agents than other cells in the immune system [62, 63]. Tamoxifen as an adjuvant has produced some counter-intuitive results in trials of adjuvant therapy as well. Originally the drug was assumed to work as a competitive anti-oestrogen however we now know that tamoxifen has multiple and complex biological actions. It can provoke transforming growth factor beta through acting on stromal fibroblast, it can reduce the circulating levels of insulin like growth factor via a number of pathways, and it can encourage apoptosis and inhibit angiogenesis [64-66].

There is still no adequate explanation for the unpredictable and often extremely prolonged latent intervals between treatment, relapse and death. Mathematical models do not demonstrate a constant proportional hazard for relapse and death following primary treatment in the presence or absence of adjuvant systemic therapy. The pattern of hazard rates after local therapy are quite extraordinary, demonstrating a peak at about three years after initial surgery which then falls to a baseline level, followed by a second peak seven or eight years later [67, 68]. Furthermore the results of adjuvant systemic therapy are not what could have been predicted, with endocrine approaches achieving the same degree of success as chemotherapy in spite of the fact that only about a third of primary breast cancers retain the oestrogen receptor. In particular tamoxifen demonstrates a significant effect in post-menopausal women in the absence of an oestrogen receptor in the primary tumour [69].

In the advanced disease setting, the major determinants of survival are site of relapse, receptor status, disease-free interval and quality of life. While aggressive therapies may offer a more rapid response, and perhaps a greater likelihood of response, overall survival does not seem to have been influenced by chemotherapeutic regimen or treatment intensity. The rationale for the myeloablative approach is that we haven't been able to give enough drug.

Our suggestion is that this will not be achieved using killing strategies. All the evidence points to the preservation if not the generation of a subset of less responsive cells operating in an impaired host environment. We are on the way to the development of regulation-based strategies. These need to be both conceptual and pragmatic, leading from the head, to the lab and to the clinic.

As Skipper, Blumenson and Slack and others developed a mathematical basis for the killing paradigm, we must elaborate an instability mathematics [8, 70]. It will have to take into account both the tumour cell (the sole focus of the current model), and the microenvironment. That should lead to a function-dependent rather than morphology driven series of cell culture, and environment culture systems.

In this model, what would be the criteria for a successful (high dose) therapy? First there would have to be evidence of a change in natural history. That amounts to a break in the disease-free and overall survival curves, or a change in pattern of relapse as has been demonstrated in the childhood leukemias, and germ cell tumours. Second, relapsing and remitting populations should have elucidated differences in regulatory pathways. Third, there should be evidence that the abnormal pathways have been restored, bypassed or otherwise stabilized in those patients achieving remission. Fourth, unstable alternative clones or pathways should not have emerged.

Thus while safer and cheaper killing strategies may bring further small improvements in disease-free survival, the quantum leap in our treatment will come when approaches become more « biological ». It is hard to find an example in biology where eradication alone is sufficient to control an abnormal population or behaviour. Where we have succeeded in controlling aberrant proliferation, it has been accomplished by a combination of population reducing procedures, regulatory initiatives and environmental change. There is little to suggest that control of breast cancer will be otherwise.

References

1. Bitran JD, Samuels B, Klein L, et al. Tandem high-dose chemotherapy supported by hematopoietic progenitor cells yields prolonged survival in stage IV breast cancer. *Bone Marrow Transplant* 1996; 17: 157-62.
2. Holland KH, Dix SP, Geller RB, et al. Minimal toxicity and mortality in high-risk breast cancer patients receiving high-dose cyclophosphamide, thiotepa, and carboplatin plus autologous marrow-stem-cell transplantation and comprehensive supportive care. *J Clin Oncol* 1996; 14: 1156-64.
3. Peters WP, Ross M, Vredenburgh JJ, et al. The use of intensive clinic support to permit outpatient autologous bone marrow transplantation for breast cancer. *Semin Oncol* 1994; 21, suppl: 25-31.
4. Schipper H, Goh CR, Wang TL. Rethinking cancer: should we control rather than kill? Part 1. *Can J Oncol* 1993; 3: 207-16.
5. Schipper H, Goh CR, Wang TL. Rethinking cancer: should we control rather than kill? Part 2. *Can J Oncol* 1993; 3: 220-4.
6. Schipper H, Goh CR, Wang TL. Shifting the cancer paradigm: Must we kill to cure? *J Clin Oncol* 1995; 13: 801-7.
7. Furth J, Kalim MC. The transmission of leukemia of mice with a single cell. *Am J Cancer* 1937; 31: 276-82.
8. Skipper HE. Historic milestones in cancer biology: a few that are important in cancer treatment. *Semin Oncol* 1979; 6: 506-14.
9. McGrath MS, Shiramizu B, Meeker TC, Kaplan LD, Herndier B. AIDS-associated polyclonal lymphoma. Identification of a new HIV-associated disease process. *J Acquir Immune Defic Syndrome* 1991; 4: 408-15.
10. Urba WJ, Longo DL. Cytologic, immunologic and clinical diversity in non-Hodgkins lymphoma: therapeutic implications. *Semin Oncol* 1985; 12: 250-267.
11. Krueger GR, Papadakis T, Schaefer HJ. Persistent active Epstein-Barr virus infection and atypical lymphoproliferation. Report on 2 cases. *Am J Surg Pathol* 1987; 11: 972-81.

12. Judson IR. Understanding anticancer drug resistance: Opportunities for modulation and impact on new drug design. *Eur J Cancer* 1992; 28: 285-9.
13. Fojo AT, Ueda K, Slamon DS, Poplack DG, Gottesman MM, Pastan I. Expression of a multi-drug resistance gene in human tumors and tissues. *Proc Natl Acad Sci USA* 1987; 84: 265-9.
14. Bates SE. Clinical applications of serum tumor markers. *Ann Intern Med* 1991; 115: 623-38.
15. Leutz A, Graf T. Relationships between oncogenes and growth control. In: Sporn MB, Roberts AB, eds. *Peptide growth factors and their receptors*, Vol II. Heidelberg: Springer-Verlag, 1991: 655-703.
16. Reed JC, Tsujimoto Y, Alpers JD, Croce CM, Nowell PC. Regulation of BCL-2 proto-oncogene expression during normal human lymphocyte proliferation. *Science* 1987; 236: 1295-9.
17. Aaronson SA. Growth factors and cancer. *Science* 1991; 254: 1146-53.
18. Feizi T. Demonstration by monoclonal antibodies that carbohydrate structures of glycoproteins and glycolipids are onco-developmental antigens. *Nature* 1985; 314: 53-7.
19. Sachs L. The molecular control of blood cell development. *Science* 1987; 238: 1374-9.
20. Rowley JD. Principles of molecular biology of cancer: Chromosomal abnormalities. In: DeVita VT, Jr., Hellman S, Rosenberg SA, eds. *Cancer: Principles and Practice of Oncology*. 3rd ed. Philadelphia: Lippincott, 1989: 81-7.
21. Collard JG, van de Poll M, Scheffer A, *et al*. Location of genes involved in invasion and metastasis on human chromosome 7. *Cancer Res* 1987; 47: 6666-70.
22. Whitmore WF, Jr. The natural history of prostatic cancer. *Cancer* 1973; 32: 1104-12.
23. Fisher B, Montague E, Redmond C, *et al*. Comparison of radical mastectomy with alternative treatments for primary breast cancer: a first report of results from a prospective trial. *Cancer* 1977; 39: 2827-34.
24. Norton L. Biology of residual breast cancer after therapy: a kinetic interpretation. *Prog Clin Biol Res* 1990; 354A: 109-32.
25. Fisher B, Saffer EA, Deutsch M. Influence of irradiation of a primary tumor on the labeling index and estrogen receptor index in a distant tumor focus. *Int J Radiat Oncol Biol Phys* 1986; 12: 879-85.
26. Fisher B, Gunduz N, Saffer E. Influence of the interval between primary tumor removal and chemotherapy on kinetics and growth of metastasis. *Cancer Res* 1983; 43: 1488-92.
27. DeWys WD. Studies correlating the growth rate of a tumor and its metastases and providing evidence of tumor-related systemic growth-retarding factors. *Cancer Res* 1972; 32: 374-9.
28. Trosko JE, Jone C, Chang CC. Inhibition of gap junctional-mediated intercellular communication *in vitro* by aldrin, dieldrin and toxaphene: a possible cellular mechanism for their tumor-promoting and neurotoxic events. *Molecular Toxicology* 1987; 1: 83-93.
29. Trosko JE. Mechanisms of tumor promotion: Possible role of inhibited intercellular communication. *Eur J Cancer Clin Oncol* 1987; 23: 599-601.
30. Sporn MB, Roberts AB. Autocrine secretion - 10 years later. *Ann Intern Med* 1992; 117: 408-14.
31. Wolf DA, Kohlhuber F, Schulz P, Fittler F, Eick D. Transcriptional down-regulation of c-myc in human prostate carcinoma by the synthetic androgen mibolerone. *Br J Cancer* 1992; 65: 376-82.
32. Huang H, Ye Y, Chen S, *et al*. Use of all-trans retinoic acid in the treatment of acute promyelocytic leukemia. *Blood* 1988; 72: 567-72.
33. Warrel RP, Frankel SR, Miller WH, *et al*. Differentiation therapy of acute promyelocytic leukemia with tretinin (all-trans retinoic acid). *N Engl J Med* 1991; 324: 1385-93.
34. Alcalay M, Zangrilli D, Pandolfi PP, *et al*. Translocation breakpoint of acute promyelocytic leukemia lies within the retinoic acid receptor alpha locus. *Proc Natl Acad Sci USA* 1991; 88: 1977-81.
35. Rouslahti E. Control of cell motility and tumour invasion by extracellular matrix interactions. *Br J Cancer* 1992; 66: 239-42.
36. Oren M. The involvement of oncogenes and tumor suppressor genes in control of apoptosis. *Cancer Metastasis Rev* 1992; 11: 141-8.
37. Robertson LE, Chubb S, Meyn RE, *et al*. Induction of apoptotic cell death in chronic lymphocytic leukemia by 2-chloro-2'-deoxyadenosine and 9-B-D-arabinosyl-2fluoroadenine. *Blood* 1993; 81: 143-50.
38. Lowe SW, Ruley HE, Jacks T, Houseman DE. p-53-Dependent apoptosis modulates the cytotoxicity of anticancer agents. *Cell* 1993; 74: 957-67.
39. Yin Y, Tainsky MA, Bischoff FZ, Strong LC, Wahl GM. Wild-type p53 restores cell cycle control and inhibits gene amplification in cells with mutant p53 alleles. *Cell* 1992; 70: 937-48.

40. Chin KV, Ueda K, Pastan I, Gottesman MM. Modulation of activity of the promotor of the human MDR1 gene by Ras and p53. *Science* 1992; 255: 459-62.
41. Bourhis J, Bosq J, Wilson GD, *et al*. Correlation between p53 gene expression and tumor-cell proliferation in oropharyngeal cancer. *Int J Cancer* 1994; 57: 458-62.
42. Mintz B, Illmensee K. Normal genetically mosaic mice produced from malignant teratcarcinoma cells. *Proc Natl Acad Sci USA* 1975; 72: 3585-9.
43. Brambilla E, Moro D, Gazzeri S, *et al*. Cytotoxic chemotherapy induces cell differentiation in small-cell lung cancers. *J Clin Oncol* 1991; 9: 50-61.
44. Roge J, Druet P, Marche C, de Roissard P, Camilleri JP. Alpha-chain disease: cured with antibiotics (letter). *Br Med J* 1975; 4: 225.
45. Wotherspoon AC, Doglioni C, Diss TC, *et al*. Regression of primary low-grade B-cell gastric lymphoma of mucosa-associated lymphoid tissue type after eradication of *Helicobacter pylori*. *Lancet* 1993; 342: 575-7.
46. Hussell T, Isaacson PG, Crabtree JE, Spencer J. The response of cells from low-grade B-cell gastric lymphomas of mucosa-associated lymphoid tissue to *Helicobacter pylori*. *Lancet* 1993; 342: 571-4.
47. Cooper IA, Wolf MM, Robertson TI, *et al*. Randomized comparison of MACOP-B with CHOP in patients with intermediate-grade non-Hodgkin's lymphoma. *J Clin Oncol* 1994; 12: 769-78.
48. Fisher RI, Gaynor ER, Dahlberg S, *et al*. Comparison of a standard regimen (CHOP) with three intensive chemotherapy regimens for advanced non-Hodgkin's lymphoma. *N Engl J Med* 1993; 328: 1002-6.
49. Gordon LI, Harrington D, Andersen J, *et al*. Comparison of a second generation combination chemotherapeutic regimen (m-BACOD) with a standard regiment (CHOP) for advanced diffuse non-Hodgkin's lymphoma. *N Engl J Med* 1992; 327: 1342-9.
50. Eddy DM. High-dose chemotherapy with autologous bone marrow transplantation for the treatment of metastatic breast cancer. *J Clin Oncol* 1992; 10: 657-70.
51. Seidman AD, Scher HI, Gabrilove JL, *et al*. Dose-intensification of MVAC with recombinant granulocyte colony-stimulating factor as initial therapy in advanced urothelial cancer. *J Clin Oncol* 1993; 11: 408-14.
52. Ihde DC, Deisseroth AB, Lichter AS, *et al*. Late intensive combined modality therapy followed by autologous bone marrow transplantation in extensive stage small cell lung cancer. *J Clin Oncol* 1986; 4: 1443-54.
53. Elias AD, Ayash L, Wheeler C, *et al*. High dose combination alkylating agents supported by autologous marrow (ABMT) with chest radiotherapy for responding limited stage (LD) small cell lung cancer (SCLC). *Proc Amer Soc Clin Onc* 1992; 11: 296 (abstract).
54. Sullivan KM, Fefer A, Witherspoon R, *et al*. Graft-*versus*-leukemia in man: Relationship of acute and chronic graft-versus-host disease to relapse of acute leukemia following allogeneic bone marrow transplantation. *Prog Clin Biol Res* 1987; 244: 391-9.
55. Kapoor N, Copelan EA, Klein J, Tutschka PT. Graft-versus-host disease: Effects on long term disease-free survival in marrow transplantation for haematological malignancies. *Bone Marrow Transplant* 1989; 4 (Suppl 4): 153-5.
56. Billard C, Sigaux F, Castagne S, *et al*. Treatment of hairy cell leukemia with recombinant Alpha interferon: II *In vivo* down-regulation of Alpha interferon receptors on tumor cells. *Blood* 1986; 67: 821-6.
57. Quesada JR, Hersh EM, Manning J, *et al*. Treatment of hairy cell leukemia with recombinant alpha-interferon. *Blood* 1986; 68: 493-7.
58. Apperley JF, Rassool F, Parreira A, *et al*. Philadelphia-positive metaphases in the marrow after bone marrow transplantation for chronic granulocytic leukemia. *Am J Hematol* 1986; 22: 199-204.
59. Westbrook CA. The role of molecular techniques in the clinical management of leukemia: Lessons from the Philadelphia chromosome. *Cancer* 1992; 70: 1695-700.
60. Price CGA, Meerabux J, Murtagh S, *et al*. The significance of circulating cells carrying t(14; 18) in long remission from follicular lymphoma. *J Clin Oncol* 1991; 9: 1527-32.
61. Lambrechts AC, Hupkes PE, Dorssers LCJ, van't Veer MB. Clinical significance of t (14; 18) - positive cells in the circulation of patients with stage III or IV follicular Non-Hodgkin's lymphoma during first remission. *J Clin Oncol* 1994; 12: 1541-6.

62. Rose DP, Davis TE. Ovarian function in patients receiving adjuvant chemotherapy for breast cancer. *Lancet* 1977; 1: 1174-6.
63. Colletta AA, Benson JR, Baum M. Alternate mechanisms of action of antioestrogens. *Breast Cancer Res Treat* 1994; 31: 5-9.
64. Benson JR, Wakefield LM, Sporn MB, *et al*. Secretion of TGFß isoforms by primary cultures of human breast tumour fibroblasts *in vitro* and their modulation by tamoxifen (Abstr.). *Breast Cancer Res Treat* 1993; 27: 163.
65. Hunyh HT, Tetenes E, Wallace L, Pollack M. *In vivo* inhibition of insulin-like growth factor I gene expression by tamoxifen. *Cancer Res* 1993; 53: 1727-30.
66. Gagliardi A, Collins DC. Inhibition of angiogenesis by anti-oestrogens. *Cancer Res* 1993; 53: 533-5.
67. Baum M, Badwe RA. Does surgery influence the natural history of breast cancer?. In: Wise L, Johnson HJ, eds. *Breast Cancer: Controversies in management*. Armonk, New York: Futura Publishing, 1996: 61-9.
68. Oliver RTD. Does surgery disseminate or accelerate cancer? *Lancet* 1995; 346: 1506-7.
69. Nolvadex Adjuvant Trial Organisation. Controlled trial of tamoxifen as a single agent in the management of early breast cancer. *Br J Cancer* 1987; 54: 608-11.
70. Goldberger AL. Non-linear dynamics for clinicians: chaos theory, fractals, and complexity at the bedside. *Lancet* 1996; 347: 1312-4.

High dose sequential chemotherapy in poor prognosis breast cancer patients

J.M. Extra, C. Cuvier, M. Espie, P. Cottu and M. Marty

Department of Medical Oncology, Saint Louis Hospital, Paris, France

Abstract

The rather well established relation between dose, dose-intensity, relative dose intensity and the efficacy of conventional chemotherapy in breast cancer patients has lead to the systematic study of dose-densified and dose intensive regimens [1]. One of the possible approaches has been single dose intensification most commonly with hemopoietic stem cell support, while dose-densification - through increased doses and shorter intervals - currently leading to High Dose Sequential Therapy with stem cell support has been the other one. We review here the main results achieved with the latter as well as anticipated developments.

Dose-densified chemotherapy

Although there is no unequivocal definition of dose densification, we will use the following: an increase in the relative dose intensity through higher doses and shorter intervals with or without the support of chemoprotective agents and hemopoietic growth factors (HGF) allowing for identical courses to be repeated from 4 to 6 times without changes in the the dose-intensity (*i.e* dose reductions or prolonged intervals).

Single agent dose-densification

While the maximum tolerated dose of a majority of agents is well defined when they are given every 3 to 4 weeks, the data concerning administration at shorter intervals are still rare.
Table I depicts the MTD of some agents when given with short interval.

Table I. Recommended dose and interval for dose-densification of single agent therapy.

Agent	Dose (mg/sqm)	Interval (days)	RDI (mg/sqm/w)	Reference
Cyclophosphamide	1500-3000	14	750-1500	2, 3
Epirubicin	110	14	53	4
Cisplatinum	70	7	70	5
Paclitaxel	250	14	125	6
Docetaxel	75-->100	14	37.5-50	unpublished

Dose-densified combination chemotherapy

Table II summarizes some of the dose-densified regimens which have been reported with anthracyclins and cyclophosphamide. Obviously other strategies including increased doses with HGF support every 3 weeks and/or sequential regimens have been used. The following conclusions can be drawn:
• Only agents responsible for predominant neutropenia of short duration (cyclophosphamide, thiotepa, anthracyclins, taxanes) appear suitable for such dose densification.
• 2 drugs regimens appear easier to use for dose densification than 3 (or more) drugs combinations.
• The use of accelerated chemotherapy with HGF is often limited by cumulative thrombocytopenia and/or mucositis.
• RDI of 1.4-2.5 as compared to classical AC or EC have been achieved.
• In general high response rates have been reported while progression-free survival is often not depicted.

Table II. Dose densified combinations of anthracyclins and cyclophosphamide.

Reference	Doxorubicin	Epirubicin	Cyclophosphamide	HGF	Interval
7	100		500	Yes	14 days
8	40		1 000	Yes	14 days
9		75	1 200	No	14 days
10		75	500	Yes	10 days

Dose densified epirubicin and cyclophosphamide

The experience obtained with a combination of cyclophosphamide (1,200mg/m^2) and epirubicin (75mg/m^2) given every 14 days without HGF, whatever the blood cell counts (except for febrile neutropenia) for 6 courses will be reviewed [9]. This regimen has been used as initial chemotherapy for inflammatory breast cancer (90 patients) (group 1) or as first line chemotherapy for the metastatic progression (120 pts, of whom 53 (group 3) were relapsing). When given to patients with inflammatory breast cancer or with metastatic disease at presentation surgery (mastectomy for IBC, lumpectomy or mastectomy for metastatic patients was performed immediately following induction; finally all patients received maintenance chemotherapy for 6 months, and loco-regional radiotherapy when they had been operated.
When haematological toxicity is shown in *Table III*: neutropenia and thrombocytopenia were

more frequent in metastatic patients, in particular in those relapsing after initial therapy. Febrile neutropenia requiring hospitalization for parenteral antibiotics occurred in less than 15% of the cycles (median duration of hospitalization: 3.5 days). No patients received HGF; no toxic death was observed. Finally little no dose modification was necessary and few cycles had to be delayed so that median RDI is 100% in patients with IBC and 96% in patients with metastatic breast cancer.

Table III. Incidence of myelosuppression and related complications with dose densified cyclophosphamide and epirubicin (% of cycles).

	Inflammatory breast cancer (90pts, 540 cycles)	Metastatic at presentation (67pts, 392 cycles)	Metastatic relapse (53)
N pts	90	67	53
N cycles	540	392	256
Grade 3-4 neutropenia	75%	82%	89%
Thrombocytopenia (grade 3-4)	2%	6%	10%
Febrile neutropenia	6%	8%	12.5%

Among non haematological side-effects, nausea and vomiting were controlled with 5-HT$_3$ receptor antagonists (with or without corticosteroids) in 73% of the patients, no renal, hepatic or cardiac toxicity was observed.

87/90 pts with IBC experienced a complete response of inflammatory symptoms, 64 (71%) had a clinical response of their breast tumor (14% complete) and 87 had mastectomy with axillary clearance; at pathological examination of the breast: 13 (14.9%) had no residual tumor and 53 (61%) had a major response (< 30% tumor cells in the tumor bed); 25 (29%) had no nodal involvement; 36 (41%) had involvement of 1 to 3 nodes. Median Relapse-free survival was 50 months and 5 years relapse-free survival is 47%.

Response rate in metastatic patients was 58.5% (17% complete responses) apparently not influenced by previously received therapy; median progression-free survival was 16.5 months, and median overall-survival was 36 months in both groups of metastatic patients.

Thus dose-densified chemotherapy with cyclophosphamide and epirubicin can be given without HGF support with an acceptable safety profile; it does not impact on tolerance of further surgery, radiotherapy and maintenance chemotherapy; in inflammatory breast cancer a complete response of inflammatory symptoms is achieved in 97% of the patients and major pathological response of breast tumor and regional nodes is achieved in local control is achieved in 76 and 70% of the patients respectively; long term relapse-free survival is achieved in 47% of the patients. When patients with metastatic breast cancer, whether at presentation or as their first relapse are concerned, median progression-free survival (16.5 months) and overall survival (3 years) are almost doubled as compared to « classical » chemotherapy regimens and compare favourably with those reported with late intensification in patients with response to induction regimen [11].

These results, with other, give an excellent rationale for intensive sequential chemotherapy with stem cell support in high risk breast cancer.

Intensive sequential chemotherapy

This approach is based upon sequential cycles of accelerated high dose chemotherapy with HGF and Peripheral Blood Stem Cells (PBSC) support. PBSC are collected following the first cycle(s) and priming with HGF and are reinfused in the following cycles. Different chemotherapy regimens have been used in terms of agents, alternating regimens, interval between cycles, number of cycles and subsequent treatment. Such regimens can be classified as double intensification or multicycle intensive therapy with PBSC support.

Double intensification

The high number of PBSC collected after chemotherapy and HGF priming and the shorter duration of pancytopenia and related complications when PBSC reinfusion is used following myelosuppressive chemotherapy (as compared to autologous marrow transplant) has made possible the use of double intensification.

A tandem intensification with high dose melphalan (140 to 180 mg/m^2), followed (median = 25 days) by CTCb (cyclophosphamide 6.000 mg/m^2, thiotepa 500 mg/m^2, and carboplatin 800 mg/m^2), each regimen with PBSC and G-CSF support has been studied in patients who responded to induction chemotherapy [12]. No toxic death was observed; duration of pancytopenia was 6 days following melphalan and 24 days following CTCb which required an hospitalization of 25 days. This clearly indicates that multicycle chemotherapy cannot be considered using such regimen.

The randomized study presented by Bezwoda *et al.* [13] is the most mature trial of such an approach despite the atypical therapeutic arms. It compared two cycles of high-dose CNV (cyclophosphamide 2.4 g/m^2, mitoxantrone 35 to 45 mg/m^2, and etoposide 2.5 g/m^2) supported by either ABMT or PBSC, *versus* six to eight cycles of conventional-dose CNV (cyclophosphamide 600 mg/m^2, mitoxantrone 12 mg/m^2, and vincristine 1.4 mg/m^2) as first-line treatment in 90 patients with metastatic breast cancer. Response rates were significantly different: HD-CNV 95% (51% CR) *versus* 53% with CNV. Duration of response and survival were significantly longer with HD-CNV. Yet CNV does not appear an optimal regimen with less than 6 months progression-free survival while PFS and OS with HD-CNV do not appear longer than that reported with dose densified, early or late-intensification regimens.

Other authors [14] have reported the poor feasibility of tandem intensification with more intensive regimens.

Multicycle intensive chemotherapy

This is still an experimental approach, although its feasibility with some chemotherapy regimens is established. *Table IV* summarizes some of the proposed schedules. In general PBSC are collected following the first cycle and the quantities allow for 2 reinfusions (each > 2.10^6 CD34$^+$/kg). The planned interval between cycles is 14 days, but can be increased to 20 days when the patient has not recoverd from severe toxicity.

With the last regimen studied in 17 patients with metastaic breast cancer the following data were observed: PBSC collection (guided by CD34+ cell counts) was performed at day 11 (median) following the first cycle. One apheresis collected 13.6 10^6/kg CD34$^+$ (> 4 in 88% of the patients). 16/17 pts completed the 4 courses (one developed haemorrhagic cystitis following cycle 3 despite prophyllactic mesna in all patients): duration of grade IV neutropenia following cycles 1, 2, 3 and 4 (3 and 4 with PBSC reinfusion) was 4, 5, 8 and 7 days; an hospitalization was required for febrile neutropenia and parenteral antibiotics in 37% of the cycles (median duration 4 days); no patient developed grade IV thrombocytopenia following cycle 1, but the incidence increased thereafter (14%, 24%, 50% respectively with a duration of 1-13 days and 43% of the patients received platelet transfusions; mucositis was observed in 50% of the patients; no cardiac toxicity (monitored by Left Ventricular Ejection Fraction Test) was observed. The actual RDI was 90% (75-98%). 8/12 pts achieved a response. Responding patients received 6 months maintenance chemotherapy. Progression free surival in this population is currently > 6 months.

Table IV. Regimens in high dose sequential chemotherapy with PBSC support in patients with advanced breast cancer. CPM : cyclophosphamide ; LPAM : melphalan ; TTP : thiotepa ; EDOX : epirubicin.

Reference	Cycle 1	Cycle 2	Cycle 3	Cycle 4
15	CPM : $3g/m^2$	CPM : $3g/m^2$	TTP : 5-700 mg/m^2	TTP : 5-700 mg/m^2
16	CPM : $5g/m^2$	LPAM : $180mg/m^2$	TTP : $700mg/m^2$	
17	CPM : $3g/m^2$ Edox : $100mg/m^2$	CPM : $3g/m^2$ Edox : $100mg/m^2$	CPM : $3g/m^2$ Edox : $100mg/m^2$ CPM : $3g/m^2$ Edox : $100mg/m^2$	

Questions associated with intensive sequential chemotherapy with stem cell support

A number of questions are still to be answered.

Some are related to the therapeutic procedures: optimal chemotherapy regimen (alternating or identical cycles; optimal agents - including the taxanes - and doses); optimal number of cycles; optimal period for PBSC collection (*in vivo* purging) and processing (positive or negative selection). One can expect phase I-II trials to answer them.

Obviously the major one addresses the true efficacy of such an approach: only randomized studies with an optimal comparator can be expected to answer them.

Conclusions

Multicycle dose-densified or intensive chemotherapy with PBSC support has been shown to be an acceptable approach in the treatment of high risk breast cancer. Indeed studies with dose-densified chemotherapy have been conducted on an outpatient basis with minimal toxicities when RDI (1.7-3) as compared to established regimens are concerned; the efficacy is strongly supported by progression-free and overall survival achieved in inflammatory and metastatic breast cancer. These results prompt studies of intensive sequential chemotherapy with stem cell support. Yet the possible benefits will have to be established not only through comparison with established regimens but also with regimens incorporating the newer active cytotoxic such as the taxanes but also with Early or Late Intensification.

References

1. Osborne CK. Dose Intensity As A Therapeutic Strategy In Breast Cancer. *Breast Cancer Res Treat* 1991; 20 Suppl: S11-4.
2. Capizzi RL. Protection of normal tissues from the cytotoxic effects of chemotherapy by amifostine (Ethyol): clinical experiences. *Semin Oncol* 1994; 21 (5 Suppl 11): 8-15.
3. Gilewski T, Theodoulou M, Currie V, Crown J, Seidman A, Hudis C, Caravelli J, Yao TJ, Norton L. Short-interval high-dose cyclophosphamide (CPA) and recombinant granulocyte colony stimulating factor (GCSF) in metastatic breast carcinoma: A Phase I study. *Proc Annu Meet Am Soc Clin Oncol* 1993; 12: A83.
4. Fountzilas G, Skarlos D, Giannakakis T, Athanasiades A, Bafaloukos D, Kalogera-Fountzila A, Bamia C, Pavlidis N, Kosmidis P. Intensive chemotherapy with high-dose epirubicin every 2 weeks and prophylactic administration of filgrastim in advanced breast cancer. *Eur J Cancer* 1994; 30A (7): 965-9.
5. Vermorkken J et al. To be published.
6. Hudis C, Seidman A, Baselga J, Raptis G, Lebwohl D, Gilewski T, Moynahan M, Sklarin N, Fennelly D, Crown J, et al. Sequential high dose adjuvant doxorubicin (A), paclitaxel (T), and cyclophosphamide (C) with G-CSF (G) is feasible for women patients (pts) with resected breast cancer (BC) and greater than or equal to 4 (+) lymph nodes (LN). *Proc Annu Meet Am Soc Clin Oncol* 1994; 13: A62.
7. Dodwell D, Ferguson J, Howell A, Seymour A, Richards M. Intensification of Adriamycin and cyclophosphamide treatment for advanced breast cancer with rGCSF: effect on peripheral blood stem cells. *Br J Cancer* 1992; 66 (Suppl XVII): 9.
8. Swain S, Honig S, Egan E, Walton L, Berg C. A Phase I, Dose-Intensity Trial For Node-Positive Breast Cancer Patients Using Adjuvant Cyclophosphamide (C), Doxorubicin (A) And Granulocyte Colony-Stimulating Factor (Gcsf). *Proc Annu Meet Am Assoc Cancer Res* 1992; 33: A1533.
9. Marty M, Extra JM, Espie M, Giacchetti S, Dieras V. High (H) relative dose-intensity (RDI) cyclophosphamide (C) epirubicin (E) induction phase in patients (pts) with inflammatory or metastatic breast cancer (BC). *Proc Annu Meet Am Assoc Cancer Res* 1993; 34: A1188.
10. Lalisang R, Wils J, Nortier J, Burghouts J, Hupperets P, Erdkamp F, Schouten H, Blijham G. A comparative study of dose escalation vs interval reduction to obtain dose intensification of epirubicin (E) and cyclophosphamide (C) with G-CSF (filgrastim) for patients with metastatic breast cancer (BC). *Proc Annu Meet Am Soc Clin Oncol* 1994; 13: A42.
11. Vahdat L, Raptis G, Fennelly D, Crown J. High-dose chemotherapy of metastatic breast cancer: a review. *Cancer Invest* 1995; 13 (5): 505-10.
12. Ayash LJ, Elias A, Wheeler C, Reich E, Schwartz G, Mazanet R, Tepler I, Warren D, Lynch C, Gonin R, et al. Double dose-intensive chemotherapy with autologous marrow and peripheral-blood progenitor-cell support for metastatic breast cancer: a feasibility study. *J Clin Oncol* 1994; 12 (1): 37-44.
13. Bezwoda WR, Seymour L, Dansey RD. High-dose chemotherapy with hematopoietic rescue as primary treatment for metastatic breast cancer: a randomized trial. *J Clin Oncol* 1995; 13 (10): 2483-9.
14. Ho AD, Mason J, Mulroney C, Corringham RE. Sequential high-dose chemotherapy with alternating regimens and stem cell support for patients with metastatic breast cancer. *Proc Annu Meet Am Soc Clin Oncol* 1994; 13: A188.
15. Vahdat L, Crown J, Reich L, Hudis C, Gilewski T, Hamilton N, Seidman A, Moore M, Harrison M, Yao TJ, et al. Granulocyte colony-stimulating factor (G-CSF) and peripheral blood progenitors (PBP) facilitate rapidly cycled courses of high-dose chemotherapy (HDC) in patients with metastatic breast cancer (MBC). *Proc Annu Meet Am Soc Clin Oncol* 1993; 12: A199.
16. Raptis G, Vahdat L, Hamilton N, Fennelly D, Norton L, Crown J. High complete remission (CR) rate with accelerated multicycle high-dose chemotherapy (HDC) in patients (pts) with metastatic breast cancer (MBC). *Proc Annu Meet Am Soc Clin Oncol* 1995; 14: A954.

Breast Cancer. Advances in biology and therapeutics.
F. Calvo, M. Crépin, H. Magdelenat, eds. John Libbey Eurotext © 1996, pp. 251-256.

Summary of clinical results of vinorelbine (Navelbine®) in the treatment of breast cancer

Gabriel N. Hortobagyi

The University of Texas MD Anderson Cancer Center, Houston, Texas, USA

The vinca alkaloids have been an important component of cytotoxic therapy for hematologic malignancies and solid tumors. Vinblastine and vindesine have been used for the treatment of breast cancer with moderate efficacy [1]. The development of vinorelbine, a nor-vinblastine derivative, added a new dimension to vinca alkaloid treatment [2]. This agent appeared to be equivalent to, and in many cases superior to, the traditional vinca alkaloids in pre-clinical tumor systems, with enhanced therapeutic index. Among the advantages is the relative sparing of axonal microtubules, an effect that is thought to be responsible for the limited neurotoxic potential demonstrated in clinical trials. Early clinical trials demonstrated that vinorelbine had marked anti-tumor activity against several solid tumors, especially breast cancer [3-9] and non-small cell lung cancer [10], with an excellent toxicity profile [2]. These studies suggested that a weekly schedule of administration, utilizing 30 mg/m^2 per week, was effective and well tolerated. Extensive clinical experience demonstrated that the real administered dose intensity was 22.5 mg/m^2 per week in most reported studies. The clinical development of vinorelbine was concentrated on two common malignancies: breast cancer and non-small cell lung cancer. In this paper, we will concentrate on the existing data of single-agent vinorelbine, and vinorelbine-based combinations for the management of breast cancer.

Single-agent activity

Utilizing the weekly intravenous schedule of administration, vinorelbine has been evaluated in first-line therapy of breast cancer in several studies *(Table I)* [3-5, 7, 11-13]. In this setting, the activity of vinorelbine is comparable to that of the most effective anti-tumor agents used for the management of this disease. In fact, the reported efficacy in first-line is comparable to the results of commonly used combination therapy programs, including cyclophosphamide, methotrexate and 5-fluorouracil (CMF) [14]. Vinorelbine has also been tested in patients previously exposed to chemotherapy *(Table II)* [8, 9, 11, 15-17]. In this setting, the activity was more modest, but major objective regressions were observed in 16 to 40% of patients. Antitumor activity persisted in anthracycline-refractory breast cancer. In fact, the only prospective randomized trial in anthracycline-resistant breast cancer was the comparison of vinorelbine and melphalan [18]. While the activity of both drugs in this group of patients was modest, vinorelbine was clearly superior, in terms of response rate, time to progression and survival, without compromising quality of life.

Table I. Activity of single-agent vinorelbine in first-line therapy of metastatic breast cancer.

Author [Ref.]	No. of patients (evaluable)	No. of responses : CP+PR	Overall response rate (95% CI)	Median response duration in weeks	Median survival in weeks
Canobbio [5]	26 (19)	9	52% (30%-74%)	22	not available
Fumoleau [3]	157 (145)	10+50	41% (33%-49%)	34	73
Garcia-Conde [4]	54 (50)	2+24	50% (36%-64%)	36	65
Bruno [7]	68 (63)	5+23	44% (32%-56%)	18	50
Romero [12]	45 (44)	3+15	41% (26%-50%)	36	not reached
Twelves [13]	34	2+15	50%	23	40
Weber [11]	60	9+12	35% (23%-48%)	34	67

CR: complete remission; PR: partial remission; CI: confidence intervals.

Table II. Activity of single-agent vinorelbine in second-line chemotherapy of metastatic breast cancer and beyond.

Author [Ref.]	No. of patients (evaluable)	No. of responses : CP+PR	Overall response rate (95% CI)	Median response duration in weeks	Median survival in weeks
Marty [59]	33 (25)	2+8	30%	21	not available
Tresca [8]	50 (38)	2+6	20%	34	not available
Degardin [17]	100 (100)	1+15	16% (8%-23%)	20	79-94
Weber [11]	47	3+12	32% (20%-47%)	34	62
Gasparini [16]	70 (67)	3+21	36% (24%-47%)	29	58
Toussaint [15]	68 (30)	0+12	40%	23	40

CR: complete remission; PR: partial remission; CI: confidence intervals.

Safety profile

The dose-limiting toxicity of vinorelbine is rapidly reversible myelosuppression, especially neutropenia [4, 11, 16, 19, 20]. Thrombocytopenia and anemia are much less common, and other toxic effects, including nausea, vomiting, mucositis, anorexia, and alopecia, are less common and seldom severe. When administered through a peripheral vein, injection-site reactions, including phlebitis, have been reported in up to 26% of patients [21]. This symptom can be prevented in most patients by rapid administration over 6-10 minutes, or by the use of central venous catheters. Peripheral neuropathy has been described in 20% of patients; this effect is usually minor, and certainly much less severe than the neuropathy observed with other vinca alkaloids or with other tubulin-active agents (*i.e.*, the taxanes). No effects over fertility, and no teratogenic or carcinogenic effects have been demonstrated.

Table III. Antitumor activity of vinorelbine-containing combination chemotherapy for metastatic breast cancer.

Source [Ref.]	In combination with	No. of patients (evaluable)	No. of CR+PR (%)	Median response duration in months	Median survival in months
Spielmann [29]	Doxorubicin	97 (89)	21+53 (74%)	12	30
Hochster [28, 36]	Doxorubicin	62 (58)	7+27 (59%)	not available	not available
Blajman [24]	Doxorubicin	53 (45)	(34%)	not available	not available
Chadjaa [32]	Epirubicin	30 (30)	6+12 (60%)	6	8
Ferrero [31]	Mitoxantrone	33 (32)	8+10 (56%)	not available	not available
Feuvret [26]	Mitoxantrone	24 (20)	5+4 (45%)	7.5	not available
Spielmann [40]	Mitoxantrone	31 (25)	0+9 (36%)	2.2	not available
Froudarakis [23]	5-Fluorouracil	16 (16)	0+5 (31%)	not available	not available
Dieras [22]	5-Fluorouracil	63 (63)	10+32 (67%)	12	18
Vogel [33]	5-Fluorouracil	57 (47)	0+22 (46%)	not available	not available
Ibrahim [30, 35]	Paclitaxel	38 (38)	3+14 (45%)	5+	5+
Van Praagh [27, 34] (neoadjuvant)	Epirubicin Methotrexate	36 (36)	3+24 (74%)	not available	not available
FNOG [25] (neoadjuvant)	Mitoxantrone	41 (25)	1+12 (52%)	not available	not available
Wendling [41]	Mitoxantrone, Cisplatin	25 (20)	5+11 (75%)	not available	not available

Combination chemotherapy

Vinorelbine has been successfully combined with several anti-tumor agents active in the management of breast cancer *(Table III)* [22-36]. The most successful combinations included anthracyclines. First-line chemotherapy with vinorelbine and doxorubicin was reported to produce a response rate of 74%, with a 24% complete remission rate [29]. Remission duration, time to progression and survival were clearly comparable to those obtained with other leading anthracycline-containing regimens, such fluorouracil, doxorubicin, cyclophosphamide (FAC), and others. Combinations of vinorelbine with epirubicin were similarly effective [27, 32]. A randomized trial that compared FAC to vinorelbine-doxorubicin showed no difference in response rate, time to progression or survival [24]. An updated analysis of this trial, as well as confirmatory trials of this comparison, are awaited.

Combinations of vinorelbine with 5-fluorouracil have also shown a high degree of efficacy [22, 23, 33]. The response rates were similar to those of other first-line chemotherapy programs, and even in previously treated patients, the activity of this regimen was substantial. Mucositis can be a significant toxic effect of this combination, although modest reductions in dose can reduce the severity of this toxic effect considerably. More recently, vinorelbine has been combined with both docetaxel and paclitaxel [30, 35, 37]. While the optimal way to combine these two classes of agents remains to be determined, combinations of vinca alkaloids with taxoids appear promising and well tolerated. Vinorelbine-containing combinations were also evaluated in the neoadjuvant setting [25, 27, 34]. The two regimens described had high overall clinical response rates, and more importantly, a greater than 20% pathologically confirmed complete remission rate. Although intertrial comparisons are fraught with danger, this degree of pathologically confirmed complete remission rate is considerably higher than what has been described after other regimens, such as FAC or FEC, in the recent past [38, 39]. Furthermore, since these regimens appeared well-tolerated, additional evaluation in the preoperative setting is appropriate.

Vinorelbine-based combination chemotherapy programs are currently under evaluation in the adjuvant treatment of primary breast cancer. Since this evaluation is optimally done in the context of prospective randomized trials, we will need several additional years of patient accrual and follow-up before we can determine the contribution of these regimens to the multidisciplinary management of the disease.

Vinorelbine is an important addition to the management of breast cancer. It is an effective and well-tolerated drug that can be used as single-agent therapy in first-line and second-line therapy of breast cancer. Vinorelbine-based combinations appear promising for successful palliative management of metastatic disease, and as primary chemotherapy for high-risk primary breast cancer.

References

1. Yau JC, Yap HY, Buzdar AU, Hortobagyi GN, Bodey GP, Blumenschein GR. A Comparative Randomized Trial of Vinca Alkaloids in Patients With Metastatic Breast Carcinoma. *Cancer* 1985; 55 (2): 337-40.
2. Rowinsky EK, Noe DA, Trump DL, Winer EP, Lucas VS, Wargin WA, Hohneker JA, Lubejko B, Sartorius SE, Ettinger DS, *et al.* Pharmacokinetic, Bioavailability, and Feasibility Study of Oral Vinorelbine in Patients With Solid Tumors. *J Clin Oncol* 1994; 12 (9): 1754-63.
3. Fumoleau P, Delgado FM, Delozier T, Monnier A, Gil Delgado MA, Kerbrat P, Garcia-Giralt E, Keiling R, Namer M, Closon MT, *et al.* Phase II trial of weekly intravenous vinorelbine in first-line advanced breast cancer chemotherapy. *J Clin Oncol* 1993; 11: 1245-52.
4. Garcia-Conde J, Lluch A, Martin M, Casado A, Gervasio H, De Oliveira C, De Pablo JL, Gorostiaga J, Giron GC, Cervantes A, *et al.* Phase II trial of Weekly IV Navelbine in First-Line Advanced Breast Cancer Chemotherapy. *Ann Oncol* 1994; 5 (9): 854-7.
5. Canobbio L, Boccardo F, Pastorino G, Brema F, Martini C, Resasco M, Santi L. Phase II study of Navelbine in advanced breast cancer. *Sem Oncol* 1989; 16 (2), Suppl 4: 33-6.
6. Romero A, Rabinovich M, Vallejo C, *et al.* Promising preliminary results of weekly Navelbine as first line chemotherapy for metastatic breast cancer. [Abstract] *Proc Amer Soc Clin Oncol* 1993; 12: 76 (abst 107).
7. Bruno S, Lira-Puerto V, Texeira L, *et al.* Phase II trial with Navelbine in the treatment of advanced breast cancer patients. [Abstract] *Ann Oncol* 1992; 3 (Suppl 1): 126 (abst 268a).
8. Tresca P, Fumoleau P, Roche H, *et al.* Vinorelbine, a new active drug in breast carcinoma: results of an ARTAC phase II trial. [Abstract] *Breast Cancer Res Treat* 1990; 16: 123.
9. Marty M, Leandri S, Extra JM, *et al.* A phase II study of vinorelbine in patients with advanced breast cancer. [Abstract] *Proc Amer Assoc Cancer Res* 1989; 30: 256 (abst 1017).
10. Depierre A, Lemarie E, Dabouis G, Garnier G, Jacoulet P, Dalphin JC. Efficacy of Navelbine in Non-Small Cell Lung Cancer. *Semin Oncol* 1989; 16 (2 (Suppl 4)): 26-9.
11. Weber BL, Vogel C, Jones S, Harvey H, Hutchins L, Bigley J, Hohneker J. Intravenous vinorelbine as first-line and second-line therapy in advanced breast cancer. *J Clin Oncol* 1995; 13 (11): 2722-30.
12. Romero A, Rabinovich MG, Vallejo CT, Perez JE, Rodriguez R, Cuevas MA, Machiavelli M, Lacava

JA, Langhi M, Romero Acuna L, *et al*. Vinorelbine as first-line chemotherapy for metastatic breast carcinoma. *J Clin Oncol* 1994; 12(2): 336-41.

13. Twelves CJ, Dobbs NA, Curnow A, Coleman RE, Stewart AL, Tyrrell CJ, Canney P, Rubens RD. A phase II, multicentre, UK study of vinorelbine in advanced breast cancer. *Cancer* 1994; 70 (5): 990-3.
14. Henderson IC. Harris JR, Hellman S, Henderson IC, Kinne DW, editors. Breast Diseases. 2nd ed. Philadelphia: J.B. Lippincott Company; 1991; 22, *Chemotherapy for Metastatic disease*. p. 604-65.
15. Toussaint C, Izzo J, Spielmann M, Merle S, May-Levin F, Armand JP, Lacombe D, Tursz T, Sunderland M, Chabot GG, *et al*. Phase I/II Trial of Continuous Infusion Vinorelbine for Advanced Breast Cancer. *J Clin Oncol* 1995, 12 (10): 2102-12.
16. Gasparini G, Caffo O, Barni S, Frontini L, Testolin A, Guglielmi RB, Ambrosini G. Vinorelbine Is an Active Antiproliferative Agent in Pretreated Advanced Breast Cancer Patients: A Phase II Study. *J Clin Oncol* 1994; 12 (10): 2094-101.
17. Degardin M, Bonneterre J, Hecquet B, Pion JM, Adenis A, Horner D, Demaille A. Vinorelbine (navelbine) as a salvage treatment for advanced breast cancer. *Ann Oncol* 1994; 5 (5): 423-6.
18. Jones S, Winer E, Vogel C, *et al*. A Multicenter, Randomized Trial of IV Navelbine vs. IV Alkeran in Patients With Anthracycline-Refractory Advanced Breast Cancer. [Abstract] *Proc Am Soc Clin Oncol* 1994; 13: 103 (Abst. 216).
19. Smith GA. Current Status of Vinorelbine for Breast Cancer. *Oncol* 1995; 9 (8): 767-73.
20. Jones S, Winer E, Vogel C, Laufman L, Hutchins L, O'Rourke M, Lembersky B, Budman D, Bigley J, Hohneker J. Randomized comparison of vinorelbine and melphalan in anthracycline-refractory advanced breast cancer. *J Clin Oncol* 1995; 13 (10): 2567-74.
21. Hohneker JA. A summary of vinorelbine (Navelbine) safety data from North American clinical trials. *Sem Oncol* 1994; 21 (5: Suppl 10): 42-6.
22. Dieras V, Pierga J, Extra J, *et al*. Results of a combination of Navelbine and fluorouracil in advanced breast cancer with a group sequential design. [Abstract] *Ann Oncol* 1992; 3 (suppl 5): 46 (abst 178).
23. Froudarakis M, Catimel G, Guastalla JP, *et al*. Phase II study of Navelbine and 5-fluorouracil as second line chemotherapy in metastatic breast carcinoma. [Abstract] *Ann Oncol* 1992; 3 (suppl 5): 88 (abst 343).
24. Blajman C, Balbiani L, Block J, *et al*. Navelbine plus adriamycin vs FAC in advanced breast cancer. [Abstract] *Proc Amer Soc Clin Oncol* 1993; 12: 92 (abst 170).
25. French Northern Oncology Group. Mitoxantrone and vinorelbine as a primary treatment of locoregional breast cancer. [Abstract] Proc IVth International Congress on anticancer chemotherapy 1993; 223 (abst S7).
26. Feuvret L, Antoine E, Vuillemin E, *et al*. Mitoxantrone, 5-fluorouracile, and vinorelbine in highly refractory advanced breast cancer: a new effective regimen. [Abstract] Proc IVth International Congress on anticancer chemotherapy 1993; 150 (abst p. 49).
27. Van Praagh I, Pivoteau N, Cure H, *et al*. Tolerance and efficiency of a regimen vinorelbine-epirubicin-methotrexate in first line neoadjuvant and metastatic breast cancer. [Abstract] *Ann Oncol* 1992; 3 (suppl 5): 99 (abst 383).
28. Hochster H, Vogel C, Blumenreich M, *et al*. A multicenter phase II study of Navelbine and doxorubicin as first line chemotherapyof metastatic breast cancer. [Abstract] *Proc Amer Soc Clin Oncol* 1994; 13: 100 (abst 203).
29. Spielmann M, Dorval T, Turpin F, Antoine E, Jouve M, Maylevin F, Lacombe D, Rouesse J, Pouillart P, Tursz T, *et al*. Phase II Trial of Vinorelbine/Doxorubicin as First-Line Therapy of Advanced Breast Cancer. *J Clin Oncol* 1994; 12 (9): 1764-70.
30. Ibrahim N, Hortobagyi GN, Valero V, *et al*. Phase I Study of Vinorelbine (Navelbine) and Paclitaxel by Simultaneous 3-Hour Infusion for Untreated Metastatic Breast Cancer. [Abstract] *Proc Am Assoc Cancer Res* 1995; 36: 242 (Abst. 1443).
31. Ferrero JM, Wendling JL, Hoch M, *et al*. Mitoxantrone-Vinorelbine as First Line Chemotherapy in Metastatic Breast Cancer: A Pilot Study. [Abstract] *Proc Am Soc Clin Oncol* 1993; 12: 108 (Abst. 234).
32. Chadjaa M, Izzo J, May-Levin F, *et al*. Preliminary Data on 4'Epiadriamycine-Vinorelbine: A New Combination in Advanced Breast Cancer. [Abstract] *Proc Am Soc Clin Oncol* 1993; 12: 88 (Abst. 152).

33. Vogel C, Hochster H, Blumenreich M, *et al.* A US Multicenter Phase II Study of IV Navelbine and 5-Fluorouracil as First Line Treatment of Patients With Advanced Breast Cancer. [Abstract] *Proc Am Soc Clin Oncol* 1995; 14: 91 (Abst. 62).
34. Chollet P, Charrier S, Brain E, *et al.* Neoadjuvant Chemotherapy in Breast Cancer. High Pathological Response Rate Induced by Intensive Anthracycline-Based Regimen. [Abstract] *Proc Am Soc Clin Oncol* 1995; 14: 130 (Abst. 218).
35. Ibrahim NK, Hortobagyi GN, Valero V, *et al.* Phase I Study of Vinorelbine (Navelbine) and Paclitaxel (Taxol) by Simultaneous 3-Hour Infusion With G-CSF Support, for Untreated Metastatic Breast Cancer. [Abstract] *Breast Cancer Res Treat* 1996; 37: (Suppl) 44 (Abst. 107).
36. Hochster HS. Combined doxorubicin/vinorelbine (Navelbine) therapy in the treatment of advanced breast cancer. [Review]. *Sem Oncol* 1995; 22 (2: Suppl 5): 55-9.
37. Fumoleau P, Delacroix V, Perrocheau G, *et al.* Docetaxel in Combination With Vinorelbine as 1st Line CT in Pts With MBC: Preliminary Results on 22 Entered Pts. [Abstract] *Breast Cancer Res Treat* 1995; in press.
38. Feldman LD, Hortobagyi GN, Buzdar AU, Ames FC, Blumenschein GR. Pathological assessment of response to induction chemotherapy in breast cancer. *Cancer Res* 1986; 46: 2578-81.
39. Hortobagyi GN. Multidisciplinary management of advanced primary and metastatic breast cancer. [Review]. *Cancer* 1994; 74 (1: Suppl): 416-23.
40. Spielmann M, Brain E, Sari C, *et al.* Salvage Chemotherapy with combination of mitoxantrone and vinorelbine in resistant to anthracyclines advanced breast cancer. [Abstract] Proc IVth International Congress on anticancer chemotherapy 1993; 61 (abst 14).
41. Wendling JL, Nouyrigat P, Vallicioni D, *et al.* Cisplatinum-Mitoxantrone-Vinorelbine as First Line Chemotherapy for Metastatic Breast Cancer: a Pilot Study. [Abstract] *Proc Am Soc Clin Oncol* 1995; 14: 142 (Abst. 266).

Breast Cancer. Advances in biology and therapeutics.
F. Calvo, M. Crépin, H. Magdelenat, eds. John Libbey Eurotext © 1996, pp. 257-264.

Docetaxel in the treatment of breast cancer: current status, ongoing trials and future directions

M.J. Piccart, A. Di Leo, A. Awada and D. de Valeriola

Chemotherapy Unit, Jules Bordet Institute, rue Héger-Bordet, 1, 1000 Brussels, Belgium

Abstract

This paper summarizes the clinical experience with docetaxel in patients with advanced breast cancer, with special emphasis on the activity of this drug in anthracycline-resistant disease and in liver metastases.
New clinical developments for docetaxel, such as its combination with other chemotherapeutic agents or its administration in the adjuvant setting, are also briefly discussed.
The rapid move of this very active agent to front line therapy of breast cancer may have a positive impact on the natural history of this disease in the coming years.

Introduction

In Europe, 135 000 new breast cancer cases are diagnosed each year and 58,000 deaths from this disease are annually registered. This disease is well known for its early metastatic spread and therefore, innovative systemic treatments are badly needed. In the past 5 years, a new class of chemotherapeutic agents, the taxanes (paclitaxel and docetaxel), have demonstrated unusually high activity in phase II trials. This review will focus on the most recent results obtained with docetaxel and the future directions of its clinical development.

Current status of docetaxel as a single agent in metastatic breast cancer

Five phase II studies with docetaxel, given at the dose of 100 mg/m^2 every 3 weeks, as first-line treatment for metastatic disease have been performed. Overall, 154 patients have been entered and 86 objective responses (12 CRs) have been observed, for an overall response rate of 56% (95% CI: 52-69%) [1, 2].

A pooled analysis of four trials in which docetaxel has been tested, using the same dose and schedule, as second-line treatment for metastatic disease gave the following results: among 162 patients, 64 objective responses (4 CRs) were documented for an overall response rate of 40% [2-4]. Among the 162 cases treated with docetaxel as second-line, 134 patients had previously received doxorubicin and 79 had a primary resistance to this drug defined as progressive disease while receiving a doxorubicin-containing regimen given in the adjuvant or in the metastatic setting. Response rates to docetaxel were 37% and 34% for the whole population of patients pretreated with doxorubicin and for the subgroup with a primary doxorubicin resistance, respectively. While a slight decrease in activity is observed when the drug is given to pretreated patients, the percentage of tumor remissions remains still high, suggesting that docetaxel might be the most active drug in the treatment of patients whose disease has escaped to anthracycline control.

The activity of docetaxel seems to be particularly striking in patients with liver metastases, who represent a cohort with a poor prognosis: the average survival from diagnosis of liver metastases is in the range of six to nine months. In the pooled analysis of the five trials evaluating docetaxel as first-line therapy for metastatic breast cancer, patients with liver involvement had a response rate to docetaxel of 62%. Noteworthy, among a small cohort of 16 patients with liver lesions equal or larger than 2 cm in diameter, 4 complete and 8 partial remissions were observed [2]. These interesting data of docetaxel activity on liver disease were confirmed when the four trials testing docetaxel as second-line were analyzed together: among patients with liver metastases, a 45% objective response rate was documented; interestingly, patients with anthracycline failure and liver lesions experienced a 30% remission rate [2-4].

Docetaxel in comparison with other active agents for the treatment of metastatic breast cancer

Table I gives an overview of the ongoing phase III programs of docetaxel in the treatment of metastatic breast cancer. These trials should clarify up to which extent the activity of this new taxane is superior to the one of the most active standard drug, doxorubicin, or some routinely used second-line regimens such as mitomycin C + vinblastine. The impact of docetaxel on the quality of life of patients with metastatic disease will also be compared to the one of conventional drugs. Finally, a direct comparison between the two taxanes, paclitaxel and docetaxel, will also be informative in these aspects.

Docetaxel in combination with other drugs

Preclinical data in mammary models have shown that a synergism between docetaxel and other chemotherapeutic agents may exist; interestingly, the level of activity does not seem to be largely influenced by the sequence of drug administration [5].

A growing number of clinical pilot studies are currently focusing on the combination of docetaxel with other drugs. *Table II* summarizes these combinations, of which a number might prove useful, later on, for breast cancer patients.

Table I. Ongoing phase III clinical programs of docetaxel in metastatic breast cancer patients after failure to a first-line chemotherapy regimen.

	Study design	Target population
R {	Docetaxel 100 mg/^{2} in 1 hour q 3 wks Doxorubicin 75 mg/^{2} q 3 wks	CMF failures
R {	Docetaxel 100 mg/^{2} in 1 hour q 3 wks Mitomycin C + vinblastine q 4 wks	Anthracyclines failures
R {	Docetaxel 100 mg/^{2} in 1 hour q 3 wks Paclitaxel 175 mg/^{2} in 3 hours q 3 wks	Anthracyclines failures

The interesting observation, up to now, is that relatively high and effective doses of docetaxel, ranging from 75 to 100 mg/m^2, can be given within most of these combinations. The only dose limiting toxicities observed so far are febrile neutropenia and mucositis, the latter being dose-limiting only when docetaxel is combined with fluorouracil or vinorelbine. An important issue to examine in the clinic when docetaxel is combined to other drugs is the optimal sequence between the other agent and docetaxel. The experience gained with paclitaxel in combination with cisplatin or doxorubicin, has shown that pharmacokinetics and side effects may change according to the sequence of administration [6]. So far, the clinical results obtained with docetaxel, in particular concerning its combination with cisplatin, do not support a clear correlation between drug sequencing and drug pharmacokinetics [7]; however, this area deserves further investigation.

Docetaxel in sequence with other drugs

The very high antitumor activity of docetaxel as a single agent, at the dose of 100 mg/^{2}, might be somewhat compromised if the drug is given at 75 mg/^{2} [8], although only a randomized clinical trial would give a definitive answer in this regard.

Because the dose-response issue might be a critical one, especially in the adjuvant setting, it is tempting to explore, in advanced disease, sequential or alternating treatment approaches, where one tries to optimize both drug dose and schedule through the sequential administration of full dose single agent docetaxel and full dose single agent doxorubicin or a doxorubicin-based combination.

This sequential or alternating approach could also delay the onset or reduce the incidence of several drug toxicities such as the docetaxel-induced fluid retention syndrome. A number of these sequential treatment regimens are currently being investigated with docetaxel.

Table II. Ongoing trials of docetaxel in combination with other drugs.

Drugs	Current doses (mg/m^2)	Days	Interval (days)	Dose-limiting Toxicity	Comments
Docetaxel Cyclophosphamide Doxorubicin	60 600 60	- - -	- - -	Febrile neutropenia	Drugs are given sequentially
Doxorubicin Docetaxel	60 50 60 85	1 1	21 21	Febrile neutropenia	22 responses out of 26 cases at the highest feasible dose-level
Docetaxel Fluorouracil (bolus)	60 300	1 1,5	21 21	Febrile neutropenia Mucositis	Active in breast and gastric cancers
Docetaxel Fluorouracil (cont. infusion)	85 1 000	1 1-5	21 21	Febrile neutropenia Mucositis	Fluorouracil at end of docetaxel
Cyclophosphamide Docetaxel	700 75	1 1	21 21	Febrile neutropenia	Docetaxel 1 hour after cyclophosphamide
Docetaxel Ifosfamide	85 5 000	1 1	21 21	Febrile neutropenia	Responses in sarcoma, melanoma and lung cancer
Docetaxel Vinorelbine	75-100 20-22.5	1 1 and 5	21 21	Febrile neutropenia Mucositis	Vinorelbine 20 mg/^{2} and docetaxel 85 mg/^{2} are the recommended doses for phase II studies
Docetaxel Cisplatin	75 75-100	1 1	21 21	Febrile neutropenia	Active in lung and head & neck cancers

Forthcoming combinations with: carboplatin, gemcitabine, topo I inhibitors, epirubicin, oxaliplatin, etoposide

Docetaxel in induction regimens before high dose chemotherapy with peripheral blood progenitor cell support

In the past years, high-dose chemotherapy with peripheral blood progenitor cell support has been proposed as an innovative strategy to be investigated in the treatment of both early and metastatic breast cancer. Phase II studies have shown that this treatment approach is feasible and an interesting level of antitumor activity has been reported in highly selected patients with metastatic disease. Recently, the first trial comparing, in a randomized fashion, a high-dose with a conventional-dose treatment as first-line therapy of advanced breast cancer has been reported [9]. Two cycles of high-dose treatment with cyclophosphamide, mitoxantrone and etoposide have been compared to a conventional-dose regimen containing cyclophosphamide, mitoxantrone and vincristine. Although this study shows a survival advantage for the high-dose arm, there is still room for improvement. One way for ameliorating results could consist in using docetaxel in the induction treatment before consolidation with high-dose chemotherapy. This choice is supported by the high percentage of tumor responses observed when docetaxel is given as a first-line treatment: a significant « tumor debulking » through 3 to 4 cycles of docetaxel might be obtained, while reserving the other drugs (alkylating agents, mitoxantrone) for the high-dose consolidation treatment. Furthermore, the administration of docetaxel as an induction therapy lasting no more than 3 to 4 cycles, should avoid the onset of cumulative toxicities such as the fluid retention syndrome. Based on this rationale, a phase III study of high dose chemotherapy will be activated in Belgium very soon.

Incorporating docetaxel in the adjuvant setting

Docetaxel being clearly one of the most if not the most active drug for the treatment of metastatic breast cancer, the forthcoming development of this drug is in the adjuvant setting. This rapid upfront move is also supported by the noticeable activity observed with docetaxel in anthracycline-resistant patients and in liver metastases. The last point seems to be worth-mentioning, because it has been reported that the regimens currently used as adjuvant treatment improve patients outcome mainly by reducing the incidence of local, regional or distant soft-tissue relapses, while first recurrences in bone or viscera appear to be much less influenced [10].
Some multicentric trials incorporating docetaxel in the adjuvant treatment of stage II breast cancer are already ongoing and should determine the role of this drug in the early stage of the disease.

Coping with the fluid retention syndrome and other side effects of taxotere

The fluid retention syndrome (FRS) is the most peculiar toxicity encountered so far with docetaxel. It is clear that the onset of this phenomenum is dependent on the cumulative dose of docetaxel given, with a high probability of occurrence (60%) after the cumulative dose of 400 mg/m2 has been reached. Lower extremities, as well as the pleural and peritoneal cavity, are the targets of this syndrome and diuretics or capillary-protectors have not been found to have a significant impact on the natural history of the syndrome. It is suspected that this syndrome is caused by an abnormal transcapillary filtration of proteins but no information on its etiology is available. There is now compelling evidence that a pre- and post-medication with dexamethasone or methylprednisolone is able to prevent or at least delay the onset of FRS; in particular, a randomized study, where patients were allocated to receive or not receive methylprednisone shortly before and for 3 days after docetaxel administration, has demonstrated that peripheral fluid retention or pleural effusions occured after mean docetaxel cumulative doses of 550 mg/m2 and 296 mg/m2, respectively (p = 0.003) [11].
Besides the FRS, other side-effects may be observed with docetaxel. The most common events are neutropenia (91% of patients, with infectious episodes in 20% of cases), alopecia (83%), asthenia (68%), dermatological effects (64%), neurosensory effects (48%), nausea (44%), diarrhea (43%), mucositis (43%) and hypersensitivity reactions (31%) [12]. It is worth mentioning that patients with altered liver function tests (SGOT and/or SGPT > 1.5 and alkaline phos-

phatase > 2,5 x upper limit of normal) have a 25-30% reduction in docetaxel clearance and, according to a retrospective analysis, a much higher probability of severe myelosuppression. Indeed, it has been shown that the incidence of febrile neutropenia is 13% in patients with liver function tests within the normal range *versus* 24% in case of altered hepatic function; toxic deaths were noted in 1,7% *versus* 11,9% of cases, if liver function tests were abnormal. Clearly, more clinical experience is needed in this setting and one may want to deliver the first two cycles of docetaxel to patients with abnormal liver function tests with a dose-reduction of 25%, and thereafter, in case of a favourable response, to administer the drug at full dose. One study is ongoing to support this proposal.

Different strategies, as the utilization of granulocyte-CSFs, are ongoing for ameliorating docetaxel-induced neutropenia. Based on some preliminary data coming from the combination of amifostine with paclitaxel, which suggest that neurotoxicity might be attenuated by this « chemoprotector » [13], a pilot experience is ongoing within the Investigational Drug Branch of the EORTC Breast Cancer Cooperative Group: all patients will receive the first cycle of docetaxel without amifostine and the subsequent cycles with amifostine; this study design will help to clarify the effect of this compound on docetaxel toxicity and pharmacokinetics.

Developing projects

A considerable amount of preclinical and early clinical projects are focusing on different developmental strategies for docetaxel.

Laboratory data suggest that there is not a complete cross-resistance between docetaxel and paclitaxel and preliminary clinical data have shown, among 24 patients pretreated with paclitaxel, one CR and 2 PRs induced by docetaxel [14]. If these data are confirmed, one can foresee the possibility of combining these taxanes or to deliver one drug when the other one has already failed.

A further area of research is represented by the combination of docetaxel, as well as of other chemotherapeutic agents, with angiogenesis inhibitors, which have the potential to arrest tumor spread. This family of compounds is quite heterogeneous because it includes a wide range of molecules with alternative mechanisms of action. Early data suggest that these drugs are optimally tolerated, without a clear relationship between dose-escalation and increase in toxicity. Furthermore, there is the hope that these drugs, representing a non-cytotoxic « tumourostatic » approach, may offer an ideal complement for those patients having achieved a marked tumor shrinkage with potent cytotoxic drugs, such as docetaxel [15].

Recent data also suggest that monoclonal antibodies blocking the epidermal growth factor receptor or the neu (c-erbB-2) receptor may synergize with cytotoxics such as doxorubicin, cisplatin and paclitaxel. This might also be demonstrated with docetaxel, in which case such a new combination would deserve to be tested clinically in breast or ovarian cancers expressing such receptors [16].

Finally, at least two different mechanisms of *in-vitro* resistance to docetaxel have been identified; one, similar to the mechanism of doxorubicin-resistance, is based on the expression of a multidrug resistance protein which acts as an efflux pump, and the second relates to the formation of altered microtubular components which do not properly interact with docetaxel [17, 18]. Attempts should now be made to elucidate in vivo mechanisms of docetaxel resistance and to identify predictive markers associated with a high or a low probability of response to this drug.

Conclusions

Docetaxel represents a clear step forward in the treatment of advanced breast cancer, through its significant impact on anthracycline-resistant disease. A rapid move of this very active drug in the first-line treatment of metastatic breast cancer and in the adjuvant setting is taking place and carries the hope of a significant improvement in the management of this disease for the near future.

Acknowledgements

The authors want to thank the foundation Les Amis de l'Institut Jules Bordet for supporting the clinical research fellowship of Doctor A. Di Leo, M.D. and the Foundation J. Houtart for supporting the research activities of Doctor D. de Valeriola, M.D.

References

1. Trudeau ME. Docetaxel (taxotere): an overview of first-line monotherapy. *Semin Oncol* 1995, 22: 17-21.
2. Taxotere® (docetaxel): International Product Monograph. 2nd edition, 1996: 29-36.
3. Van Oosterom AT. Docetaxel (taxotere): an effective agent in the management of second-line breast cancer. *Semin Oncol* 1995, 22: 22-8.
4. Piccart MJ, Raymond E, Aapro M, Eisenhauer EA and Cvitkovic E. Cytotoxic agents with activity in breast cancer patients previously exposed to anthracyclines: current status and future prospects. *Eur J Cancer* 1995, 31A: S1-S10.
5. Bissery MC, Nohynek G, Sanderink GJ. Docetaxel (taxotere Rm): a review of preclinical and clinical experience. Part 1: preclinical experience. Anticancer Drugs 1995, 6: 339-68.
6. Sledge GW Jr, Robert N, Sparano JA. Paclitaxel (taxol)/doxorubicin combinations in advanced breast cancer: the Eastern Cooperative Oncology Group experience. *Semin Oncol* 1994, 21: 15-8.
7. Schellens JHM, Ma J, Bruno R, Paccaly D, Vergniol JC, Planting AST, de Boer-Dennert M, Van der Burg MEL, Storer G, Verweij J. Pharmacokinetics of cisplatin and taxotere (docetaxel) and WBC DNA-adduct formation of cisplatin in the sequence taxotere/cisplatin and cisplatin/taxotere in a phase I/II study in solid tumor patients. *Proc. Am Soc Clin Oncol* 1994, 13: 323.
8. Taguchi T, Mori S, Abe R. Late phase II clinical study of RP 56976 (docetaxel) in patients with advanced recurrent breast cancer. *Jpn J Cancer Chemother* 1994, 21: 2625-32.
9. Bezwoda WR, Seymour L, Dansey RD. High-dose chemotherapy with hematopoietic rescue as a primary treatment for metastatic breast cancer: a randomized trial. *J Clin Oncol* 1995, 13: 2483-9.
10. Goldhirsch A, Gelber RD, Price KN, Castiglione M, Coates AS, Rudenstam CM, Collins J, Lindtner J, Hacking A, Marini G, Byrne M, Cortes-Funes H, Schnurch G, Brunner KW, Tattersall MHN, Forbes J, Senn HJ. Effect of systemic adjuvant treatment on first sites of breast cancer relapse. *Lancet* 1994, 343: 377-81.
11. Piccart MJ, Klijn J, Paridaens R, Nooij M, Mauriac L, Coleman R, Awada A, Selleslags J, Van Vreckem A, Van Glabbeke M. Steroids do reduce the severity and delay the onset of docetaxel induced fluid retention: final results of a randomized trial of the EORTC Investigational Drug Branch for Breast Cancer (IDBBC). *Eur J Cancer* 1995, 31A: S75.
12. Cortes JE, Pazdur R. Docetaxel. *J Clin Oncol* 1995, 13: 2643-55.
13. Schuchter L, Dipaola R, Greenberg E. A phase I study of amifostine and escalating doses of taxol in patients with advanced cancer. *Eur J Cancer* 1995, 31A: 958.
14. Ravdin P, Valero V, Burris III H, Von Hoff DD, Hortobagyi G. Docetaxel therapy in anthracycline/anthracenedione or paclitaxel resistant metastatic breast cancer. *Proc. American Society Clinical Oncology* 1995, 14: 94.

15. Folkman J. Clinical applications of research on angiogenesis. *Semin. Med.* 1995, 333: 1757.
16. Dillman RO. Antibodies as cytotoxic therapy. *J Clin Oncol* 1994, 12: 1497-515.
17. Bissery MC, Vrignaud P, Riou JF, Lavelle F. *In vivo* isolation and characterization of a docetaxel resistant B16 melanoma. *Proc. American Association Cancer Research* 1995, 36: 316.
18. Fellous A, Fromes Y, Veitia R, Mazie JC, Bissery MC. Docetaxel sensitive and refractory pancreatic tumors contain different polypeptides related to brain microtubule associated proteins. *Proc. American Association Society Clinical Oncology* 1995, 14: 87.

In vivo evaluation of docetaxel (Taxotere®) and vinorelbine (Navelbine®) as single agents and in combination in mammary tumor models

M.C. Bissery, P. Vrignaud and F. Lavelle

Rhône-Poulenc Rorer SA, Centre de Recherche de Vitry-Alfortville, Vitry-sur-Seine, France

Docetaxel (RP 56976, Taxotere®) is a semi-synthetic compound, prepared from a non cytotoxic precursor, 10-deacetyl baccatin III extracted from the needles of the yew tree *Taxus baccata L.*. It promotes tubulin polymerization and stabilizes the formed microtubules [1]. Vinorelbine (Navelbine®) is a semi-synthetic vinca alkaloid. It inhibits the polymerization of tubulin into microtubules [2]. Both compounds have now demonstrated clinical antitumor activity in first line breast cancer with an overall response rate of 61% and 41% for docetaxel and vinorelbine, respectively [3-5]. This paper reports the preclinical evaluation of docetaxel and vinorelbine as single agents and in combination in mammary tumors models in mice.

Material and methods

Drugs

Docetaxel (RP 56976, NSC 628503) was first dissolved in ethanol, then polysorbate 80 was added and the final dilution of docetaxel was obtained with 5% glucose in water (5/5/90; v/v/v). The pH of the solution was 5 and it was injected i.v. under 0.4 ml per mouse. Vinorelbine was obtained from Laboratoire Pierre Fabre Oncologie (Boulogne, France). It was prepared in 5% glucose in water. The pH of the final solution ranged between 5 and 6. The volume of injection was 0.2 ml per mouse i.v.

Mice

Females C3H/HeN were bred at Charles River (Cléon, France) from strains obtained from Charles River Laboratories, Wilmington, MA, USA. Mice were over 18 g at start of chemotherapy. Swiss nu/nu were bred at IFFA CREDO (L'Arbresle, France) from strains obtained from The Jackson Laboratories, Bar Harbor, ME, USA. They were supplied food (UAR reference 113, Epinay-sur-Orge, France) and water *ad libitum*.

Tumor models

The murine tumors used for *in vivo* evaluation were: mammary adenocarcinoma 13/C (MA13/C), 16/C (MA16/C), and 17/A (MA17/A) [6]; mammary carcinoma 44 (MA 44) obtained from Dr T.H. Corbett. The human tumor xenografted in nude mice was Calc-18 established from a 10^7 cells implant (cells were obtained from Dr. J.F. Riou) [7] and passaged subcutaneously. The murine tumors were maintained in the mouse strain of origin *i.e.*, C3H/HeN (MA16/C, MA13/C, MA17/A, MA44). The human tumor was maintained in nude mice. Solid tumors were transplanted as s.c. fragments. For chemotherapy trials, tumors were transplanted in the strain of origin or in the appropriate F1 hybrid.

In vivo solid tumor evaluation

The methods of protocol design, chemotherapy techniques, and data analysis have been presented in detail [8, 9]. Briefly, for efficacy trials, i.v. chemotherapy was started between day 3 and day 24 after tumor implantation. Mice were weighed at least 3 times a week. Solid tumors were measured with a caliper twice or three times weekly, depending on the tumor growth rate, until the tumor reached 2,000 mg or until the animal died. Solid tumor weights (mg) were estimated from two dimensional tumor measurements (mm):

$$\text{Tumor weight} = \frac{\text{length} \times \text{width}^2}{2}$$

Antitumor activity was evaluated at the highest non toxic dose (HNTD) which is the highest dosage that can be administered without causing death or undue toxicity. A dosage producing a weight loss nadir or drug-related deaths of $\geq$ 20% was considered as excessively toxic. Animal body weights included tumor weights.

The end points for assessing solid tumor activity were as follows [8, 9]:

Tumor growth inhibition (T/C value)

$$\text{T/C (\%)} = \frac{\text{Median tumor weight of the Treated (T)}}{\text{Median tumor weight of the Control (C)}} \times 100$$

According to the National Cancer Institute (NCI) standards, a T/C $\leq$ 42% is the minimum level for activity. A T/C < 10% is considered as a high antitumor activity level which justifies further development (Decision Network-2 level, DN-2).

Tumor growth delay (T-C value)

The tumor growth delay assays are based on the median time (in days), required for the treatment group (T) and the control group (C) tumors, to reach a predetermined size (usually 750 to 1,000 mg). Tumor-free survivors are excluded from these calculations and tabulated separately. This value allows the quantitation of the tumor cell kill.

Determination of the tumor doubling time (Td)

Td is estimated from the best fit straight line from a log linear growth plot of the control group tumors in exponential growth (100 to 1,000 mg range).

Calculation of tumor cell kill

For s.c. growing tumors, the total cell kill is calculated from the following formula:

$$\log \text{ cell kill} = \frac{\text{T-C value in days}}{3.32 \times Td}$$

where T-C is the tumor growth delay in days as defined above, and Td is the tumor volume doubling time in days.

Regression of advanced stage primary site tumor

A complete regression is a regression below the limit of palpation.

Determination of therapeutic synergism and combination toxicity index

The methods used for the determination of therapeutic synergism and the calculation of the combination toxicity index are described in detail in [10]. A combination is considered to have therapeutic synergism if it is therapeutically superior to the optimum use of either agent alone. In all trials presented, comparisons between the single agents and the combinations were made at the maximum tolerated dose. The combination toxicity index represents the sum of the fractions of the lethal dose 10 of each single agent. A CTI of 1 indicates that only 50% (or any other ratios, 70:30, 40:60...) of the LD10 of each agent can be used in combination without incurring additional toxicity whereas a CTI of 2 indicates that 100% of the LD10 dose of each single agent can be used in combination.

Results

Efficacy of docetaxel as a single agent

Docetaxel was evaluated i.v. using intermittent schedules against 5 mammary tumors, 4 of them from mouse (MA16/C, MA13/C, MA17/A, MA44) and 1 of them from human origin (Calc-18). Full dose response trials were carried out and the highest non toxic dose (HNTD) was defined as the dosage that did not produce lethality or excessive body weight loss (20%). Results are reported in *Table I*.
- *Mammary 16/C:* This tumor is a fast growing (Td ≅ 1.4 days) metastatic adenocarcinoma. It is highly sensitive to doxorubicin. Mice bearing early stage MA16/C were treated using a Q2D x 3 schedule. At the highest non toxic dose (15 mg/kg/injection), docetaxel was found highly active with a 0% T/C corresponding to a 2.4 log cell kill. It was also tested against advanced stage MA16/C (tumor burden ranging from 126-395 mg with a median of 190 mg) using the same schedule. The highest non toxic dose was 10.8 mg/kg/injection and produced 100% complete regressions.
- *Mammary 13/C:* This doxorubicin-sensitive adenocarcinoma has a 2.5-3.5 days tumor doubling time. Docetaxel was administered on a Q2D x 3 schedule to mice bearing early stage MA13/C. The highest non toxic dose (14.2 mg/kg/injection), produced a 0% T/C with a 4.3 log cell kill. At an advanced stage (the tumor burden ranged between 200-320 mg), the highest non toxic dose 15 mg/kg/injection administered on a Q3D x 3 schedule, yielded 60% complete regressions with a 2.5 log cell kill.
- *Mammary 17/A:* This tumor is an adenocarcinoma with approximately a 1.6 days tumor doubling time and marked sensitivity to doxorubicin. At the highest non toxic dose 15 mg/

kg/injection, administered on day 4, 6 and 8 post tumor implantation, docetaxel was found highly active with a 0% T/C and a 2.8 log cell kill.
- *Mammary 44:* This tumor is a highly metastatic and invasive carcinoma with approximately a 2 days tumor doubling time and with marginal sensitivity to doxorubicin. Docetaxel was administered on day 3, 5, 7 post tumor implantation. At the highest non toxic dose 22 mg/kg/injection, the T/C was 39% which is a very minor activity.
- *Human mammary Calc-18:* This model is a slow growing adenocarcinoma with a 5.9 days tumor doubling time. It was established in mice with 10^7 cells per mouse and propagated subcutaneously with tumor fragments afterwards. Using a Q3D x 3 schedule, docetaxel was found highly active on palpable Calc-18, and yielded a 2.1 log cell kill at the highest non toxic dose (32.2 mg/kg/injection).

Table I. *In vivo* antitumor activity of docetaxel.

Breast Tumor (Subcutaneous)	Highest Non Toxic IV Dose (mg/kg/injection)	Schedule (d)	Total Dose (mg/kg)	T/C Value (%)	T-C (days)	Log Cell Kill	CR
Murine							
MA16/C early	15.0	3,5,7	45.0	0	12.6	2.4	
MA16/C advanced	10.8	7,9,11	32.4	-	14.3	2.9	5/5
MA13/C early	14.2	3,5,7	42.6	0	36.0	4.3	
MA13/C advanced	15.0	24,27,30	45	-	26.5	2.5	3/5
MA17/A early	15.0	4,6,8	45.0	0	17.7	2.8	
MA44 early	22.0	3,5,7	66.0	39	-	-	
Human							
Calc-18 advanced	32.2	7,10,13	96.6	-	40.8	2.1	

Abbreviations: IV, intravenous; T, median tumor weight of treated animals; C, median tumor weight of control animals; T/C, tumor growth inhibition (T/C ≤ 42% active; T/C < 10% highly active); T-C, tumor growth delay; CR, complete regressions.

Efficacy of vinorelbine as a single agent

Vinorelbine was evaluated i.v. using single or multiple intermittent administration against 4 murine early stage mammary tumors (MA16/C, MA13/C, MA17/A and MA44). Dose response studies were carried out, and the results are reported at optimal dosage in *Table II*.
- *Mammary 16/C:* At the HNTD, 5 mg/kg/injection administered using an intermittent schedule, vinorelbine was found highly active with a 0% T/C and a 4.3 log cell kill.
- *Mammary 13/C:* Using a single bolus administration, the HNTD of vinorelbine was 17.7 mg/kg/injection. It produced a 0% T/C corresponding to a 2.8 log cell kill.
- *Mammary 17/A:* A very good activity was also obtained with this tumor at the HNTD of 6.7 mg/kg/injection administered on a Q2Dx3 schedule. The T/C was 0% and the corresponding log cell kill was 3.0.
- *Mammary 44:* This tumor was the less sensitive of the 4 models. At the HNTD (6.3 mg/kg/injection) administered on days 3, 5 and 7, the T/C was 23% with a 0.8 associated log cell kill.

Table II. *In vivo* antitumor activity of vinorelbine.

Breast Tumor (Subcutaneous)	Highest Non Toxic IV Dose (mg/kg/injection)	Schedule (d)	Total Dose (mg/kg)	T/C Value (%)	T-C (days)	Log Cell Kill
Murine						
MA16/C	5.0	4,8,12,18	20.0	0.0	17.3	4.3*
MA13/C	17.7	5	17.7	0.0	22.9	2.8
MA17/A	6.7	3,5,7	20.1	0.0	12.9	3.0
MA44	6.3	3,5,7	18.9	23.0	4.9	0.8

Abbreviations and activity rating, see legend in Table I.
* The very high activity observed in this trial should be viewed with caution as the duration of treatment was three thimes greater than in the other trials.

Efficacy of docetaxel and vinorelbine in combination

This combination was evaluated using mammary 13/C and mammary 16/C.

Mammary 13/C

A first trial was performed against palpable mammary 13/C tumor. Docetaxel was administered on day 11 and 18, and vinorelbine was administered on day 11. The HNTD of docetaxel was 35 mg/kg/injection and produced 50% tumor free survivors 195 days post tumor implantation. The tumor growth delay for the mice that developed tumors was 51.6 days. The HNTD of vinorelbine was 10.5 mg/kg in the trial and produced a 21.7 days tumor growth delay. When the two agents were combined, the tumor growth delay of the highest non toxic combination was 55.6 days and produced 12.5% tumor free survivors on day 195. This optimal combination contained 31.5 mg/kg/injection of docetaxel and 15.3 mg/kg/injection of vinorelbine. This corresponded to a 1.8 combination toxicity index. Because of the great number of cures, the combination was evaluated against the same tumor model but at a more advanced stage.
In this second trial, docetaxel was administered on day 24 and 31 against measurable mammary 13/C tumors ranging from 380-450 mg, and vinorelbine was administered on day 24 only. The highest non toxic dose of docetaxel (37 mg/kg/injection) induced 100% complete regressions and 40% of the mice were cured on day 210 post tumor implantation. The tumor growth delay for the mice that developed tumors was 67.5 days. The body weight loss at nadir was 11.5%. Vinorelbine, at its highest non toxic dose 15 mg/kg/injection produced a similar body weight loss at nadir. Sixty percent complete regressions were obtained with a corresponding tumor growth delay of 25.3 days. When administered in combination simultaneously, the optimal dosage was 29.6 mg/kg/injection of docetaxel and 12 mg/kg/injection of vinorelbine. This corresponded to a 1.55 combination toxicity index. This combination produced 11% body weight loss (day 35), 100% complete regression and 40% cures. The tumor growth delay on the tumors that regrew was 75.8 days.

Mammary 16/C

Using an intermittent schedule day 4 and 11, docetaxel highest non toxic dose was 30 mg/kg/injection and yielded a tumor growth delay of 17.4 days. Vinorelbine using the same schedule yielded a 10.1 day tumor growth delay at the highest non toxic dose, 10 mg/kg/injection. The body weight loss at nadir were 10 and 3% for docetaxel and vinorelbine, respectively. When combined simultaneously, it was possible to administer 36 mg/kg/injection of docetaxel and 12 mg/kg/injection of vinorelbine without incurring additional toxicity, which corresponded to a combination toxicity index of 2. The associated body weight loss was 11% with a 17 day host recovery time. This combination produced 40% tumor free survivors on day 130 post tumor implantation and a tumor growth delay of 20.5 days for the tumor that regrew.

Table III. *In vivo* combination therapy of docetaxel with vinorelbine.

Agent IV	HNTD (mg/kg/injection) IV	Schedule (d)	Total Dose (mg/kg)	T-C (d)	CR	Tumor free survivors	Log Cell Kill	CTI at* LD10
Mammary adenocarcinoma MA13/C								
docetaxel	35	11,18	70	51.6		4/8	7.8	
vinorelbine	10.5	11	10.5	21.7		0/8	3.3	
docetaxel +	31.5	11,18	63	55.6		1/8	8.4	1.8
vinorelbine	15.3	11	15.3					
Tumor doubling time = 2 days; Time for control median tumor to reach 750 mg = 19 days								
Mammary adenocarcinoma MA13/C								
docetaxel	37	24,31	74	67.5	5/5	2/5	5.8	
vinorelbine	15	24	15	25.3	3/5	0/5	2.2	
docetaxel +	29.6	24,31	59.2	75.8	5/5	2/5	6.5	1.55
vinorelbine	12	24	12					
Tumor doubling time = 3.5 days; Time for control median tumor to reach 750 mg = 25.5 days								
Mammary adenocarcinoma MA16/C								
docetaxel	30	4,11	60	17.4		0/5	4.4	
vinorelbine	10	4,11	20	10.1		0/5	2.6	
docetaxel +	36	4,11	72	20.5		2/5	5.1	2
vinorelbine	12		24					
Tumor doubling time = 1.2 days; Time for control median tumor to reach 1000 mg = 10.6 days								

Abbreviations, see legend in Table I. The CTI was calculated at the LD10; this differs somewhat from the evaluation in [15] where the CTI was calculated at the HNTD.

Discussion and conclusion

Docetaxel and vinorelbine are new chemical entities with unique mechanism of action. Docetaxel used as a single agent has demonstrated antitumor activity against a wide spectrum of transplantable murine and human tumors [8, 11-14] especially in the case of breast tumors including regressions of advanced stage disease in murine models (MA16/C, MA13/C) and long tumor growth delay in human tumor xenograft Calc-18. Vinorelbine was also found highly active against these same murine models treated at an early stage.
The docetaxel-vinorelbine combination was the most intriguing combinations as both compounds share the same target, *i.e.*, the tubulin-microtubule system, either inhibiting the tubulin

polymerization in the case of the vinca alkaloids or inhibiting the microtubule depolymerization in the case of taxoids. The combination toxicity indexes at the LD10 were 1.55 to 2 indicating that 77-100% of the optimal dose of each agent could be administered without increasing the toxicity to vital normal cells. This was very surprising but was found to be a common feature among inhibitors of tubulin polymerization, *i.e.*, vincristine, vinblastine and vinorelbine [15]. All of the above data were generated using simultaneous administration. However it should be noted that spacing the administration of the two compounds by 24 hours, lead to a dose reduction for the optimal combination [15].

In conclusion, although docetaxel and vinorelbine are potent agents when used in monotherapy, the above results suggest that their combination could have a key role to play in the case of breast cancer treatment. In clinical trials, both compounds have demonstrated antitumor activity in first line breast cancer with an overall response rate of 61% for docetaxel and 41% for vinorelbine [3-5]. Their combination is currently being evaluated in clinical trials [16].

Acknowledgements

The authors gratefully acknoweldge the technical assitance of the staff of the Experimental Therapeutic Laboratory, M. Avazeri, G. Baudry, M.C. Brias, R. Bernier, D. Huet, J. Pelette, R. Poulet and A. Selingue, and L. Ramdani for the preparation of the manuscript.

References

1. Guéritte-Voegelein F, Guénard D, Lavelle F, *et al.* Relationships between the structure of Taxol analogues and their antimitotic activity. *J Med Chem* 1991; 34: 992-8.
2. Binet S, Chaineau E, Fellous A, Lataste H, Krikorian A, Couzinier JP, Meiniger V. Immunofluorescence study of the action of navelbine, vincristine, and vinblastine on mitotic and axonal microtubules. *Int J Cancer* 1990; 46: 262-6.
3. Chevallier B, Fumoleau P, Kerbrat P *et al.* Docetaxel is a major cytotoxic drug for the treatment of advanced breast cancer: a phase II trial of the Clinical Screening Cooperative Group of the European Organization for Research and Treatment of Cancer (ENG). *J Clin Oncol* 1995; 13: 314-22.
4. Fumoleau P, Chevallier B, Kerbrat P *et al.* A multicentric phase II study of the efficacy and safety of docetaxel as first-line treatment of advanced breast cancer: Report of the Clinical Screening Group of the EORTC. *Ann Oncol* 1996; 7: 165-71.
5. Fumoleau P, Delgado FN, Delozier T *et al.* Phase II trial of weekly intravenous vinorelbine in first line advanced breast cancer chemotherapy. *J Clin Oncol* 1993; 11: 1245-52.
6. Corbett TH, Griswold DP Jr, Roberts BJ, *et al.* Biology and therapeutic response of a mouse mammary adenocarcinoma (16/C) and its potential as a model for surgical adjuvant chemotherapy. *Cancer Treat Rep* 1978; 62:1471-88.
7. Gioanni J, Courdi A, Lalanne CM, *et al.* Establishment, characterization, chemosenstivity, and radiosensitivity of two different cell lines derived from a human breast cancer biopsy. *Cancer Res* 1985; 45: 1246-58.
8. Bissery MC, Guénard D, Guéritte-Voegelein F, *et al.* Experimental antitumor activity of Taxotere (RP 56976, NSC 628503), a Taxol analogue. *Cancer Res* 1991; 51: 4845-52.
9. Corbett TH, Leopold WR, Dykes DJ, *et al.* Toxicity and anticancer activity of a new triazine antifolate (NSC 127755). *Cancer Res* 1982; 42: 1707-15.
10. Corbett TH, Roberts BJ, Trader MW, *et al.* Response of transplantable tumors of mice to anthracenedione derivatives alone and in combination with clinically useful agents. *Cancer Treat Rep* 1982; 66: 1187-200.
11. Dykes DJ, Waud WR, Bissery MC, *et al.* Response of human tumor xenografts in athymic nude mice to Taxotere. *Investigational New Drugs* (in press).

12. Boven E, Venema-Gaberscek E, Erkelens CAM, *et al*. Antitumor activity of Taxotere (RP 56976, NSC 628503), a new Taxol analog, in experimental ovarian cancer. *Annals of Oncology* 1993; 4: 321-4.
13. Nicoletti MI, Lucchini V, D'Incalci M, *et al*. Comparison of paclitaxel and docetaxel activity on human ovarian carcinoma xenografts. *Eur J Cancer* 1994; 30A: 691-6.
14. Braakhuis BJM, Kegel A, Welters MJP. The growth inhibiting effect of docetaxel (Taxotere,) in head and neck squamous cell carcinoma xenografts. *Cancer Letters* 1994; 81: 151-4.
15. Bissery MC, Vrignaud P, Lavelle F. Preclinical profile of docetaxel (Taxotere): efficacy as a single agent and in combination. *Sem Oncol* 1995; 22 (6) Suppl 13: 3-16.
16. Fumoleau P, Delecroix V, Gentin M, *et al*. Docetaxel (D) in combination with vinorelbine (V) as first line CT in PTS with MBC: Phase I dose finding study. *EJC* 1995; 31A Suppl 5: S195 (abstract 938).

Breast Cancer. Advances in biology and therapeutics.
F. Calvo, M. Crépin, H. Magdelenat, eds. John Libbey Eurotext © 1996, pp. 273-278.

Clinical data of Navelbine-Taxotere association in breast cancer patients

P. Fumoleau[1], V. Delecroix[1], G. Perrocheau[1], O. Borg-Olivier[2], C. Maugard[1], R. Fety[1], N. Azli[2], J.P. Louboutin[1] and A. Riva[2]

[1]*Centre René Gauducheau, ICERC, Nantes ;* [2]*Rhône-Poulenc-Rorer, Antony, France*

Introduction

Breast cancer is the leading cancer site in women in the European community, with an estimated 135,000 new cases per year and 58,000 recorded deaths per year. Improved screening techniques and their increasingly widespread availability over the past years have generally led to earlier detection and more successful treatment of primary breast tumours. Nevertheless, 40-60% of women with breast cancer go on to develop advanced or metastatic disease [1]. The natural course of metastatic breast cancer is highly variable but the average survival time is 18 to 24 months. Established drug treatments do not markedly affect survival and are essentially palliative [2, 3].

Up to a third of patients with advanced breast cancer respond to hormonal manipulation. However, for patients who do not respond, and for those who have hormone-independent or aggressive cancer types or who experience rapid progression, anti cancer chemotherapy is required. Many cytotoxic agents have demonstrated activity in advanced breast cancer, the most active and commonly used agents being cyclophosphamide, fluorouracil, doxorubicin, methotrexate and mitomycin C, either as single-agent or in combination regimens [4]. Doxorubicin containing regimens induce higher response rate with prolonged median duration of response between 10 and 18 months, but the median survival time of 18 to 26 months is modestly superior to the most commonly used combination CMF (cyclophosphamide, methotrexate, fluorouracil) [5, 6]. So, there is clearly a need to develop new anticancer agents, new combinations and new strategies in order to try to improve the chemotherapy results in breast cancer.

Recently, paclitaxel has been demonstrated to produce good results in breast cancer [7, 8]. Paclitaxel promotes polymerisation of tubulin, increasing microtubule assembly and stabilising any microtubules already formed. This prevents the reorganisation of the microtubule network required to form the spindle during mitosis and, therefore disrupts the distribution of chromosomes into daugther cells, preventing cell replication [9].

Taxotere (docetaxel) is another effective anticancer agent of the same chemical class as paclitaxel. In *in vivo* comparisons with paclitaxel, docetaxel has been shown to be 2.5 to 5 times more active against various cancer cell lines [10] and to have equal or superior activity against a number of freshly explanted and cloned human cancer specimens, including breast cancer [11]. Following 5 phase I studies, the recommended schedule and dose for phase II studies with docetaxel was 100 mg/m^2, 1-hour infusion, every three weeks. Docetaxel has been investigated as a single agent in five phase II studies of first-line treatment of metastatic breast cancer. These studies involved a total of 209 patients, 188 of whom were evaluable for response. Response rates, which are summarised in *Table 1*, are grouped according to the starting dose of docetaxel, since some patients were treated at the reduced initial dose of 75 mg/m^2. Using the recommended dose of 100 mg/m2 with a relative dose intensity of 0.91, the median response duration was 8.3 months, the median time to progression was 21 weeks and the median survival was 16.4 months.

Table I. Docetaxel therapy as first line treatment for metastatic breast cancer (response rates).

Dose of docetaxel	Study	Number of evaluable patients	Response rate (%)
75 mg/m^2	NCIC [12]	15	40
	EORTC-CSG2 [13]	31	52
	Total	**46**	**48**
100 mg/m^2	MSKCC [14]	34	56
	NCIC [12]	32	56
	EORTC-CSG1 [15]	31	68
	EORTC-CSG3 [16]	37	68
	EORTC-ECTG [17]	8	38
	Total	**142**	**61**

Vinorelbine (navelbine) is a unique semi synthetic vinca-alkaloid (VA) derivative of vinblastine synthesised by P. Potier in the late 1970s from catharantine and vindoline extracted from vinca rosea leaves. Like other VA, navelbine induces cytotoxicity by inhibiting microtubules assembly; however, navelbine appears to be more specific in that it preferentially affects microtubules of the mitotic spindle 18]. In contrast to vincristine which depolymerizes microtubules at concentrations of 5 µm, navelbine do not induce this effect below 30 µm indicating that this drug may have a reduced potential for causing neurotoxicity [19]. Following phase I studies, the recommended schedule and dose for phase II studies with navelbine was 30 mg/m^2, short weekly infusion. Navelbine has been investigated as a single agent in six phase II studies of first-line treatment of metastatic breast cancer *(Table II)*. From these studies, it appears clearly that navelbine with a response rate between 40-60% is an active drug in the treatment of advanced breast cancer. With this weekly schedule, the delivered dose intensity is between 21 and 23 mg/m^2.

Table II. Navelbine therapy as first line treatment for metastatic breast cancer (response rates and dose intensity).

Author (ref)	Number of evaluable patients	Response rate (%)	Dose intensity mg/m^2/w
Fumoleau [20]	145	41	21
Canobbio [21]	30	60	23
Bruno [22]	68	44	22.5
Garcia-Conde [23]	54	50	23
Weber [24]	65	40	-
Romero [25]	22	41	22

Docetaxel in combination with navelbine: results of a phase I dose finding study [26]

Background

Both docetaxel and navelbine have produced a high degree of activity in previously untreated patients with metastatic breast cancer. In addition, preclinical experience on the combination of docetaxel and navelbine on mice bearing s.c. transplantable tumors showed a therapeutic synergism. Moreover, the combination toxicity index (CTI, *i.e.* sum of the fractions of the LD_{10} of each agent used in the combination) of vinorelbine and docetaxel was 2, indicating that the maximum tolerated dose of each agent could be administered without additional toxicity [27].
Therefore a combination chemotherapy in breast cancer patients as first-line chemotherapy (CT) for metastatic disease has been developed to exploit the maximum benefit with these 2 drugs.
Thus a phase I dose finding study combining these 2 agents was conducted at Centre René Gauducheau (Nantes) from June 1994.
At the time of the present report, 29 patients have been entered across all planned dose levels. The objectives of this phase I study were:
- *primarily*, to determine the dose limiting toxicity (DLT), the maximum tolerated dose (MTD) and the recommended dose for phase II and III studies of docetaxel in combination with vinorelbine as first line chemotherapy in metastatic breast cancer patients previously untreated with chemotherapy for metastatic disease.
- *Secondarily*, to asses the safety profile of the combination and the pharmacokinetic of docetaxel and vinorelbine when used in combination.

Patients, methods and results

At day 1 and 5, navelbine was administered first as a 30 minutes IV infusion followed by docetaxel over 1 hour IV infusion, day 1, every 3 weeks to patients previously untreated with CT for metastatic breast cancer. Premedication with 3 days steroids + Daflon 500 mg [2g/day] was used from study entry and maintained during all the treatment.

Eligible patients had metastatic breast cancer with measurable and/or evaluable disease, WHO PS ≤ 2, normal liver, renal and hematologic functions, no prior CT for advanced disease (adjuvant CT allowed provided 12 months interval between the end of CT and study entry). Entered patients were required to have neurologic examination, including nerve conduction studies, by the same neurologist at baseline and then every 2 cycles up to the end of study. To date, 29 patients received 142 cycles. The total number of cycles, the median cumulative dose of docetaxel and vinorelbine administered by dose level and percentage of cycle with dose reduction are presented on *Table III*.

Table III. D. docetaxel, V. Vinorelbine.

Dose levels	D/V mg/m^2	Pts Ent/Ev	Total n° of cycles	Median number of cycles	Median cumulative dose of D mg/m^2	Median cumulative dose of V mg/m^2	Dose reduction (D and/or V) (% cycles)
I	60/20	3/3	18	6 (6)	360	240	0
II	75/20	6/6	34	6 (4-6)	450	240	9
III	75/22.5	4/4	19	4 (3-6)	270	145	53
IV	85/20	10/10	43	6 (4-6)	510	240	5
V	100/20	6/6	28	6 (1-6)	525	240	39

Overall tolerance is presented on *Table IV*.

Table IV. D. docetaxel; V, Vinorelbine; *FN, febrile neutropenia; **DLT, Dose Limiting Toxicity: FN>3 days and/or G3,4 non hematoxicities; °M, mucositis; °°PN, peripheral neuropathy.

Dose levels	D/V mg/m^2	Pts Ent/Ev	Total n° of cycles	G 4 Neutro % Cy	FN* % Cy	G 3-4 M° % Cy	G >1 PN°° % pts	DLT** Pts	DLT (type)	CR/PR Metas 15 eval	CR/PR Ev 13 eval
I	60/20	3/3	18	83	0	0	0	0	-	0/1	2/2
II	75/20	6/6	34	85	9	0	0	0	-	4/4	2/2
III	**75/22.5**	4/4	19	98	37	21	0	3	FN + FN/M°	0/1	2/3
IV	85/20	10/10	43	100	11	3	0	1	FN	4/6	1/4
V	**100/20**	6/6	28	100	11	4	0	4	FN + FN/M°	1/3	2/2

Symptomatic peripheral neuropathy was never observed. The premedication used in the study reduced the incidence and severity of fluid retention.

Two maximum tolerated dose were reached: the first at dose level III (dose limiting toxicity being febrile neutropenia + mucositis or febrile neutropenia alone) and the second at dose level V (dose limiting toxicity being febrile neutropenia + mucositis or febrile neutropenia alone or mucositis alone). So the recommended dose (level IV) for phase II studies is docetaxel 85 mg/m^2 day 1 and navelbine 20 mg/m^2 day 1 and day 5 every 3 weeks.

The premedication used in the study reduced the incidence and severity of fluid retention.

Responses were observed at all dose levels and at all sites and presented in *Table V*. This activity is to be confirmed during phase II studies.

Table V. D. docetaxel; V. Vinorelbine.

Dose levels D/V mg/m^2	Metas. disease Nb eval pts	CR	PR	RR	Eval. disease Nb eval pts	CR	PR	PR
60/20	1	0	0	0/1	2	0	2	2/2
75/20	4	0	4	4/4	2	0	2	2/2
75/22.5	1	0	0	0/1	3	0	2	2/3
85/20	6	2	2	4/6	4	0	1	1/4
100/20	3	0	1	1/3	2	0	2	2/2

Conclusions

Once the activity of the combination of docetaxel and vinorelbine has been confirmed during a phase II study, this chemotherapy could be advantageous to patients with first line metastatic breast cancer when further anthracycline containing therapy can not be used, and also as second line treatment for patients who have failed previous anthracycline containing treatments.

References

1. Jensen OM, Esteve J, Moller H et al. Cancer in the European Community and its member states. Eur J Cancer 1993; 26: 1167-256.
2. Harris JR, Morrow M, Bonadonna G. Cancer of the breast. In De Vita T Jr, Hellman S, Rosenberg SA (eds): Cancer Principle and Practice of Oncology, 4th edition, Philadelphia: JB Lippincot Co. 1993; 1264-332.
3. Leonard RCF, Rodger A, Dixon JM. Metastatic breast cancer BMJ 1994; 309: 1501-4.
4. Henderson IC. Chemotherapy for metastatic disease. In Harris JR, Hellman S, Henderson IC, Kinne DW (eds): Breast diseases, 2th edition, Philadelphia: JB Lippincot Co. 1991; 604-5.
5. Mouridsen HT. Systemic therapy of advanced breast cancer. Drugs 44 (Suppl. 4): 17-28, 1992.
6. Sledge GW and Antman KH. Progress in chemotherapy for metastatic breast cancer. Sem in Oncol 1992 19: 317-332.
7. Holmes FA, Walter RS, Theriault RL et al. Phase II trial of Taxol, an active drug in the treatment of metastatic breast cancer. J Natl Cancer Inst 1991; 83: 1797-805.
8. Reichman BS, Seidman AD, Crown JPA et al. Paclitaxel and recombinant human granulocyte colony stimulating factor as initial chemotherapy for breast cancer. J Clin Oncol 1993; 11: 1943-51.
9. Rowinsky EK, Cazenae LA, Donehower RC. Taxol: A novel investigational antineoplastic agent. J Natl Cancer Inst 1990; 82: 1247-59.
10. Ringel I, Horwitz SB. Studies with RP 56976 (Taxotere): A semi-syntetic analogue of taxol. J Natl Cancer Inst 1991; 83: 288-91.
11. Hanauske A-R, Degen D, Helsenbeck SG et al. Effect of Taxotere and Taxol on in vitro colony formation of freshly explanted human tumor cells. Anti-Cancer Drugs 1992; 3: 121-4.
12. Trudeau ME, Eishenhauer EA, Higgins BP et al. Docetaxel in patients with metastatic breast cancer. A phase II study of the National Cancer Institute of Canada Clinical Trials Group. J Clin Oncol 1996; 14: 422-8.
13. Dieras V, Fumoleau P, Chevallier B et al. Second EORTC-Clinical Screening Group (CSG) phase

II trial of Taxotere (docetaxel) as first line chemotherapy for advanced breast cancer. *Proc Am Soc Clin Onco* 1994, 13: 78 (Abs 115).
14. Hudis CA, Seidman AD, Crown JP. Phase II and pharmacologic study of docetaxel as initial chemotherapy for metastatic breast cancer. *J Clin Oncol* 1996; 14: 58-65.
15. Chevallier B., Fumoleau P, Kerbrat P *et al.* Docetaxel is a major cytotoxic drug for the treatment of advanced breast cancer. A phase II trial of the Clinical Sceening Group of the European Organisation for Research and Treatment of Cancer. *J Clin Oncol* 1995; 13: 314-22.
16. Fumoleau P, Chevallier B, Kerbrat P *et al.* A multicentre phase II study of the efficacy and safety of docetaxel as first-line treatment of advanced breast cancer: Report of the Clinical Screening Group of the EORTC. *Ann Oncol* 1996; 7: 165-71.
17. Ten Bokkel-Huinink WW, Van Oosterom AT, Piccart M *et al.* Taxotere in advanced breast cancer: a phase trial of the EORTC early clinical trials group. *Proc Am Soc Clin Onco* 1993, 12: (Abs 81).
18. Fellous A, Ohayon R, Vacassin T *et al.* Biochemical effects of Navelbine on tubulin and associated proteins. *Sem Oncol* 1989; 16 (supp 4): 9-14.
19. Binet S, Fellous A, Lataste H *et al.* *In situ* analysis of the action of Navelbine on various type of microtubules using immunofluorescence. *Sem Oncol* 1989; 16 (supp 4): 5-8.
20. Fumoleau P, Delgado FN, Delozier T *et al.* Phase II trial of weekly intravenous vinorelbine in first line advanced breast cancer chemotherapy. *J Clin Oncol* 1993; 11: 1245-52.
21. Cannobio L, Boccardo F, Pastorino G *et al.* Phase II study of navelbine in advanced breast cancer. *Sem Oncol* 1989; 16 (supp 4): 33-6.
22. Bruno S, Lira-Puerto V, Texeira L *et al.* Phase II trial with vinorelbine in the treatment of advanced breast cancer. *Proc ECCO* 6 1991 (Abs 268a).
23. Garcia-Conde J, Lluch A, Casado A *et al.* Phase II trial with vinorelbine in the advanced breast cancer previously untreated. Breast *Cancer Research and Treatment* 1992; 23: 142 (Abs 52).
24. Weber B, Vogel C, Jones S *et al.* A us multicenter phase II trial of Navelbine in advanced breast cancer. *Proc Am Soc Clin Onco* 1993, 12: 61 (Abs 46).
25. Romero A, Rabinovich MG, Vallejo JCT *et al.* Vinorelbine as first line chemotherpy for metastatic breast carcinoma. J Clin Oncol 1994; 11: 336-41.
26. Fumoleau P, Delecroix V, Perrocheau G *et al.* Docetaxel in combination with Vinorelbine as 1st line chemotherapy in patients with metastatic breast cancer: Final results. *Proc Am Soc Clin Onco* 1996, 15: 142 (Abs 232).
27. Bissery MC, Azli N, Fumoleau P. Docetaxel in combination with vinorelbine: Preclinical-Clinical correlation. *Proc Am Soc Clin Onco* 1996, 15: 487 (Abs1550).

Breast Cancer. Advances in biology and therapeutics.
F. Calvo, M. Crépin, H. Magdelenat, eds. John Libbey Eurotext © 1996, pp. 279-280.

A short history of drug discovery

Pierre Potier

Institut de chimie des Substances Naturelles (ICSN), Gif-sur-Yvette, France

Nature has always been an inexhaustible source of inspiration for man, especially in the area of therapeutics. Up until the end of the 18th century, most medicinal drugs were of natural origin. This is still true today for more than 60% of drugs, be they from normal or genetically modified plants, microorganisms or animals. Navelbine and Taxotere, two anticancer drugs discovered in our Institute, are no exceptions to this fact.

The discovery of Navelbine

The discovery of antitumor alkaloids isolated from the Madagascan periwinkle by the « insulin team » at the University of Western Ontario in London (Canada) and American scientists at Eli Lilly (Indianapolis) goes back almost forty years ! But it was only in 1974 that the chemical synthesis of these structurally complex natural molecules was achieved in our laboratory at the CNRS's Institut de Chimie des Substances Naturelles in Gif-sur-Yvette. This synthesis had, for over ten years, resisted the efforts of numerous chemists throughout the world.
This success gave us access to many novel molecules in this series. It was in this manner that Navelbine was first prepared and its anticancer properties, shown to be highly interesting, were evaluated. After many long years of research and development, this substance has now been commercialized by Pierre Fabre Laboratories in practically every country in the world except Japan (though this too is imminent). Navelbine is used alone or in association with other chemotherapeutic drugs for the treatment of breast, non-small-cell lung cancers and various other tumors.

The discovery of Taxotere

The yew, *Taxus baccata*, is a well known tree in our regions. Except for the red, fleshy skin covering the seeds, all parts of this tree have been known since Antiquity to be toxic. But it is by chance that the anticancer properties of the Pacific yew *(T. brevifolia)* were discovered by Americans. Among the numerous problems which complicated the development of the substance responsible for its anticancer activity (Taxol) were its low natural abundance (0.1 to 0.2 g/kg of trunk bark from trees one or more hundreds of years old) and low solubility in excipients used for injections. As a result, many tens of thousands of trees had to be felled to produce enough Taxol to permit its development and to treat patients.

We attacked this problem in 1979 and we had the chance to discover a precursor of Taxol (10-deacetylbaccatine III) in the leaves (needles) of our European yew and this in relatively large quantities (0.5 to 1 g/kg of fresh leaves). This precursor was transformed chemically into Taxol, thereby assuring unlimited supplies of this compound starting from an inexhaustible and renewable natural source, the leaves.

During the course of our synthesis of Taxol, we had the good luck of isolating an intermediate which was found to be twice as active as Taxol. It was named Taxotere and was developed in close collaboration with our colleagues of Rhône-Poulenc Rorer and several medical doctors in hospitals, both in France and elsewhere in the world.

These two discoveries are excellent examples of the fruitful collaboration which can be developed among chemists, biologists and doctors both from the public and private sectors. I hope that these examples will not be the only ones. Other molecules currently under study in our laboratory may some day lengthen this list of two for the moment.

Breast Cancer. Advances in biology and therapeutics.
F. Calvo, M. Crépin, H. Magdelenat, eds. John Libbey Eurotext © 1996, pp. 281-288.

The expression levels of episialin in human carcinomas are sufficiently high to potentially interfere with adhesion and promote metastasis

J. Hilkens, H.L. Vos, J. Wesseling, J. Peterse, J. Storm, M. Boer, S.W. van der Valk and M.C.E. Maas

Division of Tumor Biology, The Netherlands Cancer Institute, Antoni van Leeuwenhoekhuis, Plesmanlaan 121, 1066 CX Amsterdam, The Netherlands

Abstract

Episialin (also designated MUC1, EMA, CA 15-3, PEM) strongly reduces cell-cell adhesion when present at a high density on the entire cell surface. As a consequence several cellular processes are affected. For example, cytolysis of cells that overexpress episialin by cytotoxic T cells and LAK cells is strongly diminished. Other membrane associated mucins, such as epiglycanin and CD43, also have anti-adhesive effects and have a very similar protective function against immune cells; overexpression of epiglycanin on mouse cells even allows allotransplantation. Overexpression of episialin in several other types of human tumors has been observed. However, quantitation of the expression levels has been very difficult.

Here, we will review the impact of episialin overexpression on the behavior of tumor cells, and the mechanism of the anti-adhesion effect of episialin. Subsequently, we will show that the levels of episialin that significantly reduce the adhesion in vitro *are also found in primary human breast carcinomas and metastases, and thus are likely to account for decreased tumor cell-stroma contacts in those tumors that express episialin aberrantly at the tumor cell-stroma boundary.*

Introduction

The mucins can be subdivided into the classical mucins, which form the mucus layer in *e.g.* the gastrointestinal tract, and the membrane associated mucins (MAMs), which are produced by a large variety of cell types, and which are, in contrast to the secreted mucins, anchored in the plasma membrane. The common characteristic of both types of mucins is a long threonine, serine and proline rich protein backbone which consists of tandem repeats. This domain is heavily O-glycosylated and constitutes the actual mucin domain. Here, we will mainly discuss one of the MAMs, episialin/MUC1.

Episialin (also designated MUC1, EMA, PEM, CA 15-3 antigen, etc.) is a transmembrane molecule with a large extracellular domain and a cytoplasmic domain of 69 amino acids. The extracellular domain mainly consists of a region of nearly identical repeats of 20 amino acids. The repeats, that comprise most of the extracellular domain, are heavily O-glycosylated and constitute the mucin domain (for review see [1]). The mucin domain has an extended structure [2] which becomes very rigid by the addition of numerous O-linked glycans. As a result, the mucin domain of episialin protrudes high above the cell surface. Indeed, we have identified episialin on the plasma membrane of mammary tumor cells as long thread-like structures. Episialin is mainly localized at the apical side of glandular epithelial cells. Immunohistochemical studies using various monoclonal antibodies (mAbs) revealed that episialin is also present on the trophoblast, at the luminal surfaces of certain cell layers lining other body cavities, such as the mesothelium, and on certain hematopoietic cells, in particular plasma cells.

Immunohistochemical studies have suggested that episialin is highly overexpressed in most breast carcinomas relative to normal breast epithelium. We have quantitated the apparent overexpression of episialin in carcinomas at the RNA level by *in situ* hybridization. Episialin mRNA expression in most primary breast carcinomas was found to be more than ten times higher than in adjacent normal glandular epithelium.

To investigate the effect of overexpression of episialin on cellular interactions, we have transfected episialin cDNA into various cell lines: SV40 transformed mammary epithelial cells (HBL-100), A375 melanoma cells, mouse L-cells and MDCK cells. Cell aggregation experiments revealed that the cell-cell adhesion of the transfectants overexpressing episialin was strongly reduced relative to the episialin negative-controls [3]. Episialin-negative revertant cells, bulk selected with the cell sorter to avoid clonal outgrowth as much as possible, exhibited normal aggregation properties. The presence of episialin on only one of a pair of aggregating cells is already sufficient to interfere with this process. Mouse L cells transfected with both E-cadherin and episialin cDNAs, showed that episialin could override the intercellular adhesion mediated by E-cadherin [4].

High levels of episialin expression often result in altered growth characteristics: A375 cells grow partly in suspension and MDCK cells fail to form epithelial sheets and show a more fibroblastic morphology. However, HBL-100 cells expressing high levels of episialin did not show a clearly altered morphology and did not show as many non-adherent cells as the A375 transfectants, probably because the HBL-100 cells express high levels of (high affinity) integrin receptors. The effect of episialin in A375 transfectants could be reversed by a mAb that induced activation of the $\beta 1$ integrins, indicating that there is a balance between adhesion mediated by integrins and anti-adhesion caused by episialin.

The mechanism by which episialin diminishes adhesion

We have several lines of evidence that the anti-adhesion effect of episialin is caused by non-specific steric hindrance because: 1. MAb induced clustering of the episialin molecules at one side of the cell (capping) could restore cellular adhesion of both transfected and non-adherent breast carcinoma cell lines. After capping, the adhesion molecules are available to their ligands again, indicating that the affinity of the adhesion molecules is not affected by episialin overexpression [5]. 2. Mutant episialin molecules without a cytoplasmic tail can still prevent adhesion, which again can be reversed by capping with a mAb against episialin. This means that the endodomains of episialin and the adhesion molecules do not compete for cytoplasmic components (*e.g.*: components of the actin cytoskeleton), and that signalling events via the endodomain of episialin are not relevant for the anti-adhesive effect. 3. Episialin reduces adhesion mediated via different types of adhesion molecules (*e.g.* integrins and cadherins), showing that inhibition of adhesion is non-specific. 4. Episialin prevents binding of cells to immobilized mAbs, directed against cell surface components. The binding of soluble mAbs to the same cells is not affected however, indicating that episialin hampers the accessibility of receptors to immobilized ligands in general. 5. Shed episialin, as is present in conditioned medium, does not affect the extent of the anti-adhesion property, suggesting that specific association of unidentified components with this domain is not relevant for this effect.

Based on these observations, we hypothesized that the non-specific episialin-mediated anti-adhesive effect is depending on the size and/or the charge of the molecule. Whereas, molecules with 15 or more repeats showed clear anti-adhesion properties, molecules containing eight repeats showed a reduced anti-adhesion effect and molecules with only three tandem repeats did not exert such an effect at all [4], indicating that the extent of the episialin-mediated anti-adhesive effect is strongly dependent on the length of the molecule. Removal of most or all of the sialic acid and sulphate residues from the wild type molecule had only a minor effect on the anti-adhesion property of episialin, indicating that charge repulsion is not the major mechanism for the anti-adhesion effect. Thus, the episialin-mediated anti-adhesive effect is mainly caused by steric hindrance.

Episialin interferes with various cellular functions that require adhesion

LAK cell and allogeneically stimulated T cell mediated cytolysis of target cells overexpressing episialin is inhibited. Because episialin strongly diminishes cell-cell adhesion, even when only a pair of interacting cells express episialin, we assumed that the molecule may also reduce conjugate formation between cytotoxic effector cells and the target cell and thus reduce cytolysis. To study the possible interference of episialin with immune cytolysis, we used several independently derived episialin cDNA-transfected A375 melanoma cell clones (ACA$^+$ cells) and episialin negative revertant cultures from the same clones (ACA$^-$). The ACA$^+$ cells hardly formed any conjugates with IL-2 activated large lymphocytes (LAK cells), whereas 20% of the reverted cells formed conjugates with these lymphocytes. In addition, a high percentage conjugates (60%) was formed between alloreactive cytotoxic T lymphocytes (CTL) and parental A375 cells, whereas the percentage conjugates with episialin positive cells was strongly diminished. Both experiments show that episialin affects cell-cell interaction in this situation as well, which should have a profound effect on cytolysis by these cells. Therefore, we measured the lysis of the ACA$^+$ and ACA$^-$ cells by the LAK cells and alloreactive CTL with time, in a ^{51}Cr release assay. The kinetics of lysis of episialin-negative melanoma cells by the LAK cells was comparable to that of K562 cells, the standard target of LAK cells, whereas lysis of the ACA$^+$ cells was much slower. Maximal lysis of the ACA$^-$ cells was reached after 120 min incubation, whereas 50% maximal lysis of the episialin-positive transfectants was not even reached after 180 min [6].

From these results we can conclude that episialin transfected cells are partly protected against cytolysis *in vitro*. The less efficient killing of episialin expressing cells might be crucial to the survival of metastasizing cells (see next paragraph). A similar protective effect against cytolysis by immune cells is also provided by the ascites glycoprotein (ASGP) for rat mammary tumor cells [7] and epiglycanin [8] and CD43 [9].

It should be noted that the protective effect of episialin on cytolysis is independent of the observation that this molecule also can elicit an immune response [10], although episialin may also interfere with the response evoked against itself.

Effect of episialin expression on experimental metastases formation in vivo. We have injected sets of ACA$^+$ and ACA$^-$ cells into the tail vein of Balb/c nude mice, of 4 weeks and 3-5 months old. The young mice were killed after 6-7 weeks, the older mice after 8-10 weeks and they were subsequently dissected. The number of macroscopic metastases in the lung were counted and/or the lungs were weighed. The lungs of the mice injected with ACA$^+$ cells contained significantly more metastases compared with the lungs of the animals injected with the ACA$^-$ cells. In several experiments the lungs of mice injected with the ACA$^+$ clones were completely overgrown with metastases, while the lungs of the ACA$^-$ control mice were almost normal in appearance (J. Hilkens, J. Storm, J. Wesseling, H.L. Vos, manuscript in preparation). The older and the younger mice showed the same difference in this respect. These results were confirmed at the microscopic level. Other tissues than lung were only rarely affected (as determined at the macroscopical and microscopical level) with the exception of the brain. Almost all animals examined so far that showed a large number of lung nodules, also showed several brain metastases. Injection of mixtures of ACA$^+$ and ACA$^-$ cells showed that the lung nodules preferentially developed from ACA$^+$ cells confirming that the episialin positive melanoma cells develop more metastases in this experimental system than episialin negative cells. In this respect it is important to note that the *in vitro* growth rate of the revertants and transfectants did not differ. A certain threshold level of episialin seems to be necessary, since cells with intermediate levels of episialin do not form more nodules than episialin negative cells.

We conclude that most *i.v.* injected episialin positive A375 melanoma cells metastasize more efficiently than episialin negative cells, which may be the result of a difference in sensitivity to the residual cellular immune defense in the nude mice (most likely mediated by NK cells). However, we can not exclude other possible explanations such as a difference in adhesive properties between the episialin transfectants and revertants. A possible function of episialin as a ligand for selectins seems unlikely in this model system, because the ACA$^+$ cells are unable to bind to activated human umbilical cord endothelial cells (in contrast, we observed an anti-adhesive effect). The presence of selectin-binding structures on the O-linked carbohydrates of episialin will strongly depend on the cell type, however, and this mechanism might be operative in other *in vivo* settings. In this respect it is interesting that it was recently shown by Spicer *et al.* [11] that mammary tumors developing in episialin null mice were growing significant slower than mammary tumors developing in episialin positive mice. Metastases formation was also reduced in the episialin null mice, however, this difference did not reach significancy.

Is the episialin expression in human breast carcinomas sufficient to induce an anti-adhesion effect?

As we discussed above, episialin is overexpressed in human breast carcinoma cells relative to normal breast epithelium cells. The question arises whether these levels are sufficiently high to have the same biological impact on the human tumor cells as on the cells of the experimental systems described above. If adhesion of the human carcinoma cells *in vivo* is indeed reduced by episialin overexpression this may have the same effect as loss of E-cadherin function and/or reduced integrin expression. Both phenomena have been implicated in increased invasion and metastasis and correlated with poor prognosis [12-16]. To compare the expression levels of episialin in primary breast carcinoma cells with those in ACA19$^+$ tumors in nude mice (ACA$^+$ cells formed more experimental metastases than ACA19$^-$, we determined the relative mRNA levels in both tumors by *in situ* hybridization using a probe representing a non-repeat sequence in the episialin cDNA. *Figure 1* shows that the number of grains in the section of a primary human breast tumor is approximately the same as in a section of a ACA19$^+$ tumor growing subcutaneously in a nude mouse.

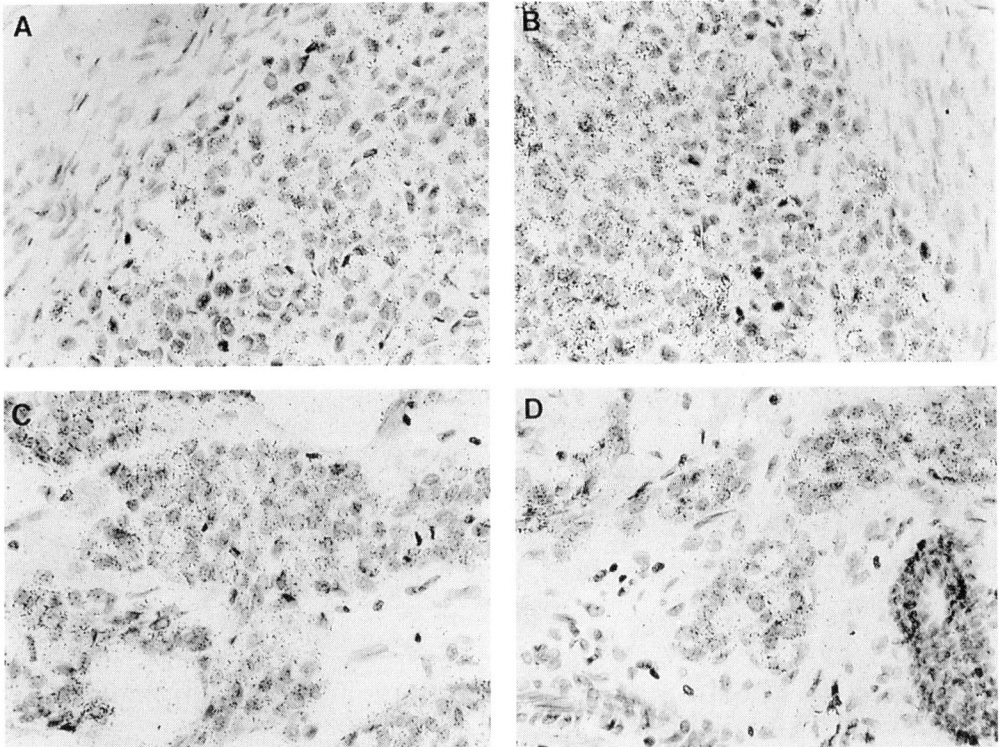

Figure 1. Comparison of the mRNA expression of episialin in a section of a primary breast carcinoma and a subcutaneous tumor of ACA19$^+$ cells in a nude mouse. The number of grains, representing the episialin mRNA expression in the section of a primary human breast tumor is approximately the same as in the section of the ACA19$^+$ tumor.

Next, we compared the expression levels of episialin on metastasizing cells in pleural and ascites fluids freshly obtained from breast and ovarian cancer patients with that on ACA19$^+$ cells growing *in vitro* using FACS analysis. *Figure 2* shows the episialin expression level in a short term culture of breast and ovarian cancer cells from pleural and ascites fluids relative to the expression in ACA19$^+$ cells. The expression level of episialin in a proportion of the ovarian and breast cancer cells is the same or even higher than in the ACA19$^+$ cells. The effusions also contained many mesothelial cells which have only a low expression of episialin. Moreover, the cancer cells tested were often derived from spheroids which frequently also contained negative or low positive cells in the center. In most cases we found that the expression levels of episialin on at least a proportion of the carcinoma cells growing in pleura or ascites fluids are higher than those on the episialin transfected melanoma cells that give rise to the enhanced experimental metastasis, and which were less sensitive to LAK cells and T cells (see above).

These observations strongly suggest that episialin is expressed at sufficiently high levels to be potentially able to affect metastasis of human cancer cells.

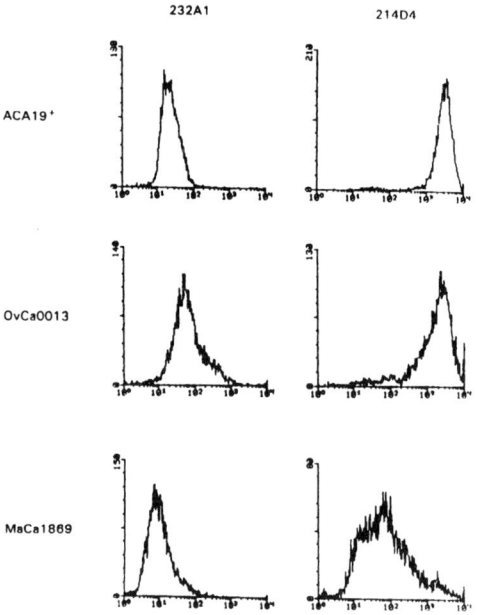

Figure 2. Episialin expression in ascites and pleural cells from a patient with ovarian carcinoma (OVCA0013) and a patient with breast carcinoma (MaCa 1869) compared with episialin expression in ACA19+ cells. The cells were stained with mAb 214D4 directed against an epitope in the repeats and mAb 232A1 directed against an unique epitope. Binding of both mAbs is independent of the glycosylation of episialin and shows the relative levels of episialin on the cells.

Episialin at the cell-stroma boundaries in human breast carcinomas induces cleft formation

The above findings urged us to investigate whether similar effects of episialin overexpression could be seen in human carcinomas. Clearly, not only the expression level itself, but also the location of the molecule is important. Expression of episialin at the apical side does not effect cellular adhesion, and thus will not influence the metastatic potential. This pattern is present in well differentiated breast carcinomas, which generally have a good prognosis. However, in many human adenocarcinomas the normal polarized architecture of the tumor cells is lost, and in these tumors the molecule is also found at those parts of the plasma membrane that are facing the stroma or adjacent cells, where it can interfere with adhesion. We showed by convential immunohistology that at these boundaries large clefts were present, which were absent at cell-stroma boundaries without episialin expression. This is remarkable because integrins are usually present at cell-stroma boundaries [17, 18]. This suggests that episialin actually prevents cell-stroma interactions.

Thus, the presence of episialin destabilizes cellular adhesion of human breast carcinomas *in vivo* as well, suggesting that upregulation of episialin may be important in invasion and metastasis. In a preliminary investigation we found a significant correlation between lymph node metastasis and cleft formation. We are presently carrying out a larger study to investigate whether these tumors have a higher propensity to metastasize.

Since there is an almost 100% correlation between cleft formation and episialin expression at the tumor stroma boundary, it is likely that the anti-adhesion effect of episialin causes this growth pattern. We have several experimental data supporting this claim: 1. *In vitro* data that episialin reduces cell-cell and cell-matrix adhesion. 2. EM studies of tumors of episialin cDNA transfected cells in nude mice, showing that episialin overexpressing cells display fewer cell-cell contacts as compared to tumors of episialin negative cells.

An extreme form of cleft formation and « inside-out » staining can be seen in some tumors where clusters of cells no longer show any cell-stoma contact and « spheroids » are formed. Spheroids with the same « inside-out » staining pattern are also present in pleural and ascites effusions of breast and ovarian carcinoma patients. It is conceivable that spheroids, covered with an episialin coat, are better equipped to survive the patient's immune defense.

Conclusion

We have shown that episialin and other membrane associated mucins have a strong effect on tumor cell growth in *in vitro* and *in vivo* experimental systems. The expression levels needed for the anti-adhesion effects of episialin are also present in human breast and ovarian carcinomas. However, the biological effect also depends on the density and affinity of the adhesion molecules. Although no direct prove has been provided, our data suggest that episialin also modulates adhesion in human primary breast carcinomas since in those regions at the tumor cell-stroma boundary where episialin is overexpressed cell-stroma contact is reduced. Haematogenic metastasis are frequently observed as spheroid-like structures with external cell membranes covered with episialin. In fact, the cells organized in these structures may more readily survive any cellular immune defense against the tumor. Reduced cell-cell adhesion mediated by episialin may contribute to the invasiveness of the tumor cells in analogy with down modulation of E-cadherin. The impact of altered cell-extra cellular matrix adhesion on invasion is more complex. In invasive tumors certain integrins are down regulated while others, depending on the tumor type, have been shown indispensable for invasion, probably to provide traction for the cells. It is conceivable that a fine tuning of adhesion and deadhesion is needed to allow the cells to become invasive, and it is likely that overexpression of episialin can interfere with this process. Since our data point the involvement of episialin in metastasis of human tumors, we assume that episialin might be a prognostic marker, which has a direct causative relation with metastasis.

References

1. Hilkens J, Ligtenberg MJL, Vos HL, Litvinov SV. Cell membrane-associated mucins and their adhesion-modulating property. *Trends Biochem Science* 1992; 17: 359-63.
2. Jentoft N. Why are proteins O-glycosylated? *Trends Biochem Science* 1990; 15: 291-4.
3. Ligtenberg MJ, Buijs F, Vos HL, Hilkens J. Suppression of cellular aggregation by high levels of episialin. *Cancer Res* 1992; 52: 2318-24.

4. Wesseling J, van der Valk SW, Hilkens J. A Mechanism for Inhibition of E-Cadherin-mediated Cell-Cell Adhesion by the Membrane-associated Mucin Episialin/MUC1. *Mol Biol Cell* 1996; in press.
5. Wesseling J, van der Valk SW, Vos HL, Sonnenberg A, Hilkens J. Episialin (MUC1) overexpression inhibits integrin-mediated cell adhesion to extracellular matrix components. *J Cell Biol* 1995; 129: 255-65.
6. Van de Wiel-van Kemenade E, Ligtenberg MJL, de Boer AJ, Buijs F, Vos HL, Melief CJM, Hilkens J, Figdor CG. Episialin (MUC1) Inhibits Cytotoxic Lymphocyte-Target Cell Interaction. *J Immunol* 1993; 151: 767-76.
7. Moriarty J, Skelly CM, Bharathan S, Moody CE, Sherblom AP. Sialomucin and Lytic susceptibility of Rat Mammary Tumor Ascites Cells. *Cancer Res* 1990; Nov; 50: 6800-5.
8. Miller SC, Codington JF, Klein G. Further studies on the relationship between allotransplantability and the presence of the cell surface glycoprotein epiglycanin in the TA3-MM mouse mammary carcinoma ascites cell. *J Natl Cancer Inst* 1982; 68: 981-8.
9. McFarland TA, Ardman B, Manjunath N, Fabry JA, Lieberman J. CD43 diminishes susceptibility to T lymphocyte-mediated cytolysis. *J Immunol* 1995; 154: 1097-104.
10. Jerome KR, Barnd DL, Bendt KM, Boyer CM, Taylor-Papadimitriou J, McKenzie IFC, Bast RC, Finn OJ. Cytotoxic T-lymphocytes derived from patients with breast adenocarcinoma recognize an epitope present on the protein core of a mucin molecule preferentially expressed by malignant cells. *Cancer Res* 1991; 51: 2908-16.
11. Spicer AP, Rowse GJ, Lidner TK, Gendler SJ. Delayed mammary tumor progression in Muc-1 null mice. *J Biol Chem* 1995; 270: 30093-101.
12. Frixen UH, Behrens J, Sachs M, Eberle G, Voss B, Warda A, Lochner D, Birchmeier W. E-cadherin-mediated cell-cell adhesion prevents invasiveness of human carcinoma cells. *J. Cell Biol* 1991; 113: 173-85.
13. Bringuier PP, Umbas R, Schaafsma HE, Karthaus HF, Debruyne FM, Schalken JA. Decreased E-cadherin immunoreactivity correlates with poor survival in patients with bladder tumors. *Cancer Res* 1993; 53: 3241-5.
14. Schipper JH, Frixen UH, Behrens J, Unger A, Jahnke K, Birchmeier W. E-cadherin expression in squamous cell carcinomas of head and neck: inverse correlation with tumor dedifferentiation and lymph node metastasis. *Cancer Res* 1991; 51: 6328-37.
15. Zutter MM, Mazoujian G, Santoro SA. Decreased expression of integrin adhesive protein receptors in adenocarcinoma of the breast. *Am J Pathol* 1990; 137: 863-70.
16. Pignatelli M, Hanby AM, Stamp GWH. Low expression of β1, α2 and α3 subunits of VLA integrins in malignant mammary tumors. *J Pathol* 1991; 165: 25-32.
17. Koukoulis GK, Virtanen I, Korhonen M, Laitinen L, Quaranta V, Gould VE. Immunohistochemical localization of integrins in the normal, hyperplastic, and neoplastic breast. *Am J Pathol* 1991; 139: 787-99.
18. Pignatelli M, Cordillo MR, Hanby A, Stamp GWH. Integrins and their accessory adhesion molecules in mammary carcinomas: loss of polarization in poorly differentiated tumors. *Hum Pathol* 1992; 23: 1159-66.

The detection of micrometastases in the lymph nodes, peripheral blood and bone marrow of patients with breast cancer using immunohistochemistry and the polymerase chain reaction

A. Schoenfeld[1, 2], K.H. Kruger[3], J. Gomm[2], H.D. Sinnett[1], J-C. Gazet[4], N. Sacks[4], H.G. Bender[5], Y. Luqmani[2] and R.C. Coombes[2]

The Cancer Research Campaign Department of Medical Oncology[1], Charing Cross and Westminster Medical School, St. Dunstan's Road, London W6 8RP, U.K. and The Departments of Surgery,Charing Cross Hospital[2] and St. Georges Hospital[3], London, United Kingdom and the Universityfrauenclinics in Frankfurt[4] and Dusseldorf[5], Germany

Immunohistochemical staining techniques have shown the presence of cancer cells in the bone marrow of approximately 20-30% of patients with operable breast cancer [1-4]. The occurrence of these micrometastases has been related to prognostic features of the primary, such as tumour size and the presence of vascular invasion, and lymph node involvement [5, 6]. In addition, the presence of bone marrow micrometastases has been strongly correlated to early recurrence and shorter overall survival [3, 6]. The risk increased with increasing number of cells detected in the bone marrow [3, 7].

However, up to 10% of patients relapse with no histological or immunohistochemical evidence of bone marrow micrometastases, following resection of the primary tumour [3, 8]. Additionally, in only 10% of patients with micrometastases at the time of surgery were metastatic cells evident on repeat aspiration, even though many of these patients subsequently developed clinically evident metastatic disease [8]. Furthermore, detection of metastatic cells in peripheral blood was rare [1, 4].

The sensitivity of immunohistochemical methods using monoclonal antibodies to epithelial antigens or cytokeratins has been estimated at approximately one cancer cell per 10^4 to 10^5 normal bone marrow cells [9, 10]. Measurement of a tissue specific gene transcript following PCR amplification, while retaining specificity, has been reported to increase the sensitivity by up to 100 times [11], with detection of a single neuroblastoma cell in 10^7 peripheral blood mononuclear cells.

We have shown that measurement of PCR amplified K19 is much superior to immunohistochemical techniques as a means of determining the presence of micrometastases in the axillary lymph nodes of patients with breast cancer [12]. However, practical considerations prevent the repeated sampling of lymph node tissue. A similar technique applied to peripheral blood or bone marrow would offer significant advantages, allowing a better assessment of the prognosis of patients with breast cancer and monitoring of the response to adjuvant chemotherapy. In this study, we have used the RT-PCR assay developed previously [12] to detect K19 mRNA transcripts in samples of peripheral blood and bone marrow from breast cancer patients. We have also analysed samples using the immunohistochemical staining technique, with an anti-keratin 19 antibody, to compare these two methods.

Materials and methods

Chemicals

MMLV reverse transcriptase was obtained from GIBCO BRL (Paisley, United Kingdom) and Taq polymerase from Penninsula Laboratories (United Kingdom). Random hexamers and dNTPs were from Pharmacia (Uppsala, Sweden) and ^{32}P dCTP (3,000 Ci/mmol) was from Amersham (United Kingdom). RNAzol was from Biogenesis (Bournemouth, United Kingdom). All other reagents were obtained from Sigma (Dorset, United Kingdom) unless indicated.

Cell lines

MCF 7 human breast cancer cells were maintained in monolayer culture in RPMI 1640 medium supplemented with 10% fetal calf serum, glutamine, penicillin and streptomycin. When required, cells were harvested by trypsinisation.

Sensitivity assay

Monolayer cultures of MCF7 cells were harvested with trypsin and, following centrifugation, washed by resuspension in PBS and then disaggregated by passing through a 26-gauge needle. Cells were counted on a haemocytometer and serial dilutions of the cell suspension prepared. Suitable volumes of media containing 5 to 500 MCF7 cells were mixed with 5×10^6 normal bone marrow cells after cell separation to give a ratio of MCF7 cells to bone marrow cells of $1:10^6$, $1:10^5$ and $1:10^4$. These preparations were then used either to prepare smears for immunohistochemistry or for RNA extraction.

Table I. Clinical data on patients with breast cancer.

	Number of patients
Total	88*
Age (years)	
Range 31 - 85	
Mean 58.2	
Menopausal status	
Pre	14
Peri and post	74
Operation	
Mastectomy	27
Wide local excision	59
Wire localization	2

* of whom: 75 had primary breast cancer.

Patients

Peripheral blood and bone marrow specimens were collected from 113 patients at Charing Cross and St. George's Hospitals in London, England and the University Clinic in Frankfurt, Germany. Clinical and pathological details are given in *Tables I* and *II*.

Table II. Pathological data on patients with breast cancer.

Parameter	Patient number
Tumour type	
Invasive ductal carcinoma	73
Invasive lobular carcinoma	8
Tubular	2
Medullary	1
Ductal carcinoma *in situ*	4
Tumour size (cm)	
0-1	16
1.1 - 2	31
2.1 - 5	29
5.1+	5
Unknown	8
Tumour Grade (Bloom and Richardson)	
Well differentiated	13
Moderately differentiated	45
Poorly differentiated	18
Unknown	12
Vascular invasion	
Present	20
Absent	17
Unknown	51
Oestrogen receptor status	
Positive	47
Negative	22
Unknown	19
Progesterone receptor status	
Positive	32
Negative	14
Unknown	42
Axillary node involvement	
None	49
1-3	14
4 or more	20
Unknown	15

There were 75 patients in this study who had untreated primary breast cancer with no evidence of distant metastatic disease by pre-operative staging. The staging included the biochemical markers of serum calcium, alkaline phosphatase and liver function tests, and the radiological investigations of a chest X-ray, liver ultrasound, isotope bone scan and skeletal survey.

In addition, there were 4 patients with ductal carcinoma *in situ*, 4 patients who had a breast carcinoma excised previously and had no evidence of recurrent disease, and 5 patients who had metastatic carcinoma of the breast with radiological evidence of bone involvement.

Positive bone marrow controls were obtained from those patients with established bone involvement of their breast cancer in whom a diagnostic marrow aspirate was required. For negative controls, bone marrows were obtained from patients undergoing a diagnostic or follow-up marrow aspirate in the haematology clinic and known not to have an epithelial malignancy.

During the course of the study, 10 patients agreed to donate a sample of peripheral blood and bone marrow.

Specimen collection

The specimens were collected from patients under general anaesthetic just before their breast operation. Under sterile conditions, a bone marrow aspirate was taken from each posterior iliac crest using a 16 Saleh needle. To minimize the risk of skin contamination, an incision was made in the skin with a scalpel before introducing the needle. Approximately 10 ml of bone marrow and venous blood was aspirated from each site in a syringe containing 1 ml of 6% EDTA as anticoagulant and then pooled.

In addition, 20 mls of peripheral blood was taken from a vein in the antecubital fossa and mixed with 1 ml of 6% EDTA. White blood cell counts were determined using a Coulter counter STKR.

Cell separation

The peripheral blood and bone marrow were processed separately under sterile conditions using the same procedure. Each sample was gently overlaid onto an equal volume of Lymphoprep (Nyegaard, Oslo, Norway), and centrifuged for 20 minutes at 500 g at room temperature. The nucleated cells, including the metastatic cancer cells, collected at the visible interface between the Lymphoprep and the serum [13].

The serum supernatant and interface were removed, diluted to a total volume of 50 ml in RPMI medium, and centrifuged for 6 minutes at 350 g at room temperature. The resulting cell pellet was gently resuspended in fresh RPMI medium and again centrifuged for 6 minutes at 350 g at room temperature. All but 2 ml of the supernatant was then removed and the cell pellet was resuspended in this, and an aliquot removed for cell counting using the Coulter counter. The sample was equally divided for subsequent analysis by either anti-cytokeratin 19 immunohistochemistry or RNA extraction and measurement of K19 mRNA expression.

For immunohistochemistry, the sample was centrifuged for 5 min and the cell pellet resuspended in a small volume (~100 µl) of the supernatant. Aliquots of this suspension (50 µl) were smeared onto two frosteal slides to form a monolayer of cells. The smears were air-dried, fixed in 100% ethanol for 1 h and then air-dried for 30 min before storage at -20° C.

The sample for RNA extraction was centrifuged for 5 min and all the supernatant discarded. The cell pellet was snap-frozen in liquid nitrogen and stored at -70° C.

Staining procedure for immunohistochemistry

The smears were equilibrated to room temperature and allowed to dry. To block endogenous alkaline phosphatase activity, slides were placed in 20% glacial acetic acid for 10 minutes, washed in water and then in 2% periodic acid for 10 minutes. The slides were rinsed sequentially in tap water and PBS, before incubation in a humidified chamber for 20 minutes with PBS buffer containing 5% bovine serum albumin and 5% goat serum. Excess fluid was wiped off the slide and the primary antibody, a mouse anti-cytokeratin 19 antibody (4.62, Sigma, United Kingdom), diluted to 5 µg/ml was added to each slide and incubation carried out at room temperature for 90 minutes.

The slides were washed in PBS and then incubated with an alkaline phosphatase conjugated goat anti-mouse antibody, (S3721, Promega, United Kingdom), which had been diluted to 1:250 in PBS/bovine serum albumin buffer containing 10% human serum. Following washing, the substrate solution, NBT/BCIP (Vector Laboratories, USA), was applied to each slide and smears then incubated for 30 minutes. The smears were dehydrated in graded alcohol and counterstained with Gill's haematoxylin, before mounting using Histomount (National Diagnostics, United Kingdom). Each slide was screened under low power light microscopy for positive cells and the morphology of each positive cell was confirmed under high power. A smear was considered to be positive if one or more stained epithelial cancer cells was observed.

Oligonucleotide primers

The primers for K19 and GAPDH were as previously described [12] and synthesized using phosphoramidite chemistry on an Applied Biosystems DNA Synthesizer. Both sets of K19 primers spanned at least one intron and sequences were designed to maximise differences with the K19 pseudogene [14-16].

RNA extraction

Total cellular RNA was extracted from the frozen peripheral blood and bone marrow samples using the acid-guanidium-phenol-chloroform technique [17] utilizing RNAzol. Following extraction, the integrity of the RNA was checked electrophoretically and quantified spectrophotometrically, and samples diluted to approximately 0.3 µg/µl in water and stored at -70° C.

Reverse transcription and PCR amplification

This was carried out exactly as described previously [12] and two 40 cycle rounds of amplification were performed. In brief, 4 µg RNA was reverse transcribed in a total reaction volume of 20 µl, and 4 µl was added to the PCR mix (100 µl) for the first amplification using the primers already described [12]. Subsequently 1 µl of the first reaction was carried over for the second amplification (in a 50 µl reaction mix) using the nested primers K6 and K7 described previously [14]. Control reactions were performed in parallel and involved using product from mock RT reactions which contained RNA but no enzyme.

Gel electrophoresis

Aliquots of chloroform extracted PCR products (20 μl) were electrophoresed at 150V for 2 hours in Tris acetate EDTA buffer on a 1.5% agarose gel containing ethidium bromide. Hae III digested ØX 174 DNA markers or the CAMBIO DNA ladder were run simultaneously. After two rounds of amplification, samples which had a discernable band corresponding to 319 bp on examination of the gel under ultra-violet light were considered as positive.

Results

Cell separation

Density gradient centrifugation resulted in an average yield of 20.4% (range 0.8-80%) for peripheral blood, and 28.2% (range 2.1-82%) for bone marrow, of the total initial number of white blood cells. The average number of cells examined was 23.0×10^6 (range $1.5 - 104 \times 10^6$) for peripheral blood and 149.2×10^6 (range $3.6 - 620 \times 10^6$) for bone marrow, and each sample was equally divided for immunohistochemical and RNA analysis.

Specificity and sensitivity of immunohistochemistry and RT-PCR for detection of K19 expression

Initial experiments were performed to determine whether K19 expression could be detected in samples from patients with no evidence of breast or other epithelial malignancy. We examined 10 paired samples of bone marrow and peripheral blood and a further 15 peripheral blood samples from such a group of unselected patients. Using immunohistochemical staining with an anti-cytokeratin 19 antibody, we were unable to detect any K19 positive cells. RT-PCR, using primers to amplify K19 mRNA, on RNA extracted from aliquots of the same samples was also performed. No signal corresponding to K19 mRNA was detected following two rounds of 40 cycles of amplification by ethidium staining of electrophoresed material. Simultaneously amplified products (of 379 bp) corresponding to a housekeeping gene, GAPDH, were clearly seen in all samples after the first PCR, confirming the presence of amplifiable cDNA and ensuring that the absence of K19 product was not due to the lack of input RNA (data not shown).

We assessed the sensitivity of both the immunohistochemical and PCR techniques by preparing smears or RNA from 5×10^6 normal bone marrow cells to which were added 5 to 500 MCF7 cancer cells. We were able to detect K19 immunopositive cells at a dilution of one MCF7 cell in 10^5 bone marrow cells on 6/7 separate occasions, but not at higher dilutions. Increasing numbers of immunopositive cells were detected as more MCF7 cells were added. Approximately 20 to 30% of the MCF7 cells added to the separated normal bone marrow cells were counted on the stained smears at all dilutions. The cytoplasmic staining appeared specifically on epithelial cells, staining over 95% of MCF7 cells, and there was no cross-reactivity with other cell types in the blood or bone marrow smears.

After two rounds of PCR amplification of RNA from the various cell preparations, a 319 bp product indicating amplification of K19 mRNA was visualized by ethidium staining at a dilution of one MCF7 cell in 10^6 bone marrow cells on 4/5 separate determinations. The staining intensity of the nested product band at 319 bp increased as expected in the preparations containing higher numbers of MCF7 cells. In most samples, a band corresponding to a ~600 bp product was also observed. We have previously shown this to be derived from contaminating DNA [12]. The intensity of this band decreased as that of the 319 bp band increased with increasing numbers of MCF7 cells. This may be the result of preferential amplification of the mRNA template due to the smaller size of the PCR product, compared to the genomic DNA template.

Detection of breast cancer cells in peripheral blood and bone marrow

In the samples from the 75 patients with primary invasive tumours and no evidence of distant metastatic disease on conventional staging, we found by a combination of the two methods K19 positivity in 20/75 (27%) peripheral blood and 27/65 (42%) bone marrow samples. By immunohistochemistry alone, we detected K19 positive cells in 4/75 (5%) peripheral blood and 14/65 (22%) bone marrow samples. The number of cells identified in each case ranged from 1 to 10 (mean 4 cells) in peripheral blood and 1 to 40 (mean 7.5 cells) in bone marrow. By RT-PCR we observed K19 expression in 19/75 (25%) peripheral blood and 23/65 (35%) bone marrow samples. This is a significantly greater percent than detected by immunocytochemistry ($p < 0.001$ and $p = 0.03$ respectively). Further analyses are presented in *Table III*. Thus in the peripheral blood, only 4/20 (20%) positives were detected by immunohistochemistry and 19/20 (95%) by RT-PCR. In the bone marrow 14/27 (52%) were detected by immunohistochemistry and 23/27 (85%) by RT-PCR. If positivity was considered in either peripheral blood or bone marrow, we detected 17 of the 36 positives (47%) by immunohistochemistry and 34/36 (94%) by RT-PCR. There was no correlation between K19 detection (either by immunochemistry or PCR) and other clinical parameters *(Table II)*.

Overall, considering both the positive and the negative samples, the concordance between peripheral blood and bone marrow samples analysed by immunohistochemistry was 79% compared with 66% by RT-PCR *(Table IV)*. However, if only those cases that were positive in either peripheral blood or bone marrow are considered, the concordance for immunohistochemistry was low (6%); 82% of the positive cases were found by analysis of the bone marrow, and only 24% from the peripheral blood. Using RT-PCR there was a better rate of concordance between peripheral blood and bone marrow samples (27%); detection of positives was also more frequent in the bone marrow (77%) than the peripheral blood (50%).

Table III. Comparison of detection rate of micrometastases in peripheral blood and bone marrow.

	Peripheral blood	Bone marrow	Peripheral blood or bone marrow
Total no. patients	75	65	75
-ve by both IH and PCR	55	38	39
+ve by either IH or PCR	20	27	36
+ve by both IH and PCR	3 (15%)	10 (37%)	15 (42%)
+ve by IH only	1 (5%)	4 (15%)	2 (5%)
+ve by PCR only	16 (80%)	13 (48%)	19 (53%)

The percentages in brackets indicate the proportion of K19 positive cells detected by that technique.

We also examined peripheral blood and bone marrow from 4 patients with *in situ* carcinoma of the breast. These samples were negative by both techniques apart from one patient who had

K19 positive cells in both blood and bone marrow. Of the group of 5 patients with radiological evidence of bone metastases, one had a single K19 positive cell in the peripheral blood detected by immunohistochemical staining and 4 had positive cells in the bone marrow. By RT-PCR we detected K19 bands in 4 of the 5 patients in both blood and bone marrow. One patient had no positive cells in blood or bone marrow by either technique.

A further 4 patients had the primary tumour excised at least one year previously and had no recorded evidence of recurrent disease. In two patients, we detected positive cells in the peripheral blood by RT-PCR; in one of these patients immunohistochemistry confirmed the presence of tumour cells in the bone marrow.

Table IV. Comparison of immunohistochemistry and RT-PCR for the detection of micrometastases.

	IH	RT-PCR
Total no of patients with K19 positive cells in either blood or bone marrow	17/75	30/65
+ve in both blood and bone marrow	1 (6%)	8 (27%)
+ve in blood only	3 (18%)	7 (23%)
+ve in bone marrow only	13 (76%)	15 (50%)

A comparison of the two sampling sites, peripheral blood and bone marrow, in the detection of K19 positive cells by immunohistochemistry and RT-PCR. The proportion of K19 positive samples found at each site is expressed as a percentage in brackets of the total number of K19 positive patients detected by that technique.

Micrometastases in axillary lymph nodes

When patients are first seen with breast cancer, over 95% will have no evidence of metastatic disease on clinical, biochemical and radiological examination. Even after apparently curative surgery, where all the local disease has been eradicated and the axillary nodes show no evidence of histological involvement by tumour, approximately 30% of women relapse with metastases within 5 years.

While several groups have used immunohistological methods to demonstrate axillary node micro-metastases that were previously missed on histological examination in a proportion of cases. A review of these studies showed that only 13% of 2,400 patients converted from node negative status to node positive. Recently, we reported that measurements of keratin 19 (K19) mRNA following RT-PCR amplification improved detection of tumour cells [12] in lymph nodes. K19 is universally expressed in breast cancers and is not present in normal lymph nodes [14].

In this extented study of 125 consecutive patients we show that this is a more sensitive way to detect micrometastases in lymph nodes.

All patients gave written informed consent to this study. Lymph nodes were collected from 125 undergoing axillary dissection for breast cancer at Charing Cross Hospital, London from January 1993 to June 1994. *Table V* shows the clinical and pathological details. Distant metastases were not detected in any patient by routine staging using isotopic bone scanning, liver ultrasound and chest x-ray.

Tumour grade pathological size and presence of vascular invasion were recorded. Oestrogen and progesterone receptor status was assessed by either the ligand binding assay or by

Table V. Clinical pathological data in the study group.

	Number of patients
Age range	24-74 y
Mean	52 y
Premenopausal	49
Postmenopausal	76
Surgery	
Wide local excision	102
(bilateral carcinoma in one patient)	
Mastectomy	23
No. nodes dissected	3-44
Mean no. of nodes	17
Tumor size (cm)	
(invasive tumours)	
0-1.0	25
1.1-2.0	60
2.1-5.0	29
> 5	2
Not known	10
Tumor type	
a) Infiltrating ductal carcinoma (IDC)	107
b) Infiltrating lobular carcinoma (ILC)	10
c) Ductal carcinoma *in situ* with microinvasion	5
d) Medullary	2
e) Mucinous	1
f) Alveolar	1
Grade	
1	10
2	61
3	36
Not known	17
Vascular invasion	
Present	45
Absent	56
Not known	25
Oestrogen receptor	
Positive	41
Negative	21
Not known	64
Progesterone receptor	
Positive	43
Negative	18
Not known	65

immunohistochemistry using the 1D5 antiserum (Dako Ltd) or progesterone receptor immunocytochemical assay (PR-ICA) (Abbott Laboratories) respectively. For K19 immunocytochemistry, we examined 4 paraffin sections from each of 46 lymph nodes from 33 patients using antiserum RCK 108 (Dako Ltd).

As a control group 28 lymph nodes were collected from 20 patients admitted for a variety of conditions but none of whom had any signs of an epithelial malignancy.
The data were analysed by the Chi-square test and the two sample t-test.
The detailed procedures have been described by our group [12]. RNA was extracted from snap-frozen lymph nodes, reverse transcribed and subjected to 40 cycles of PCR amplification using K19 and GAPDH primers (as control). PCR products were electrophoresed on a 1.5% agarose stained with ethidium bromide, blotted onto Hybond membrane and subsequently hybridised with the K19 or GAPDH probe labelled with [^{32}P]dCTP. Identity of the k19 PCR product was verified by sequencing several independent isolates by standard methods (data not shown).
RNA from all the histologically involved nodes yielded the expected 460 bp K19 PCR product. Of the 530 histologically negative nodes, 106 (20%) gave a K19 product detectable by Southern hybridisation, indicating the presence of tumour cells in 23/75 (30.6%) of the histologically staged node negative patients.
All the normal nodes had amplified GAPDH but displayed no K19 product. If all 125 patients are considered, the presence of the K19 product in lymph nodes was associated with the presence of lympho-vascular invasion in the primary ($p < 0.001$) as well as with tumour size ($p < 0.001$) and grade ($p = 0.01$) but not with receptor or menopausal status. In the histologically node-negative patients, there was no correlation with grading. There was a weak correlation with progesterone receptor ($p = 0.05$). The correlation with lympho-vascular invasion did not quite reach significance ($p < 0.06$), although there was a strong correlation with tumour size ($p < 0.001$) *(Table VI)*.

Table VI. Relationship of cytokeratin mRMA detectable in lymph nodes with other pathological characteristics.

Pathological	Keratin 19 mRNA		X^2 D.F.	p value
	positive	negative		
Tumour size				
Mean	1.96	1.59	t = 3.6	< 0.001
95% confidence for mean	1.81-2.13	1.50-1.68	563	
Tumour grade				
Well differentiated	5	47		
Moderately	56	210	4.0	ns
Poorly	32	115	2	
Vascular invasion				
Present	46	127	3.47	0.06
Absent	45	199	1	
Oestrogen receptor				
Positive	37	114	1.2	ns
Negative	27	60	1	
Progesterone receptor				
Positive	37	127	3.28	0.05
Negative	26	47	1	
Menopausal status				
Pre	37	245		
Post	70	267	1.32	ns
Peri	1	12	2	

* Two sample t-test.

Sections from 33 randomly selected nodes that were negative by histological examination but positive for K19 mRNA expression by RT-PCR were examined for presence of K19 protein by immunohistochemistry; only 3 cases (9%) were found tho have positive staining in morphologically identifiable of tumour cells. In one lymph node, only one of two sections examined had 3 positively stained tumour cells visible; the other 2 lymph nodes had small clusters of positive tumour cells.

Our results show that we can detect mRNA for the epithelial specific marker K19 in the axillary lymph nodes of almost one third of patients who have no evidence of tumour involvement on conventional histological examination. This is the expected proportion of patients at risk of early relapse.

Concerning lymph node metastases, the increased detection achieved with the RT-PCR method compared to immunohistochemistry may be due in part to the examination of a more representative proportion of the tissue as compared with a single section. This increases the chance of including tumour cells if these are relatively few as suggested by immunohistochemical data. The patients in this study had a preponderance of small carcinomas, with more than 20% having tumours less than 1 cm in size, and 85% having tumours equal or less than 2 cm in diameter. This is a particularly relevant consideration in view of the larger numbers of early stage cancers that are being diagnosed using mammographic screening techniques.

The PCR method used has significant advantages over conventional histological or immunocytochemical techniques: it also has the potential for automation and is readily applicable to other epithelial cancers, the majority of which express K19 [6]. There was a significant correlation between the presence of PCR-detected micrometastases and tumour size and vascular invasion in conventionally node negative staged patients; prognostic significance will be determined once these patients have had sufficient follow-up time.

We conclude that measurement of K19 mRNA in axillary lymph nodes by PCR amplification is a more useful means of detecting micrometastases and may have a role in identifying a group of patients who would benefit from earlier adjuvant chemotherapy and who are otherwise denied this.

Discussion

In this study, we have demonstrated that RT-PCR using K19 primers is a sensitive and specific technique for the detection of tumour cells in the peripheral blood and bone marrow of patients with breast cancer. This assay detected K19 expression from MCF7 cells serially diluted down to 1 MCF7 cell in 10^6 normal bone marrow cells. This level of sensitivity was at least 10 times greater than we achieved with immunohistochemistry and was comparable to that reported in other studies [18, 19]. RT-PCR may be capable of detecting 1 in 10^7 cells, depending on the efficiency of the primers, the abundance of the gene transcript and the design of the assay.

Detection of mRNA transcripts might be expected to be more sensitive than immunohistochemistry as multiple copies of mRNA provide a greater target, and downstream modification and translation may reduce the expression of protein. Each target may then be amplified 10^6 times before detection. In contrast, the process of smearing and immunostaining resulted in the detection of only ~30% of the added MCF7 cells. A similar proportion was observed by Osborne et al. [9]. This may be attributed to the settling or clumping of the MCF7 cells and/or the loss of cells during smearing, and necessarily compromises the sensitivity of the immunohistochemical detection.

A further disadvantage of the immunohistochemical procedure is that a trained cytologist is required to confirm the identity of stained cells. Although our monoclonal antibody to K19 appeared specific, cross reactivity of other antibodies with different cells has been described. Using antibodies to epithelial membrane antigen, occasional staining of plasma cells, early myeloid cells and degenerate cells was due to the weak expression of this antigen by those cells [20].

The specificity of RT-PCR relies on the detection of an unique or over-expressed gene in the tumour cell. Certain malignancies are characterized by unique targets; in chronic myeloid leukaemia there is a specific bcr/abl chromosomal translocation that has been exploited [21], and prostate cancer cells over-express prostate specific antigen [22, 23]. No unique markers have been identified in breast cancer cells. Although gene rearrangements on chromosome 17q have been described in some familial breast cancers, and point mutations in known oncogenes are frequently associated with sporadic breast cancer, no consistent genetic alteration has been found. We have therefore used an epithelial-specific marker, K19, as this has been reported to be present in most benign and malignant breast tissue [24] but absent in normal haematological tissue [18, 25, 26]. This was confirmed in this study in that no K19 was detected in the peripheral blood or bone marrow of patients with benign breast disease or non-epithelial malignancies.

RT-PCR improved the detection rate, compared to immunohistochemistry, of occult metastases in the peripheral blood and bone marrow of patients with breast cancer. By immunohistochemical staining, we detected bone marrow micrometastases (21%) at a similar frequency to that of other studies (16-31%) [1-4]. The RT-PCR method increased the detection rate (35%) in bone marrow samples. In addition, RT-PCR was much more effective in the detection of K19 positive cells in peripheral blood. However, RT-PCR failed to detect K19 immunopositive cells in one peripheral blood and 4 bone marrow samples. The reasons for this are not clear. It may be that these immunohistochemically detected cells were not viable [27] or « dormant » with low metabolic activity.

Both techniques detected more positives in bone marrow than peripheral blood. This may partly be a consequence of examining approximately 7 times more cells for the bone marrow compared to the peripheral blood samples. It may also be that bone marrow acts as a filter for concentrating circulating breast cancer cells and this is reflected in the propensity of breast cancer cells to form overt bone metastases.

We would conclude that immunohistochemical analysis detected only a minority of positive samples from the peripheral blood, and that sampling of bone marrow is essential for this technique to contribute useful data. RT-PCR similarly detected more positives in the bone marrow, but sampling of both the peripheral blood and bone marrow significantly improved the detection rate.

The concordance in the detection of K19 positive cells between blood and bone marrow samples by either technique was disappointingly low (immunohistochemistry (6%) and RT-PCR (27%)). A larger sample volume would probably increase the detection rate for both techniques, but may be impractical for repeated sampling. Mansi *et al.* [8] performed bone marrow sampling at 8 different sites preoperatively.

In patients with radiological evidence of bone involvement, only one patient had no positive cells by either immunohistochemistry or RT-PCR. This patient was receiving chemotherapy and was clinically in remission. The others had K19 positive cells in the bone marrow by immunohistochemical staining, and one patient had a single positive cell in the peripheral blood. These samples were positive in both blood and bone marrow by RT-PCR.

Somewhat surprisingly, one patient with *in situ* disease also had a positive result by both techniques. This patient had had a wide local excision performed with local radiotherapy to the breast, and histological examination reported microinvasion associated with the *in situ* ductal carcinoma. Although this result raises the suspicion of another, overlooked focus of invasion, mammography 6 months after surgery showed no further suspicious lesions, and the patient continues to be followed up closely.

Four patients had had breast cancer which was excised at least one year previously and had no overt metastases on routine staging. Two, however, had positive cells in their peripheral blood by RT-PCR and 1 of these had tumour cells identified immunohistochemically in her bone marrow. RT-PCR may be sufficiently sensitive to follow up patients who have had the primary excised and perhaps to monitor response to adjuvant chemotherapy.

Our study has directly compared immunohistochemistry and RT-PCR as well as the comparative merits of sampling peripheral blood and bone marrow. The study was designed to utilize a small volume of bone marrow and peripheral blood to improve the acceptability to patients and facilitate the analysis. Increasing the number of sites of bone marrow aspiration [2] or increasing the volume of peripheral blood for analysis may increase the detection of patients with occult disease up to a point and the increased sensitivity of RT-PCR will reduce the sampling error and workload.

The definitive answer to the prognostic significance of these RT-PCR detected micrometastases will require extended follow-up to assess the recurrence rate and survival of this cohort of patients. Further patients have been recruited into this study and technical improvements have been developed (unpublished results) to quantify the RT-PCR assay and simplify the routine processing of large numbers of patients.

References

1. Redding WH, Monaghan P, Imrie SF, Ormerod MG, Gazet J-C, Coombes RC, Clink H.McD, Dearnaley DP, Sloane JP, Powles TJ, and Neville, A.M. Detection of micrometastases in patients with primary breast cancer. *Lancet* 1983; 2: 1271-4.
2. Schlimok G, Funke I, Holzmann B, Götlinger G, Schmidt G, Hauser H, Swierkot S, Warnecke HH, Schneider B, Koprowski H and Reithmuller G. Micrometastatic cancer cells in bone marrow: *in vitro* detection with anti-cytokeratin and *in vivo* labeling with anti-17-1A monoclonal antibodies. *Proc Natl Acad Sci (USA)* 1987; 84: 8672-6.
3. Cote RJ, Rosen PP, Lesser ML, Old LJ, and Osborne MP. Prediction of early relapse in patients with operable breast cancer by detection of occult bone marrow micrometastases. *J Clin Oncol* 1991; 9: 1749-56.
4. Ménard S, Squicciarini P, Luini A, Sacchini V, Rovini D, Tagliabue E, Veronesi P, Salvadori B, Veronesi U, and Colnaghi M.I. Immunodetection of bone marrow micrometastases in breast carcinoma patients and its correlation with primary tumour prognostic features. *Br J Cancer* 1994; 69: 1126-9.
5. Diel I, Kaufmann M, Krempien B, Kaul S, Gorner R, Costa S and Bastert G. Immunocytochemical detection of tumor cells in bone marrow in patients with primary breast cancer. *Br J Cancer* 1990; 62: 3A.
6. Mansi JL, Easton D, Berger U, Gazet J-C, Ford HT, Dearnaley D, and Coombes RC. Bone marrow micrometastases in primary breast cancer: prognostic significance after 6 years' follow-up. *Eur J Cancer* 1991; 27: 1552-5.
7. Coombes RC, Berger U, Mansi J, Redding H, Powles TJ, Neville AM, McKinna A, Nash AG, Gazet J-C, Ford HT, Ormerod M, and McDonnell T. Prognostic significance of micrometastases in bone marrow in patients with primary breast cancer. *Nat Cancer Inst Mono* 1986; 1: 51-3.
8. Mansi JL, Berger U, Easton D, McDonnell T, Redding H, Gazet J-C., McKinna A, Powles TJ and Coombes RC. Micrometastases in bone marrow in patients with primary breast cancer: evaluation as an early predictor of bone metastases. *Br Med J* 1987; 295:1093-6.

9. Osborne MP, Wong GY, Asina S, Old LJ, Cote RJ and Rosen PP. Sensitivity of immunocytochemical detection of breast cancer cells in human bone marrow. *Cancer Res* 1991; 51: 2706-9.
10. Ellis G, Ferguson M, Yamanaka E, Livingston RB and Gown AM. Monoclonal antibodies for detection of occult carcinoma cells in bone marrow of breast cancer patients. *Cancer* 1989; 63: 2509-14.
11. Mattano LA, Moss TJ and Emerson SG. Sensitive detection of rare circulating neuroblastoma cells by the reverse transcriptase-polymerase chain reaction. *Cancer Res* 1992; 52: 4701-5.
12. Schoenfeld A, Luqmani Y, Smith D, O'Reilly S, Shousha S, Sinnett HD and Coombes RC. Detection of breast cancer micrometastases in axillary lymph nodes by using polymerase chain reaction. *Cancer Res* 1994; 54: 2986-90.
13. Dearnaley DP, Sloane JP, Ormerod MG, Steele K, Coombes RC, Clink H.McD, Powles TJ, Ford HT, Gazet J-C, and Neville AM. Increased detection of mammary carcinoma cells in marrow smears using antisera to epithelial membrane antigen. *Br J Cancer* 1981; 44: 85-90.
14. Stasiak PC, Purkis PE, Leigh IM, and Lane B. Keratin 19: predicted amino acid sequence and broad tissue distribution suggested it evolved from keratinocyte keratins. *J Invest Dermatol* 1989; 92: 707-16.
15. Savtchenko ES, Schiff TA, Jiang CK, Freedberg IM and Blumenberg M. Embryonic expression of the human 40-kD keratin: evidence from a processed pseudogene sequence. *Am J Hum Genet* 1989; 43: 630-7.
16. Bader BL, Jahn L and Franke WW. Low level expression of cytokeratins 8, 18 and 19 in vascular smooth muscle cells of human umbilical cord and in cultured cells derived therefrom, with an analysis of the chromosomal locus containing the cytokeratin 19 gene. *Eur J Cell Biol* 1988; 47: 300-19.
17. Chomczynski P and Sacchi N. Single step method of RNA isolation by acid guanidium thiocyanate-phenol-chloroform extraction. *Anal Biochem* 1987; 162: 156-9.
18. Traweek ST, Liu J and Battifora H. Keratin gene expression in non-epithelial tissues. Detection with polymerase chain reaction. *Am J Pathol* 1992; 142: 1111-8.
19. Datta YH, Adams PT, Drobyski WR, Ethier SP, Terry VH and Roth, MS. Sensitive detection of occult breast cancer by the reverse-transcriptase polymerase chain reaction. *J Clin Oncol* 1994; 12: 475-82.
20. Dearnaley DP, Ormerod MG and Sloane JP. Micrometastases in breast cancer: long term follow-up of the first patient cohort. *Eur J Cancer* 1991; 27: 236-9.
21. Lee M, Chang K, Freireich EJ, Kantajiian HM, Talpez M, Trujillo JM and Stass SA. Detection of minimal residual bcr/abl transcripts by a modified polymerase chain reaction. *Blood* 1988; 72: 893-7.
22. Moreno JG, Croce CM, Fischer R, Monne M, Vikho P, Mulholland SG and Gomella LG. Detection of haematogenous micrometastases in patients with prostate cancer. *Cancer Res* 1992; 52: 6110-2.
23. Deguchi T, Doi T, Ehara H, Ito S, Takahashi Y, Nishino Y, Fujihero S, Kawamura T, Komeda H, Horie M, Kaji H, Shimokawa K, Tanaka T and Kawada Y. Detection of micrometastatic prostate cancer cells in lymph nodes by reverse transcriptase-polymerase chain reaction. *Cancer Res* 1993; 53: 5350-4.
24. Bartek J, Taylor-Papadimitriou J, Miller N and Millis R. Patterns of expression of keratin 19 as detected with monoclonal antibodies in human breast tissues and tumours. *Int J Cancer* 1985; 36: 299-306.
25. Wu A, Ben-Ezra J and Colombero A. Detection of micrometastases in breast cancer by the polymerase chain reaction: a feasibility study. *Lab Invest* 1990; 62: 109A.
26. James PPB and Williams CJ. Detection of breast cancer in lymph nodes by reverse transcription polymerase chain reaction (RT-PCR). *Br J Cancer* 1992; 65: 14A.
27. Mansi JL, Berger U, McDonnell T, Pople A, Rayter Z, Gazet J-C and Coombes R.C. The fate of bone marrow micrometastases in patients with primary breast cancer. *J Clin Oncol* 1989; 7: 445-9.
28. Gribben JG, Neuberg D, Barber M, Moore J, Pesek KW, Freedman AS and Nadler LM. Detection of residual lymphoma cells by PCR in peripheral blood is significantly less predictive for relapse than detection in marrow. *Blood* 1994; 83: 3800-7.

Immunotherapy of breast cancer using a recombinant Vaccinia virus expressing the human *MUC1* and *IL2* genes

Nadine Bizouarne, Jean-Marc Balloul, Christian Schatz, Bruce Acres and Marie-Paule Kieny

Transgène SA, 11, rue de Molsheim, 67000 Strasbourg, France

Over the last twenty years, it has been clearly shown that most human tumours express specific tumour antigens. Some of these antigens are viral, as is the case with cervical cancer [1] which is associated with an infection by a human papilloma virus (HPV), but many tumour antigens so far characterized in man are differentiation antigens. These are usually corresponding to genes which are only expressed significantly during the foetal-embryonic period; expression regresses after birth to the point of disappearing, only persisting in some cases in a particular type of differentiated adult cell. This is indeed the case with alpha-foeto-protein (AFP) and the carcinoembryonic antigen (CEA). Nevertheless, the expression of these genes can be re-induced abnormally during tumour development.The tumour differentiation specificity of an antigen may therefore be a quantitative rather than a qualitative matter, since the antigen may be present in a localized area or on an intermittent basis (*i.e.* during the foetal-embryonic period) in healthy individuals, or exist in trace quantities, only becoming hyperexpressed or modified (altered processing) during tumourigenesis. While the antigen is normally expressed, the immune system recognizes it as part of « self »; only when it is hyperexpressed or modified does it trigger an immune response.

Most experimental anti-cancer treatments currently under evaluation seek to reinforce the cellular immunity of the host organism to the tumour, mainly by using cytokines. Results obtained from systemic administration of interleukin 2 (IL2) provide objective evidence of two facts: non-negligible general toxicity, and undeniable though limited efficacy [2-4]. Another approach consists of using live vectors to direct *in vivo* the expression of the genes coding for a specific tumour antigen and/or for a cytokine. Indeed, the release of cytokines from the infected cells should stimulate anti-tumour immunity towards the tumour antigen, which would be presented by the same cells in conjunction with MHC class I.

Poxviruses form a complex family of DNA viruses which infect both vertebrates and invertebrates. The best-known member of the poxvirus family is Smallpox virus [5]. In the eighteenth century, prophylactic immunization against smallpox was undertaken using Vaccinia virus, another closely related poxvirus. Anti-smallpox vaccination campaigns proved so successful that they have eradicated this infectious disease altogether. Genes of many pathogens have been expressed in recombinant vaccinia viruses and used for stimulating the immune response against the corresponding antigens in animal models [6-8]. A recombinant vaccinia virus expressing the Rabies virus glycoprotein gene is currently used as an oral rabies vaccine for wild animals [9].

Poxviruses hold also great potential for human clinical applications. Indeed, although Vaccinia virus has been associated with a history of mild to severe side effects during the smallpox vaccination campaigns [10], it can be attenuated by the interruption of certain genes (such as the *thymidine kinase* gene) or by expression of various cytokine genes [11-13]. Furthermore, as Vaccinia virus remains cytoplasmic and lyses all the cells that it infects, this vector is uncapable of integrating into the host genome and of causing malignancies. On a more technical side, Vaccinia virus genome will accept insertion of several kilobases of DNA coding for many genes of therapeutic value.

For these reasons, tumour-associated antigen coding sequences have also been expressed in Vaccinia virus. Lathe *et al.* [14] have used an animal model to show that tumours caused by Polyoma virus can be rejected after vaccination with a recombinant vaccinia virus expressing early genes of this virus. Estin *et al.* [15] performed anti-melanoma vaccinations in another animal model using a recombinant vaccinia virus synthesizing an antigen (p97) specific for these tumours. Meneguzzi *et al.* [16] have published encouraging results of rodent vaccination against the development of tumours induced by the Bovine Papilloma virus (BPV-1) and these results have been extended to Human Papilloma virus (HPV-16) [17]. Kaufman *et al.* [18] have constructed a recombinant Vaccinia virus expressing human CEA, and this virus has been used in humans. More recently, clinical trials of therapeutic vaccination against cervical cancer using a recombinant vaccinia virus expressing the E6 and E7 genes of HPV-16 and -18 (S. Inglis, personal communication) have been undertaken both in the United Kingdom and the United States.

In normal epithelial tissues, the mucin protein MUC1 is exported to the apical cell surface. In contrast, this antigen can be detected in abnormal quantities in the cytoplasm of epithelial cells from cancerous mammary tissue. Significant quantities of MUC1 can also be detected in other tumour epithelial tissues (pancreas, ovary, lung, etc.). Morover, the MUC1 tumour antigen presents novel epitopes which are recognized by tumour-specific antibodies [19, 20]. Indeed, the MUC1 protein is very highly glycosylated (< 50 % of the mass) while tumour associated MUC1 protein is much less so, revealing previously masked peptidic epitopes [21]. Using these tumour-specific monoclonal antibodies, the MUC1 antigen cDNA was cloned [22, 23]. The deduced amino-acid sequence includes a sub-unit of 20 amino acids which is repeated in tandem between 20 and 125 times.

Immunogenicity of a recombinant Vaccinia virus expressing the MUC1 gene

The MUC1 gene has been expressed from a recombinant vaccinia virus (VV-MUC1) [24]. Using a rat animal model, Hareuveni *et al.* [25] demonstated that vaccination with this recominant virus induced partial protection against the growth of syngeneic tumours expressing MUC1 (50-80% animals rejecting their tumour).

Similar experiments were conducted in DBA/2 mice (H2-d). Here, 30% of the mice immunized with VV-MUC1 were found to be protected against tumour (syngeneic P815-MUC1 cells) growth, whereas none of the mice immunized with the control VV were protected. The immunized mice showed moderate concentrations of MUC1-specific IgG, uncorrelated with tumour rejection. No MUC1-specific CTL response was observed in these mice [26]. More recently, we have repeated these experiments with C57/Bl6 mice (H2-b) and demonstated the induction of MHC-I restricted CTL upon vaccination with VV-MUC1 *(Figure 1)*. As expected, no activity was detected in control animals.

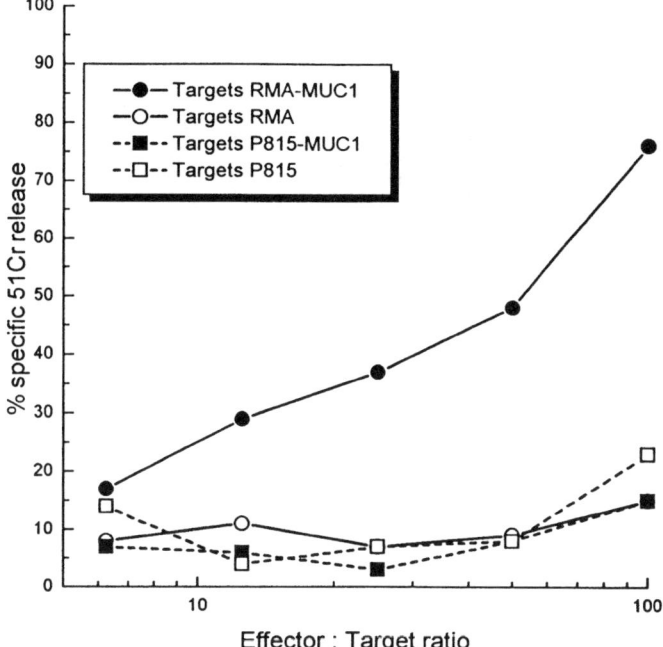

Figure 1. MHC-I -restricted, MUC1-Specific CTL activity in C57Bl/6 mice immunized with 3.10^7 pfu VVTG5058 ip.

In order to increase further both the MUC1-specific and non-specific immune responses, a cassette coding for human IL2 was added in the VV-MUC1 construction (VVTG5058). We subsequently conducted tumour protection experiments on three groups of twenty DBA/2 mice. The first group received three intramuscular administrations of buffer, the second group received three intramuscular administrations of 2×10^8 pfu of VVTG186 (VVTK⁻ without insert), and the third group received three intramuscular administrations of 2×10^8 pfu of VVTG5058. Immunizations were performed on days 0, 10 and 20. P815-MUC1 tumour cells were then implanted on day 23 in all mice. Results obtained after 43 days show that the animals immunized with VVTG5058 were best protected: 40% of mice immunized with VVTG5058 were found to reject their tumour, as opposed to 30% of mice which had received VV-MUC1 without IL2, 10% of the mice which had received VVTG186 and 8% of the mice which had received the buffer alone *(Figure 2)*. Tumour rejection appears to be triggered by a cellular mechanism as determined by adoptive transfer experiments (not shown).

In view of the potential application of this vector as a therapeutic vaccine in humans, it was of utmost importance to demonstraste its attenuation in an animal model. We therefore conducted experiments on immunocompromized (nude) mice. The animals received 10^7 pfu of VVTG5058 or wild type Vaccinia virus (VVwt) by the intramuscular (IM), intraperitoneal (IP), intravenous (IV) or intracranial (IC) routes. *Table I* shows the number of animals found dead or harbouring lesions after 20 days. These lesions were characterized by pustuliform cutaneous eruptions on the arch of the foot and the tail. These results show that VVTG5058 is substantially attenuated compared to wild-type Vaccinia virus, as no death occurred within this group.

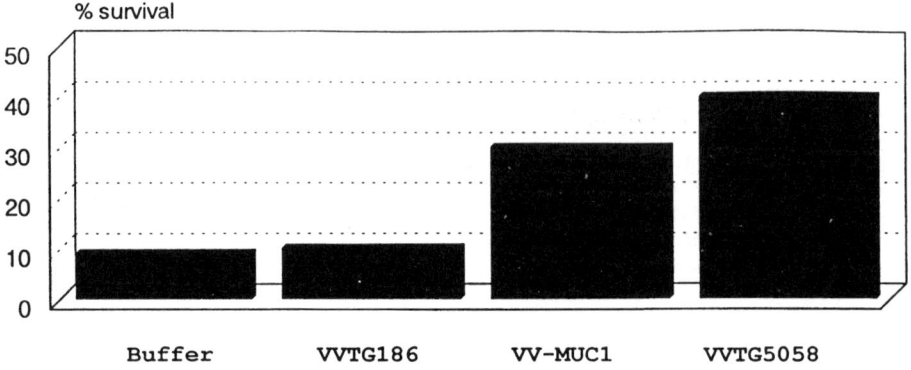

Figure 2. Tumour protection in mice.
Immunization regimen: 3.10^7 pfu VV, im, days 0, 10, 20
3.10^5 P815-MUC1, sc, day 23.

Table I. Attenuation of VVTG5058 in nude mice.

	IM		IP		IV		IC	
	VVTG5058	VVwt	VVTG5058	VVwt	VVTG5058	VVwt	VVTG5058	VVwt
A	0/5	0/5	0/5	0/5	0/5	5/5	5/5	4/4
B	0/5	0/5	0/5	0/5	0/5	2/5 dead after 20 days	0/5	4/4 dead after 3 days

A: proportion of animals presenting cutaneous lesions
B: animals dead of generalized vaccinia.
Administration of 10^7 pfu VV at day 0.

Biodistribution and *in vivo* IL2 production in mice

We have also conducted experiments on the biodistribution of VVTG5058 and on the kinetics of *in vivo* IL2 production. DBA/2 mice received intramuscular administration of 10^8 pfu of VVTG5058. Viral concentrations were measured in various organs (brain, kidney, liver, lungs, spleen, uterus/ovaries, muscle) at one, two, three, seven and ten day after administration, sacrificing two mice each time. No sign of the vaccinia virus was found in any organ except for the injection site after one, two and three days (8,000 to 1,000 pfu/mg tissue). On subsequent days, no vaccinia virus was detected.

We measured serum levels of IL2 in the same animals, using the ELISA technique. On day 1, low concentrations of IL2 (30 pg/ml) were detected. No IL2 was detected on subsequent days, which suggests that IL2 production remained localized near the injection site.

Tolerance of VVTG5058 in monkeys

VVTG5058 was administered by intramuscular injection in two groups of two monkeys (1 male, 1 female/group). One group received a single dose of vaccine corresponding to a human dose of 10^8 pfu adjusted for the animal weight (1.4×10^5 pfu/kg). The other group received a single injection of a tenth of this dose.

No instance of mortality and no clinical sign attributable to the treatment was observed except for one monkey presenting a local oedema five days after receiving an administration of the low dose (equivalent to human dose of 10^7 pfu); this regressed and disappeared after three days. Histopathological examination at the administration site revealed slight fibrosis with very slight necrosis of the muscle fibre in the monkey that suffered the local oedema. There was no sign of local irritation at either dose level.

These experiments demonstrate that VVTG5058 is safe in primates and rodents. This recombinant was also shown to be able of inducing both an humoral and a cellular immune response against the MUC1 antigen. Morover we have confirmed in further animal protection experiments the potential of this vaccine as an immunotherapeutic against MUC1 expressing tumours. All these results have prompted us to prepare a clinical grade batch of VVTG5058 and to propose a clinical evaluation of this vaccine in breast cancer patients. This phase 1 study is ongoing at Institut Curie.

References

1. Zur Hausen H, Schneider A. The role of papillomaviruses in anogenital cancer. In: *The Papovaviridae*. Eds NP Salzman et PM Howley. NY Plenium Press: 245-63.
2. Gansbacher B, Zier K, Daniels B, Cronin K, Bannerji R, Gilboa E. Interleukin 2 gene transfer into tumor cells abrogates tumorigenicity and induces protective immunity. *J Exp Med* 1990; 172: 1217-24.
3. Foa R, Guarini A, Gansbacher B. IL2 treatment for cancer: from biology to gene therapy. *Br J Cancer* 1992; 66: 992-8.
4. Bubenik J. IL-2 and gene therapy of cancer. *Int J Oncol* 1993; 2: 1049-52.
5. Behbehani AM. The Smallpox Story: Life and Death of an Old Disease. *Microbiological Reviews* 1983; 47: 455-509.
6. Panicali D, Paoletti E. Construction of poxviruses as cloning vectors: insertion of the thymidine kinase from herpex simplex into the DNA of infectious vaccinia virus. *Proc Natl Acad Sci USA* 1982; 79: 4927-31.
7. Mackett M, Smith GL, Moss B. Vaccinia virus: a selectable eukaryotic cloning and expression vector. *Proc Natl Acad Sci USA* 1982; 79: 7415-9.
8. Kieny MP, Lathe R, Drillien R, Spehner D, Skory S, Schmitt D, Wiktor T, Koprowski H, Lecocq JP. Expression of rabies virus glycoprotein from a recombinant vaccinia virus. *Nature* 1984; 312: 163-6.
9. Brochier B, Kieny MP, Costy F, Coppens P, Bauduin B, Lecocq JP, Languet B, Chappuis G, Desmettre P, Afiademanyo K, Libois R, Pastoret PP. Large-scale eradication of rabies using recombinant vaccinia-rabies vaccine. *Nature* 1991; 354: 521-2.
10. Henderson DA, Fenner F. Smallpox and vaccinia. In: Plotkin SA, Mortimer EA, eds. *Vaccines*, Philadelphia (USA): Saunders Company,1994:13-40.
11. Buller RML, Smith GL, Cremer K, Notkins AL, Moss B. Decreased virulence of recombinant vaccinia virus expression vectors is associated with a thymidine kinase-negative phenotype. *Nature* 1985; 317: 813-5.
12. Flexner C, Hügin A, Moss B. Prevention of vaccinia virus infection in immunodeficient mice by vector-derived IL-2 expression. *Nature* 1987; 330: 259-63.

13. Karupiah G, Blanden RV, Ramshaw IA. Interferon is involved in the recovery of athymic nude mice from recombinant vaccinia virus/interleukin 2 infection. *J Exp Med* 1990; 172:1495-503.
14. Lathe R, Kieny MP, Gerlinger P, Clertant P, Guizani I, Cuzin F, Chambon P. Tumor prevention and rejection with recombinant vaccinia. *Nature* 1987; 326: 878-80.
15. Estin CD, Stevenson US, Plowman GD, Hu SL, Sridhar P, Hellström I, Hellström KE. Recombinant vaccinia virus vaccine against the human melanoma antigen p97 for use in immunotherapy. *Proc Natl Acad Sci USA* 1988; 85: 1052-6.
16. Meneguzzi G, Kieny MP, Lecocq JP, Chambon P, Cuzin F, Lathe R. Vaccinia recombinants expressing early bovine papilloma virus (BPV1) proteins: retardation of BPV1 tumour development. *Vaccine* 1990; 8: 199-204.
17. Meneguzzi G, Cerni C, Kieny MP, Lathe R. Immunization against human papillomavirus type 16 tumor cells with recombinant vaccinia viruses expressing E6 and E7. *Virology* 1991; 181: 62-9.
18. Kaufman H, Schlom J, Kantor J. A recombinant vaccinia virus expressing human carcinoembryonic antigen (CEA). *Int J Cancer* 1991; 48: 900-7.
19. Burchell J, Gendler S, Taylor-Papadimitriou J, Girling A, Millis R, Lamport D. Developpment and characterization of breast cancer reactive monoclonal antibodies directed to the core protein of the human milk mucin. *Cancer Res* 1987; 47: 5476-82.
20. Keydar I, Chou CS, Hareuveni M, Tsarfaty I, Sahar E, Selzer G, Chaitchik S, Hizi M. Production and characterization of monoclonal antibodies identifying breast tumor-associated antigens. *Proc Natl Acad Sci USA* 1989; 86: 1362-6.
21. Devine PL, Warren JA, Ward BG, Mc Kenzie IFC, Layton GT. Glycosylation and the exposure of tumor-associated epitopes on mucins. *J Tumor Marker Oncol* 1990; 5: 11-26.
22. Gendler SJ, Lancaster CA, Taylor-Papadimitriou J, Dahig T, Peat N, Burchell J, Pemberton L, Lalani EN, Wilson D. Molecular cloning of human tumor-associated polymorphic epithelial mucin. *J. Biol. Chem.* 1990; 265: 15286-93.
23. Wreschner DH, Hareuveni M, Tsarfaty I, Smorodinsky H, Horey J, Zaretskey J, Kotkes P, Weiss M, Lathe R, Dion A, Keydar I. Human epithelial tumor antigen cDNA sequences: differential splicing may generate multiple protein forms. *Eur J Biochem* 1990; 189: 463-73.
24. Hareuveni M, Gautier C, Kieny MP, Wreschner D, Chambon P, Lathe R. Vaccination against tumor cells expressing breast cancer epithelial tumor antigen. *Proc. Natl. Acad. Sci USA* 1990; 87: 9498-502.
25. Hareuveni M, Wreschner DH, Kieny MP, Dott K, Gautier C, Tomasetto C, Keydar I, Chambon P, Lathe R. Vaccinia recombinants expressing secreted and transmembrane forms of breast cancer epithelial tumor antigen. *Vaccine* 1991; 9: 618-27.
26. Acres RB, Hareuveni M, Balloul JM, Kieny MP. Vaccinia virus MUC1 immunization of mice: Immune response and protection against growth of murine tumours bearing the MUC1 antigen. *J Immunother* 1993; 14: 136-43.

The *MUC1* gene as an immunogen: use of naked DNA and role of dendritic cells

Joy Burchell, Rosalind Graham, Moira Shearer, Mike Smith, Lukas Heukamp, David Miles* and Joyce Taylor-Papadimitriou

Imperial Cancer Research Fund, 44 Lincoln's Inn Fields, London WC2A 3PX;
* Immunohistology Dept, Guy's Hospital, St Thomas Street, London SE1 9RT

The immune response and cancer

In recent years, new insights into the mechanisms involved in effective antigen presentation, and the identification of tumour associated antigens have led to increased activity in the specific area of tumour immunology. As a result, the possibility that Immunotherapy may be an option for management of cancer patients is being seriously evaluated, not only in preclinical studies in model systems, but also in the clinic. The use of an antigen to induce the host immune response has the advantage that several compartments of effector cells with different functions may be recruited for tumour cell killing. In this context, it is generally assumed that cytotoxic T cells (CTLs) recognising specific peptides presented by MHC class I molecules play a crucial role, and peptides from mutated oncogenes, papilloma virus proteins, or normally silent genes such as the *MAGE* genes [1] represent candidate vaccines.

DNA based immunogens

The idea of using specific peptides comes from basic work in the field of viral immunology. The viral antigen is found intracellularly in infected cells, and endogenously derived peptides are presented by Class I molecules to T cells to induce CTLs. Helper T cells are also induced by Class II presentation of peptides derived from viral products taken up by professional antigen presenting cells (APCs). In attempting to apply the principles developed from studies on viruses to tumour antigens, the idea of introducing the DNA coding for the antigen into an appropriate cell appears logical. A direct extension of this idea is to introduce the gene coding for the antigen into a virus and recombinant viruses based on vaccinia, adenovirus and retroviruses have been developed as potential immunogens. In the last few years however, naked DNA coding for specific viral antigens has been shown to induce both cellular and humoral responses when injected intramuscularly (IM) into mice [2, 3]. Indeed in some cases, the immunity induced by the injected DNA is better than that observed using existing vaccines. It is this approach which we are trying to implement to obtain immune responses to *MUC1*.

The *MUC1* gene and its product

The *MUC1* gene codes for a surface epithelial mucin which is over expressed and aberrantly glycosylated in breast, ovarian and other carcinomas and is a candidate antigen for immunotherapy of Breast Cancer. The extracellular domain of the molecule consists largely of repeats of 20 amino acids which are rich in threonines and serines, the potential sites of O-glycosylation. The molecule is therefore highly repetitive in structure having multiple identical peptide and carbohydrate epitopes. That the cancer-associated mucin can be recognised by the immune system has been demonstrated by the fact that antibodies and CTLs specifically reactive with mucin expressing cells have been isolated from breast and ovarian cancer patients [4-6]. The CTLs appear to recognise the mucin in a non-HLA restricted fashion and preferentially kill cells expressing the underglycosylated molecule. The results suggest that the epitopes in the intact surface molecule are recognised by the T cell receptor by multiple (possibly low affinity) interactions, and that these epitopes are selectively exposed in the underglycosylated mucin. The search for Class I restricted peptide epitopes has so far been limited but certain peptides with sequences from the tandem repeats can bind to some class I alleles (A2 and A11), although whether these are produced *in vivo* is not known. Proliferative responses to the tandem repeat peptide (24 amino acids) presented by PBLs or by dendritic cells have also been observed.

Mouse models for evaluating *MUC1* based immunogens

The strategies to be used for development of a *MUC1* based vaccine will be strongly influenced by whether the important T cell responses, in particular the CTL response, is indeed mainly to the intact molecule (and therefore affected by glycosylation), or whether peptide presentation by MHC molecules is also important. *MUC1* is expressed at the apical surface of most glandular epithelial cells and in that position is less accessible to immune effector cells than the mucin expressed all around the cancer cell, which has lost polarity. On the other hand, if MHC restricted presentation is important, peptides may also be presented by Class I molecules expressed on the basolateral surface of normal epithelial cells which, if recognised, could lead to autoimmune responses with undesirable side effects. To optimise antigen presentation for tumour rejection while avoiding tissue damage, due to autoimmunity, mouse models are essential.

Syngeneic models in $H2^b$ and $H2^d$ mice have been developed where transplantable tumours have been modified to express the human *MUC1* gene [7]. RMA cells expressing the gene have been used by ourselves to test the efficacy of IM injection of *MUC1* cDNA in inducing immune responses and tumour rejection. A transgenic mouse strain expressing the human *MUC1* gene with the correct tissue specific expression is also available [8]. This latter model is particularly useful for testing for any tissue damage which could be caused by autoimmune responses.

MUC1 cDNA as an immunogen

The effectiveness of using MUC1 cDNA as an immunogen has been evaluated using the full length wild type DNA driven by the beta actin promoter in C57 Bl mice. Three injections (IM) given before challenging with MUC1-expressing RMA cells, reduced the incidence of tumours and the effect was dose dependent *(see Figure 1)*. Antibodies to the peptide backbone of the MUC1 protein could be detected after the DNA injections, thus confirming expression of the antigen, but CTLs specifically reactive with the RMA MUC1 cells were only isolated from mouse spleens after the mice had been challenged with the tumour cells [9].

In considering the mechanisms involved in MUC1 cDNA protection against tumour growth, three questions arise, namely:
1. Which components of the immune response are important for eliminating the tumour cells?
2. Are the cellular responses MHC-restricted or unrestricted?
3. Which cell type(s) is (are) expressing and presenting the antigen?

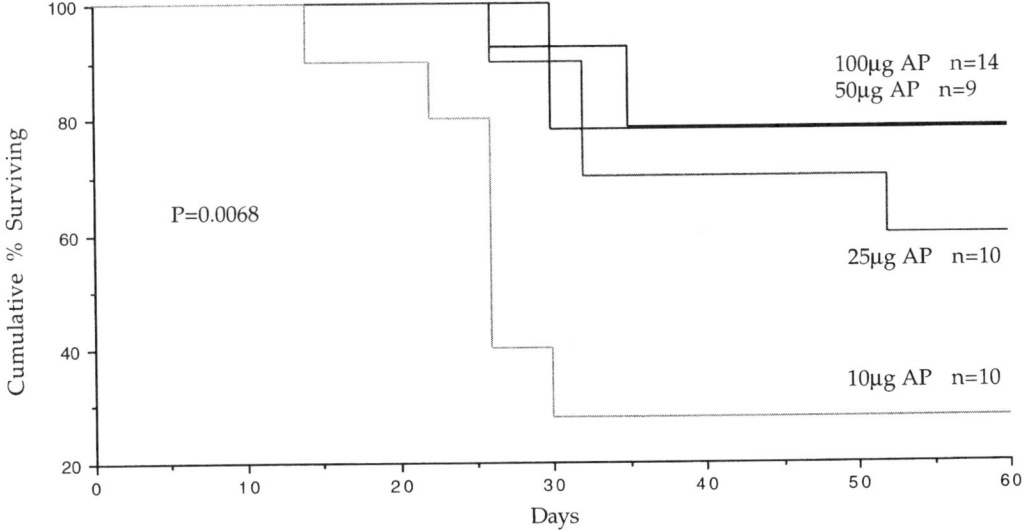

Figure 1. Dose dependence of cumulative % survival.

Undoubtedly proliferative responses of $CD4^+$ T cells can be induced using the larger 24 amino acid peptide covering the tandem repeat. Such responses have been reported in multiparous women using PBLs for antigen presentation [10]. We now find that responses can be found in most individuals if autologous dendritic cells are used to present the antigen. *Figure 2* shows an example of a response using cells from an adult female who has had one pregnancy. We have yet to determine whether the presentation of the peptide is MHC restricted and whether responses also occur in males. They can however be observed in non-parous females. A very strong proliferative response to the MUC1 peptide is also seen in T cells taken from C57Bl mice injected once with peptide pulsed dendritic cells. These results suggest stimulation of T helper cells *in vivo* in mice injected with MUC1 DNA may be achieved by dendritic cells taking up peptide expressed from muscle cells. Whether the injected cDNA is also *expressed* by the dendritic cells *in vivo* and can in this way generate MUC1 specific CTLs remains to be seen.

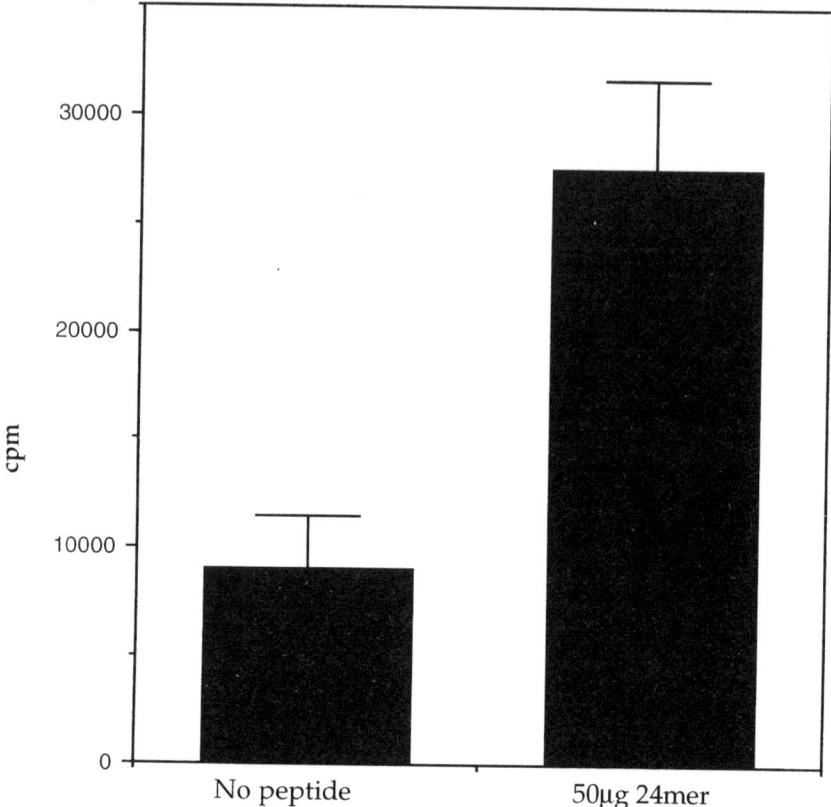

Figure 2. CD4+ T proliferative response to 24 mer (cDNA).

One way to ascertain whether CTLs are being induced by the intact molecule or *via* MHC presentation is to modify the DNA to influence processing and glycosylation and to look at the effect of such modifications on the ability to induce immune responses and tumor protection. Also, in considering the function of dendritic cells *in vivo*, some clues may be obtained using dendritic cells cultured *in vitro*, since expression of MUC1 cDNA in these cells should now be possible. We are now attempting to introduce MUC1 cDNA (and engineered mutants) into cultured mouse and human dendritic cells in order to examine the efficacy of transduced cells in inducing proliferative and cytotoxic responses *in vitro*, as well tumour rejection *in vivo*.

References

1. Coulie PG, Brichard V, Van Pel A, Wolfel T, Schneider J, Traversari C, Mattei S, De Plaen E, Lurquin C, Szikora J-P, Renauld J-C, Boon T. A new gene coding for a differentiation antigen recognised by autologous cytolytic T lymphocytes on HLA-A2 melamonas. *J Exp Med* 1994; 35-42.
2. Ulmer JB, Donnelly JJ, Parker SE, Rhodes GH, Felgner PL, Dwarki VJ, Gromkowski SH, Deck RR, DeWitt CM, Friedman A, Hawe LA, Leadner KR, Martinez D, Perry HC, Shiver JW, Montgomery DL, Liu MA. Heterologous protection against influenza by injection of DNA encoding a viral protein. *Science*. 1993; 259: 1745-9.

3. Ulmer JB, Deck RR, DeWitt CM, Friedman A, Donnelly JJ, Liu MA. Protective immunity by intramuscular injection of low doses of influenza virus DNA vaccines. *Vaccine.* 1994; 12: 1541-4.
4. Barnd DL, Lan MS, Metzgar RS, Finn OJ. Specific, major histocompatability complex-unrestricted recognition of tumour-associated mucins by human cytotoxic T cells. *Proc Natl Acad Sci USA* 1989; 86: 7159-64.
5. Jerome KR, Barnd DL, Bendt KM, Boyer CM, Taylor-Papadimitriou J, McKenzie IFC, Bast RC, Finn OJ. Cytotoxic T-lymphocytes derived from patients with breast adenocarcinoma recognize an epitope present on the protein core of a mucin molecule preferentially expressed by malignant cells. *Cancer Res* 1989; 51: 2908-16.
6. Ioannides CG, Fisk B, Jerome KR, Tatsuro I, Taylor Wharton J, Finn OJ. Cytotoxic T cells from ovarian malignant tumours can recognise polymorphic epithelial mucin core peptides. *J Immunol* 1993; 7: 3693-703.
7. Graham RA, Stewart LS, Peat NP, Beverley P, Taylor-Papadimitriou J. MUC1-based immunogens for tumour therapy: Development of murine model systems. *Tumour Targeting* 1995; 1: 211-21.
8. Peat N, Gendler SJ, Lalani E-N, Duhig T, Taylor-Papadimitriou J. Tissue specific expression of a human polymorphic epithelial mucin (MUC1) in transgenic mice. *Cancer Res* 1992; 52: 1954-60.
9. Graham RA, Burchell JM, Beverley P, Taylor-Papadimitriou J. Intramuscular immunisation with MUC1 cDNA can protect C57 mice challenged with MUC1-expressing syngeneic mouse tumour cells. *Int J Cancer* 1996; 65: 664-70.
10. Agrawal B, Reddish MA, Krantz MJ, Longenecker BM. Does pregnancy immunize against breast cancer. *Cancer Res* 1995; 55: 2257-61.

Tumour immunotherapy against MUC1 expressing tumours using mannan MUC1

V. Apostolopoulos[1], G.A. Pietersz[1], B. Acres[2], C. Osinski[1], G. Thynne[3], P.-X. Xing[1], V. Karanikas[1], H.A. Vaughan[1], L. Hwang[1], V. Popovski[1], C. Lees[1], C.S. Ong[1] and I.F.C. McKenzie[1]

[1] The Austin Research Institute, Studley Road, Heidelberg Vic 3084, Australia;
[2] Transgene, 11, rue de Molsheim, 67082 Strasbourg Cedex, France;
[3] Allamanda Medical Centre, Southport, QLD, 4215, Australia

Introduction

Tumour immunotherapy is now attracting much attention due entirely to the genetic engineering techniques now available, which lead to:- a) the capacity to produce large amounts of synthetic and recombinant materials such as tumour antigens; b) the description and availability of cytokines; c) the identification, using gene cloning techniques of genes encoding tumour antigens; d) the identification of peptides presented by Class I molecules which serve as targets for cytotoxic T cell lymphocytes (CTLs). This is real progress, and we should now be optimistic that a substantial impact in cancer therapy will be made by any or all of these advances. In this light, we are studying Mucin 1 (MUC1) - a ubiquitous mucin, which, in the normal state is found either intracellularly or in the lining of ducts, and in secretions such as breast milk. In the malignant state, MUC1 is found in very large amounts throughout the cell, and on the cell surface, and in which there is aberrant glycosylation exposing part of the protein core - which could serve as a target for antibody or non-MHC restricted killer cells [1]. We presume that the massive increase in mucin production by tumour cells should lead to some of the excess MUC1 peptides synthestised and find their way into the Class I MHC groove and be presented to CTLs. Thus, MUC1 should theoretically be a good target for immunotherapy. Two observations lend weight to the concept of targeting MUC1 in immunotherapeutic studies. Firstly, Mucin 1 is highly immunogenic - at least for antibody production in mice, and the amino acids APDTR of the repeat region are the most immunogenic of the whole MUC1 molecule, as monoclonal antibodies made to tumours, mucins such as HMFG or indeed synthetic peptides recognise APDTR [2]. Secondly, Dr O. Finn has found in the lymph nodes of patients with breast cancer can be found CTL precursors which, on stimulation *in vitro*, lead to CTLs which have non-MHC restricted activity; the target of these cells also appears to be the APDTR sequence [3]. On this basis, we and others are determining how is the best way to increase the immune response to MUC1, particularly the VNTR peptides (containing APDTR) and now describe the use of mannan MUC1 conjugates which are immunogenic in mice, monkeys and humans. The results of the studies are summarised in *Table I*.

Murine immune response to MUC1 peptides

As indicated above, synthetic peptides were able to immunise mice for anti-MUC1 antibody production - could they be used to induce cellular immunity and anti-tumour effects? We made a MUC1 synthetic peptide (Cp13-32) containing 20 amino acids of MUC1 (which spontaneously dimerises due to the formation of disulphide bonds, linked this to either KLH, or diphtheria toxoid and immunised mice. As before, antibodies were produced and cellular immunity was demonstrated by CD4$^+$ mediated DTH reactions [4]. Anti-tumour immunity examined by challenging mice with human MUC1$^+$ tumours (induced by transfecting mouse tumours with *MUC1* gene) indicated some anti-tumour effects with protection with low dose of tumour challenge (10^6 cells) [4]. This protection disappeared when 5 times the dose was used. With this immunisation protocol, no CTLs were produced. In this particular model, mice ultimately rejected MUC1$^+$ tumours (in non-immunised mice) and produced weak antibody responses, DTH and CTLs (revealed only after deglycosylation of target antigens) *(Table 1)*. On the basis of the anti-tumour responses (albeit weak) after peptide immunisation, a clinical trial was performed.

Immunogenicity of human MUC1 peptides in humans

A Phase I trial was performed using increasing doses of MUC1 peptides 150-1,000 micrograms in 13 patients, seeking evidence of toxicity, autoimmunity, and immunogenicity. For these studies, diphtheria toxoid was used as a carrier and the only toxicity noted were the severe DTH reactions to the carrier after multiple immunisations. There was no evidence of autoimmunity (which could occur due to anti-MUC1 responses in salivary gland, lung, kidney, pancreas and elsewhere - sites of MUC1 expression). There was weak immunogenicity, with small amounts of antibody produced and T cell proliferation in some of the patients [5]. No anti-tumour responses were noted, although these were not formally sought. Our conclusions were that the peptides were weakly immunogenic, but not sufficiently so to be of any benefit, and we sought to improve the immunogenicity by conjugation to mannan which will form the basis of the rest of this paper.

Murine immune responses to mannan MUC1 (MFP)

After using a number of methods to couple MUC1 to a potential carrier, conjugation to mannan under oxidising conditions by periodate was used and this generated exceedingly good cellular responses *(Table 1)* to MUC1 and poor humoral responses [6, 7]. The conjugation conditions to mannan were most important - oxidising conditions leading to cellular responses, reducing conditions leading to humoral responses - indeed, of the same type obtained using MUC1 peptides or a MUC1 fusion protein (produced as a 5 repeat synthetic peptide of 105 amino acids). The strength of the immune response was startling - mice previously susceptible to 5×10^6 tumour cells were now resistant to 5×10^7 cell challenge, little antibody was produced, DTH was again present, but this time, CD8$^+$ CTLs could be induced prior to tumour challenge and with a high frequency ($^1/8,000$). Several different tumour models have been used and in all, mannan fusion protein (MFP) given as 3 injections at weekly intervals leads to total resistance to a subsequent tumour challenge (studies with the highly malignant MUC1$^+$ DA3 metastatic tumour are in progress). In addition, the injection of mice carrying MUC1$^+$ tumours led to a rapid reversal of their growth - of importance for patients with cancer.

Table I. Immunogenicity of various MUC1 immunogens in mice[a].

	MUC1 Tumour	MUC1 Peptide Fusion Protein or HMFG	Oxidised MFP	Reduced MFP
Immunogenicity				
Antibody Production	+	+++	±	++
DTH	+++	+++	+++	+++
CTL	+ (after PAGAL)	-	++	-
Tumour Protection	++	±	+++	±
Mediators				
CD4	-	*	-	*
CD8	+	*	+	*
Cytokine secretion after immunisation				
IL-2	*	-	+	-
IL-4	*	+	-	+
IL-12	*	-	+	-
γ-IFN	*	-	+	-
CTL responses				
MHC-restricted		*	Yes	
MHC-non restricted			No	
Responding H-2 haplotypes			b, d, k, s, z	
non-responding H-2 haplotypes			Nil	
HLA responses			HLA-A2 (others not tested)	
Enhancement of responses to mannan MUC1				
Cyclophosphamide			Yes	
Adjuvants				
CFA			No	
IFA			Yes	
Aluminum hydroxide			Yes	
GM-DP			Yes	
M-DP			Yes	
Macrophage (F4/80+, 33D1-) presentation by adoptive transfer				
in vivo			Yes	
in vitro			Yes	
Dendritic cell (F4/80-, 33D1+) presentation by adoptive transfer				
in vivo			in progress	
in vivo			in progress	
Cytokines				
IL-12			Yes	
IL-7+GM-CSF			Yes	
IL-4+γ-IFN			Yes	

[a] +++, excellent; ++, very good; + good; ± weak; - nil; in progress.
CTL, cytotoxic T lymphocytes; DTH, delayed type hypersensitivity; HMFG, human milk fat globule; MFP, mannan-MUC1fusion protein; PAGAL, phenyl N-acetyl-a-D-galactosamide.

Cytokine profiles after MFP immunisation and MHC restriction

In contrast to the predominant antibody production produced with peptides, fusion protein or reduced MFP, oxidised MFP gave predominant cellular responses and little antibody - suggestive of a T_1 response. This was confirmed in cytokine studies where the former gave rise to IL-4 secretion and little T_1 cytokine, whereas the use of oxidised MFP gave rise to the production of IL-2, γ-IFN, IL-12 and no IL-4 ie. a T_1 response [7]. It was intriguing that, by simply altering the oxidising conditions, a response could be switched from T_1 to T_2. MFP induces MHC restricted CTL responses [8]. Although the descriptions of CTLs from Finn indicated these were non-MHC restricted, in all our murine studies only H-2 restricted responses could be induced and indeed, 9 strains of 5 different haplotypes could all be immunised; there were no non-responder strains. By using inbred, congenic, recombinant and mutant mice, the responses are clearly shown to be H-2 restricted and this was confirmed using cells transfected with selected Class I genes and in stabilisation studies using RMA-S cells. There is no doubt the response is MHC restricted and furthermore, non-MHC restricted responses were not seen.

These studies have recently been extended by mapping the epitopes presented by the different Class I molecule (*see Table I*). Of note, now that epitopes did not fit the usual binding rules, but nonetheless, molecular modelling studies clearly demonstrated that MUC1 is firmly bound to Class I molecules, and furthermore, provides the only example wherein peptides in the Class I groove are accessible to anti-MUC1 peptide antibodies (Apostolopoulos *et al.*, MS in preparation).

Presentation of MUC1 by HLA antigens

Using HLA-2 transgenic mice immunised with MFP, it was clearly demonstrated that HLA restricted CTLs could be induced *in vivo* and these could be detected without restimulation *in vitro*. Furthermore, such CTLs could lyse HLA-A2$^+$ MUC1$^+$ MCF7 cells *in vitro*, but not HLA-A2$^-$ MUC1$^+$ BT20 breast cancer cells. The HLA-A2 presented MUC1 epitopes have also been mapped (Apostolopoulos *et al.*, in preparation).

Clinical trials with MFP in patients with adenocarcinoma and in monkeys

Based on the foregoing, 27 patients with adenocarcinoma (predominantly breast or colon) were immunised with MFP. In contrast to the murine studies, most of the patients made high titres of antibody to MUC1 peptide; gave weak DTH responses; T cell proliferation was detected, and CTLs are in the process of being measured. Thus, human MUC1 is highly immunogenic in humans. Similar studies were performed in 4 monkeys and again significant antibody responses were noted - cellular immunity measurements are now in progress. In neither monkeys nor humans, was there evidence of autoimmunity. It appears that MUC1, while being immunogenic, does not incite autoimmune responses.

Enhancement of anti-MUC1 responses

In an endeavour to further increase the immunogenicity of MFP, we used cyclophosphamide, various adjuvants and cytokines *(Table I)* - as shown, a number of the adjuvants can increase the CTLp frequency as can cyclophosphamide and several of the cytokines, particularly in combination eg. IL-4 and γ-IFN and particularly IL-12. How these could be used in clinical studies is not clear at present.

Mode of action of MFP

At present it is not clear how MFP functions increase immune responses. Clearly mannan is important and could bind to the mannose receptor on macrophages and other cells, however, this is not the whole explanation as oxidised and reduced mannan bind equally well to macrophages and indeed, to the isolated mannose receptor expressed in transfected Cos cells, the reduced form binds better. We consider that macrophages are likely to be the major site of action of MFP rather than in dendritic cells (DC) as MFP does not bind well to DCs or to a DC tumour cell line, whereas it binds to macrophages, but the influence of dendritic cells on macrophages or their interactions are currently under examination. However, what has been shown is that peritoneal exudate cells (containing approximately 90% macrophages, 10% DCs) can be satisfactorily immunised *in vitro*, adoptively transfer immunity to mice and furthermore, one injection of such adoptively transferred cells is equivalent to 3 *in vivo* injections of MFP. We are currently examining the feasibility of sensitising human cells *in vitro* for clinical study.

Conclusion

Our studies have clearly demonstrated that mannan MUC1 (MFP) produced under oxidising conditions is a powerful immunogen for inducing CTL T cell immunity in mice - indeed, the most potent immunogen yet described, giving rise to much greater responses than those found with synthetic MUC1 peptides, whatever carrier is used. However, it should be emphasised that what we are measuring is the murine response to human MUC1, which is merely a model and an indication of what could happen in patients. As noted, when patients were immunised with human MUC1, humoral responses were noted and we are currently determining what degree of cellular immunity was found. However, at this time, other models should be used such as mice transgenic for human MUC1, and we also determining the immunogenicity of mannan conjugated with autologous MUC1 in monkeys (by cloning cynologous monkey MUC1) and also mannan-murine MUC1 in mice; these models are more relevant to the immunisation of patients than cross species immunisation with MUC1. Nonetheless, the results are encouraging and it was appropriate to perform preclinical studies before clinical studies were embarked upon. We are particularly encouraged by preliminary studies wherein MUC1 transgenic mice can be immunised against MUC1, although the CTL precursor frequency (CTLp) is substantially less than that obtained with human MUC1, although with the success in mice immunising macrophages or adoptive transfer - these approaches are likely to be the basis of further clinical trials. At this time the results are encouraging and indicate that the preclinical and clinical studies should be vigorously pursued, simultaneously monitoring immunogenicity, anti-tumour effects and the possibility of auto-immunity - which at this stage does not seem to be a problem.

Abreviations

Cp13-32 peptide, C-PAHGVTSAPDTRPAPGSTAP; CTL, cytotoxic T lymphocytes; DC, dendritic cells; DTH, delayed type hypersensitivity; HMFG, human milk fat globule; PAGAL, phenyl N-acetyl-a-D-galactosamide; MFP, mannan-MUC1 fusion protein; MUC1, Human Mucin 1.

References

1. Barnd DL, Lan MS, Metzgar RS, Finn OJ. Specific major histocompatibility complex - unrestricted recognition of tumour-associated mucins by human cytotoxic T cells. *Proc Natl Acad Sci USA* 1989; 86: 7159-63.
2. Xing PX, Reynolds K, Tjandra JJ, Tang XL, McKenzie IFC. Synthetic peptides reactive with anti-human milk fat globule membrane monoclonal antibodies. *Cancer Res* 1990; 50: 89-96.
3. Jerome KR, Domenech N, Finn OJ. Tumour-specific cytotoxic T lymphocyte clones from patients with breast and pancreatic adenocarcinoma recognise EBV-immortalized B cells transfected with polymorphic epithelial mucin cDNA. *J Immunol* 1993; 151: 1654-62.
4. Apostolopoulos V, Xing PX, McKenzie IFC. Murine immune response to cells transfected with human MUC1: immunisation with cellular and synthetic antigens. *Cancer Res* 1994; 54: 5186-93.
5. Xing PX, Michaels M, Apostolopoulos V, Prenzoska J, Bishop J, McKenzie IFC. Phase I study of synthetic MUC1 peptides in cancer. *Int J Oncol* 1995; 6: 1283-9.
6. Apostolopoulos V, Pietersz GA, McKenzie IFC. Cell-mediated immune responses to MUC1 fusion protein coupled to mannan. *Vaccine* 1995 (In Press).
7. Apostolopoulos V, Pietersz GA, Loveland BE, Sandrin MS, McKenzie IFC. Oxidative/reductive conjugation of mannan to antigen selects for T_1 or T_2 immune responses. *Proc Natl Acad Sci USA* 1995; 92: 10128-32.
8. Apostolopoulos V, Loveland BE, Pietersz GA, McKenzie IFC. CTL in mice immunised with human Mucin 1 are MHC-restricted. *J Immunol* 1995; 155: 5089-94.

Review of the epidemiologic data on hormone replacement therapy in relation to the risk of breast cancer

Lynda F. Voigt, Noel S. Weiss and Janet L. Stanford

Fred Hutchinson Cancer Research Center, 1124 Columbia Street, MP-381, Seattle, WA 98104, USA

Abstract

Over 40 epidemiologic studies of breast cancer in relation to ERT or combined therapy have been conducted, with inconsistent results. Efforts to synthesize the results of these studies are complicated by differences in design and inclusion criteria regarding menopausal status, age, and in situ *breast cancer. Most studies find that the incidence of breast cancer in women who have previously used ERT or combined therapy, or have been treated for only a few years, is not different from that of women who have not used replacement hormones. Study results are discrepant, however, with respect to recency and long-term hormone use.*

It is uncertain whether the modest increase in the risk of breast cancer with hormone use found in some epidemiologic studies reflects a causal association or rather the influence of one or more forms of bias. It has been suggested that increased surveillance of women using hormones may account for the elevated incidence of breast cancer among current hormones users found in some studies [14, 26]. However, mammography rates were only 14% higher in women currently using hormones than in women who had never used hormones in the Nurses' Health Study [8]: a difference of this size cannot account for the 46% increased risk of breast cancer associated with recent hormone use that was found in this study. Also in the Nurses' Health Study, recent long-term hormone use was associated with an increased mortality from breast cancer as well as an increased incidence.

The differences between studies may be a result of uncontrolled confounding or of differences in distribution by variables that modify the effect of hormones on breast cancer risk. For example, if an increased risk of breast cancer in truth is only associated with hormone use in lean women, study populations with predominantly lean women would tend to show more of an increased risk than would others. Misclassification of hormone exposure may also bias study results. Inaccurate recall of hormone use is a concern in studies that classify hormone use by respondent report. However, several studies have found that respondent recall of hormone type and duration corresponds well to medical record data [27, 28] and prescription records [29], and is not differential with respect to disease status [27]. Studies that rely only on prescription data have no information about compliance and may classify women as hormone users who never actually used the drug. However, this bias probably only affects classification of ever and short term use, since it is unlikely that women would continue to refill prescriptions that are not used.

If recent hormone use or long duration of use truly does increase the risk of breast cancer, the increase seems to be modest in relative terms. However, since postmenopausal hormone use is widespread and breast cancer is quite common, even small relative increases in risk have great public health importance. For example, Steinberg et al estimated that a 30% increase in relative risk would result in nearly 5,000 added cases of breast cancer per year in the US alone [6]. In an attempt to determine whether the small relative increases in breast cancer risk that have (sometimes) been observed do or do not reflect a causal relation, randomized trials of ERT and combined therapy are now underway [30]. Nonetheless, additional nonrandomized studies are also needed to identify any factors that may influence the association of hormone use on the risk of breast cancer. Until then, when women weigh the benefits and risks of long-term postmenopausal hormone therapy, they need to continue to consider the possibility that their risk of breast cancer may be unfavorably altered.

The benefits of estrogen replacement therapy (ERT) include relief of menopausal symptoms and protection against osteoporosis and heart disease [1]. Also, there is some evidence that exogenous estrogens may improve cognitive functioning and overall survival in women [1, 2]. Since most benefits of ERT wane soon after the hormone is discontinued, long-term therapy has been advocated [3]. The danger of endometrial cancer in long-term estrogen users has been substantially reduced by the addition of progestogen [1]. However, concern about whether or not exogenous sex hormones increase the risk of breast cancer remains.

Estrogen replacement therapy

Several meta-analyses have been performed to generate a combined risk estimate from epidemiologic studies of the association of ERT and breast cancer [2, 4-6]. None found an increased risk of breast cancer associated with ever use of ERT. Women who used ERT for eight or more years had a 20-30% increase in risk relative to women who had never used hormones in the three meta-analyses that examined duration [1, 4-7], but this was by no means a constant finding across the individual studies. Recency of ERT was only examined in one meta-analysis that was based on three studies. This analysis, which was heavily weighted by the Nurses' Health Study, reported a 40% increased risk of breast cancer associated with ERT use within two years of diagnosis [8]. The conclusions of two meta-analyses that examined estrogen dose are contradictory [4, 5].

Three cohort and three case-control studies published since the most recent meta-analysis also have not obtained consistent findings regarding the relationship of duration or recency of ERT to breast cancer. The Nurses' Health Study, an earlier analysis of which was included in the meta-analysis, examined data from four additional years of follow-up and observed a relative risk of 1.46 (95% Confidence interval (CI) = 1,2-1,7) for current estrogen use of five or more years duration [8]. This study found no increased risk associated with past use of estrogen of any duration or for current use that lasted less than five years. Another cohort study reported a 30% increased risk for current estrogen use (95% CI = 1.1-1.5), but found no association with past use [9]. A Canadian case-control study reported a relative risk of breast cancer of 1.4 (95% CI = 1.0-2.0) associated with current estrogen use and a risk of 1.6 (95% CI = 1.1-2.5) for ten or more years of use [10]. Three additional studies found no association with either recent estrogen use or duration of use ranging from five to twenty years [11, 12, 13]. One of these studies, however, was unable to separate unopposed estrogen use from ERT supplemented by progestogen (combined therapy) and had follow-up data for only three years [11].

Several studies have examined factors that may modify the association of ERT on the incidence of breast cancer. The authors of two meta-analyses concluded that benign breast disease had little effect on the risk of breast cancer associated with ERT [4, 5]. One meta-analysis found no evidence that family history of breast cancer influenced the risk associated with ERT [4]. However, eight of the ten studies that have stratified hormone use by weight or body mass index have found some increase in breast cancer risk associated with hormone use among thinner women, but no increase in the heaviest women [10, 12-18].

Combined therapy (estrogen supplemented with a progestogen)

Tables I and *II* summarize the findings of the studies reported to date in the literature. Two hospital-based case-control studies are not included in this table because <1% of the controls had used combined therapy [15, 25]. These studies have produced inconsistent results with respect to ever, recent and long-term use of combined therapy. A small randomized trial found no cases of breast cancer among women who used combined therapy for ten years whereas four of the 84 (4.8%) who did not use hormones developed breast cancer during the ten year trial [19]. No cases of breast cancer occurred in the women who had been randomized to combined therapy during twelve additional years of follow-up [19]. Two nonrandomized studies also found that women who used combined therapy had a decreased risk of breast cancer relative to women who did not use hormones [16, 20]. However, these results were hampered by small numbers and possibly uncontrolled confounding in one of the studies [20]. Five studies found no association of breast cancer with ever use of combined therapy [10-13, 21, 23], whereas two found an increased risk of 30-40% [22, 24]. Three of the four studies that evaluated recent use of combined therapy found no association with breast cancer [9, 12, 13]; the fourth study found a 40% increase in breast cancer incidence [8]. One study found no association of breast cancer with past use of combined therapy [13] and two found slight elevations in risk of 30-40% [9, 12]. Four studies examined duration of combined therapy. One study found no increased risk associated with combined therapy for eight or more years [13] and another no association after 15 years of combined therapy [12]. On the other hand, Schairer reported a 40% increased breast cancer risk for women who used combined therapy for four or more years [9] and Bergkvist found a four-fold increased risk for women who used combined therapy for 6-9 years relative to short term estrogen users [21].

The only study to examine factors that may modify the relationship of combined therapy with breast cancer found an increased risk associated with ever use of combined therapy in women with a prior bilateral oophorectomy and in lean women [13]. The numbers of exposed women in each of these groups, however, were small.

Table I. Cohort studies of breast cancer and estrogen replacement therapy supplemented by progestogen (combined therapy).

Reference	Dates of Cohort Inception	Duration of Follow-Up	Source of Cohort	Inclusion Criteria	Comparison Group	Measure of combined therapy	N of Cases Exposed	RR 95% CI
Nachtigall New York, US [19]	1965-1966	22 years	Chronic care facility	Post-menopausal Intact uterus and ovaries Invasive and *in situ*	Randomized trial	Evers	0	4.8 expected
Gambrell Texas, US [20]	1975-1979	9 years	Military hospital	Post-menopausal Most with intact uterus Invasive and *in situ*	Internal	Ever	11	0.2 (0.1-0.4)
Schairer (BCDP Study, US) [9]	1973-1980	16 years	Volunteers for breast cancer detection study	No menses for 3 months before interview Invasive and *in situ*	Internal	Ever Within 1 year of DX Past use 4+ years of use	72 49 37 20	1.2 (1.0-1.6) 1.2 (0.9-1.6) 1.4 (1.0-2.0) 1.4 (0.9-2.2)
Colditz (Nurses Health Study, US) [8]	1976	16 years	Female registered nurses who returned mailed questionnaire	Post-menopausal Invasive only 30-55 years of age in 1976	Internal	Within 2 years of DX	111	1.4 (1.2-1.7)
Bergkvist Sweden [21, 22]	1977-1980	6 years	Estrogen prescription records	All with estrogen prescriptions Invasive and *in situ*	Population	Ever Used Used combined only for 73-108 months	? 10	1.3 (1.1-1.6) 4.4 (0.9-22.4)
Risch, 1994 Saskatchewan, Canada [23]	1976-1987	14 years	Health registration files	43-49 years of age in 1976 Invasive and *in situ*	Internal	1 year or more of use and at least 3.5 years prior to DX		1.2 (0.8-1.3)

Table II. Population-based case-control studies of breast cancer and estrogen replacement therapy supplemented by progestogen.

Reference	Date of Study	Type of Study	Type of Interview	Source of Controls	Inclusion Criteria	Measure of Progestogen Use	N of Cases Exposed	RR 95% CI
Newcomb, 4 United-States [12]	1989-1991	Population-Based	Telephone	Drivers license and HICFA lists	Post-menopausal listed phone current drivers license (if <65 years of age) <75 years of age Invasive only	Ever Within 2 years of DX Past use 15+ years of use	138 90 48 15	1.0 (0.8-1.3) 0.9 (0.7-1.2) 1.3 (0.8-1.9) 1.1 (0.5-2.3)
Yang British Columbia, Canada [10]	1988-1989	Population-Based	Mailed questionnaire	Voters list	Post-menopausal <70 years of age Invasive and in situ	Any use 12 or more months prior to DX	22	1.2 (0.6-2.2)
Stanford Western Washington State, US [13]	1988-1990	Population-Based	In person	Random digit dialing	50-64 years of age Invasive and in situ	Any use 3 or more months prior to DX Within 3-12 months of DX Past use 8+ years of use	113 83 30 8	0.9 (0.7-1.3) 0.9 (0.6-1.2) 1.1 (0.6-2.0) 0.4 (0.2-1.0)
Palmer Toronto, Canada [16]	1982-1986	Cases from cancer treatment hospital	In person	Matched by neighborhood and age to cases	<70 years of age Invasive and in situ	Any use	4	0.6 (0.2-2.0)
Ewertz Denmark [24]	1983-1984	Population-Based	Mailed questionnaire	Population registry	<70 years of age	Sequential, ever	111	1.4 (1.9-1.9)

References

1. Grady D, Rubin SM, Petitti DB, Fox CS, Black D, Ettinger B, Ernster VL, Cummings SR. Hormone therapy to prevent disease and prolong life in postmenopausal women. *Ann Intern Med* 1992; 117: 1016-37.
2. Sherwin BB. Hormones, mood and cognitive functioning in postmenopausal women. *Obstet Gynecol* 1996; 87: 20S-26S.
3. Lobo RA. Benefits and risk of estrogen replacement therapy. *Am J Obstet Gynecol* 1995; 173: 982-90.
4. Colditz GA, Egan KM, Stampfer MJ. Hormone replacement therapy and risk of breast cancer: results from epidemiologic studies. *Obstet Gynecol* 1993; 168: 1473-80.
5. Dupont WD, Page DL. Menopausal estrogen replacement therapy and breast cancer. *Arch Intern Med* 1991; 151: 67-72.
6. Steinberg KK, Thacker SB, Smith SJ, Stroup DF, Zack MM, Flanders WD, Berkelman RL. A meta-analysis of the effect of estrogen replacement therapy on the risk of breast cancer. *JAMA* 1991; 265: 1985-90.
7. Steinberg KK, Smith SJ, Thacker SB, Stroup DF. Breast cancer risk and duration of estrogen use: the role of study design in meta-analysis. *Epidemiology* 1994; 5: 415-21.
8. Colditz GA, Hankinson SE, Hunter DJ, Willett WC, Manson JE, Stampfer MJ, Hennekens C, Rosner B, Speizer FE. The use of estrogens and progestins and the risk of breast cancer in postmenopausal women. *N Engl J Med* 1995; 332: 1589-93.
9. Schairer C, Byrne C, Keyl PM, Brinton LA, Sturgeon SR, Hoover RN. Menopausal estrogen and estrogen-progestin replacement therapy and risk of breast cancer (United States). *Cancer Causes Control* 1994; 5: 491-500.
10. Yang CP, Daling JR, Band PR, Gallagher RP, White E, Weiss NS. Noncontraceptive hormone use and risk of breast cancer. *Cancer Causes Control* 1992; 3: 475-9.
11. Schuurman AG, van den Brandt PA, Goldbohm RA. Exogenous hormone use and the risk of postmenopausal breast cancer: results from the Netherlands Cohort Study. *Cancer Causes Control* 1995; 6: 416-24.
12. Newcomb PA, Longnecker MP, Storer BE, Mittendorf R, Baron J, Clapp RW, Bogdan G, Willett WC. Long-term hormone replacement therapy and risk of breast cancer in postmenopausal women. *Am J Epidemiol* 1995; 142: 788-95.
13. Stanford JL, Weiss NS, Voigt LF, Daling JR, Habel LA, Rossing MA. Combined estrogen and progestin hormone replacement therapy in relation to risk of breast cancer in middle-aged women. *JAMA* 1995; 274: 137-42.
14. Colditz GA, Stampfer MJ, Willett WC, Hunter DJ, Manson JE, Hennekens CH, Rosner BA, Speizer FE. Type of postmenopausal hormone use and risk of breast cancer: 12-year follow-up from the Nurses' Health Study. *Cancer Causes Control* 1992; 3: 433-9.
15. Kaufman DW, Palmer JR, de Mouzon J, Rosenberg L, Stolley PD, Warshauer ME, Zauber AG, Shapiro S. Estrogen replacement therapy and the risk of breast cancer: results from the Case-control Surveillance Study. *Am J Epidemiol* 1991; 134: 1375-85.
16. Palmer JR, Rosenberg L, Clarke EA, Miller DR, Shapiro S. Breast cancer risk after estrogen replacement therapy: results from the Toronto Breast Cancer Study. *Am J Epidemiol* 1991; 134: 1386-95.
17. Weinstein AL, Mahoney MC, Nasca PC, Hanson RL, Leske MC, Varma AO. Oestrogen replacement therapy and breast cancer risk: a case-control study. *Int J Epidemiol* 1993; 5: 781-9.
18. Harris RE, Namboodiri KK, Wynder EL. Breast cancer risk: effects of estrogen replacement therapy and body mass. *JNCI* 1992; 84: 1575-82.
19. Nachtigall MJ, Smilen SW, Natchtigall RD, Nachtigall RH, Nachtigall LE. Incidence of breast cancer in a 22-year study of women receiving estrogen-progestin replacement therapy. *Obstet Gynecol* 1992; 80: 827-30.
20. Gambrell RD. Use of progestogen therapy. *Am J Obstet Gynecol* 1987; 156: 1304-13.
21. Bergkvist L, Adami HO, Persson I, Hoover R, Schairer C. The risk of breast cancer after estrogen and estrogen-progestin replacement. *N Engl J Med* 1989; 321: 293-7.
22. Persson I, Yuen J, Bergkvist L, Adami HO, Hoover R, Schairer C. Combined oestrogen-progestogen replacement and breast cancer risk (letter). *Lancet* 1992; 340: 1044.

23. Risch HA, Howe GR. Menopausal hormone usage and breast cancer in Saskatchewan: a record-linkage cohort study. *Am J Epidemiol* 1994; 139: 670-83.
24. Ewertz M. Influence of non-contraceptive exogenous and endogenous sex hormones on breast cancer risk in Denmark. *Int J Cancer* 1988; 42: 832-8.
25. LaVecchia C, Negri E, Franceschi S, Favero A, Nanni O, Filiberti R, Conti E, Montella M, Veronesi A, Ferraroni M, Decarli A. Hormone replacement treatment and breast cancer risk: a cooperative Italian study. *Br J Cancer* 1995; 72: 244-8.
26. Speroff L. Postmenopausal hormone therapy and breast cancer. *Obstet Gynecol* 1996; 87: 44S-54S.
27. Paganini-Hill A, Ross RK. Reliability of recall of drug usage and other health-related information. *Am J Epidemiol* 1982; 116: 114-22.
28. Stadel BV, Weiss N. Characteristics of menopausal women: a survey of King and Pierce Counties in Washington, 1973-1974. *Am J Epidemiol* 1975; 102: 209-16.
29. Persson I, Bergkvist L, Adami HO. Reliability of women's histories of climacteric oestrogen treatment assessed by prescription forms. *Int J Epidemiol* 1987; 16: 222-8.
30. Kirschstein R. Largest US clinical trial ever gets underway. *JAMA* 1993; 270: 1521.

Influence of percutaneous administration of estradiol and progesterone on the proliferation of human breast epithelial cells

J.M. Foidart[1], C. Colin[1], X. Denoo[1], J. Desreux[1], S. Fournier[2] and B. de Lignières[3]

[1] Department of General and Cell Biology, University of Liège, Pathology Tower, Sart Tilman, B-4000 Liège, Belgium,
[2] Laboratoires Besins-Iscovesco, 5, rue du Bourg-l'Abbé, 75003 Paris, France,
[3] Department of Endocrinology and Reproductive Medicine, Necker Hospital, 149, rue de Sèvres, 75743 Paris, France

The endocrine regulation of normal breast cells proliferation remains controversial. 17β-estradiol (E_2), in physiological concentrations, stimulates the proliferation of normal breast epithelial cells while the influence of progesterone (P) has been debated for two decades.

Depending upon the models used (animal or human, *in vitro* or *in vivo* studies), the timing of P administration, and the method of evaluation (mitotic index, PCNA, K_{i67} or ^{3}H-thymidine labeling), P is reported to stimulate, reduce or be neutral on mitotic activity and proliferation of breast epithelial cells [1-3].

Some studies suggest that progesterone and/or synthetic progestins stimulate, reduce, or have no effect on hyperplastic lesions [1-3]. Colditz *et al.* showed that the addition of progestins to estrogen therapy does not reduce the risk of breast cancer among postmenopausal women [4]. Gambrell, on the contrary, demonstrated that the incidence of breast cancer was significantly lower in estrogen-progestin users than in untreated or estrogen treated postmenopausal women [5]. Similarly, Risch and Howe [6] and Stanford et al [7], in a large cohort studies also suggested recently that progestins reduced the estrogen associated risk of breast cancer. Therefore, the therapeutical suggestions of P treatment or avoidance are based on insufficient and controversial epidemiological evidences and on a lack of adequately controlled data on the influence of P on normal breast epithelium.

A recent *in vivo*, double blind randomized trial demonstrated that percutaneous administration of estradiol and progesterone for 10-13 days prior to surgery for removal of a lump in premenopausal women had opposite effects. Increased tissue E_2 concentrations stimulated the number of cycling epithelial cells while P administration decreased the number of proliferative epithelial cells [8].

Premenopausal women with spontaneous endocrine ovarian activity, when submitted to general anesthesia and hospitalization for breast surgery, are more likely to experience stress-induced disturbances in their endogenous P and E_2 ovarian secretion that might interfere with the exogenously applied steroids.

We therefore conducted a double blind randomized clinical trial in 40 postmenopausal women who had not received any hormone replacement therapy (HRT) in order to precisely delineate the effects of P, E_2, or both, on breast epithelial cells proliferation.

Patients

Forty postmenopausal women with documented untreated menopause (FSH > 30 mU/ml; E_2 < 20 pg/ml) were enrolled in this study. Previous HRT had to be withdrawn for at least 12 weeks. They were randomly allocated to 4 treatment groups who received a hydro-alcoholic gel (2.5 g/day): (1) E_2 (1.5 mg/day); (2) P 25 mg/day; (3) P + E_2 (25 mg + 1.5 mg/day) or a (4) Placebo. Each gel formulation was daily applied on both breasts for 14 days prior to surgery for plastic surgery or removal of presumably benign lesion. The study design was approved by the University Ethics Committee and informed consent was obtained from each woman.

Study design

Surgery was performed on the 15th day. At surgery, a blood sample was taken for E_2 and P plasma level measurement by specific RIAs described previously [8].

Two samples of normal breast tissue (approximately 500 mg each) were taken in a normal area of the breast at least 5 cm away from any lesion. The first sample was stored at -20° C and processed for measurement of E_2 and P tissue concentrations. The second sample was fixed in formalin and used for measurements of the cell cycle marker (PCNA) according to a previously described protocol [8].

Automated quantitative immunostaining analysis was performed on a computer assisted image processor (SAMBA, Alcatel, Grenoble, France), as previously reported. At least 2.000 nuclei were evaluated from each tissue sample in 20 fields from each of 6 non consecutive sections from each normal specimen. Appropriate positive and negative controls were included. All analyses were performed blindly before opening the code of the trial.

Statistical analysis

Statistical analysis was performed using the Krusdal Wallis non parametric test of variance among the four treatment groups. When the null hypothesis (the four groups are identical) was rejected at the level 0.05, a multiple comparison procedure was used to determine which pairs of groups differed significantly ($p < 0.05$) («t» Student Test).

Results

Patients and treatment

Fourty four women initially enrolled effectively completed the study. Four patients were excluded because the baseline E_2 and FSH levels demonstrated persisting ovarian activity. Among the 40 remaining volunteers, 10 received a placebo, 13 received the P gel, 10 the E_2 gel and 7 the E_2 + P gel *(Table I)*.

Table I. Study population.

Groups		Placebo	P	E_2	$E_2 + P$
Age (years)	n	10	13	10	7
	m	62.7	63.3	59.3	58.1
	sd	9.9	8.9	5.3	6.7
	median	66	64	59.5	59
	min-max	47-77	51-80	50-67	50-69
Weight (kg)	m	66.4	62.2	66.2	71.6
	sd	4.9	9.2	6.5	13.4
	median	67.5	60	65	67
	min-max	55-73	48-80	57-79	57-92
Length (cm)	m	163.8	162.2	163.4	164.5
	sd	3.5	2.8	3.5	5.0
	median	164.5	162	164.5	164
	min-max	156-168	159-168	158-169	159-172

m = mean; sd = standard deviation; n = number of patients

Plasma levels

Table II shows the P and E_2 plasma levels at the time of surgery in the 40 women. A statistically significant ($p < 0.001$) difference in plasma P concentrations is observed (after logarithmic conversion) between the treatment groups. The P concentration was significantly higher in the group treated with the P gel or with the $E_2 + P$ gel than in the E_2 gel or placebo treated groups ($p < 0.001$) *(Table III)*. The group receiving E_2 (E_2 gel or $E_2 + P$ gel) also showed significantly evelated E_2 plasma levels in comparison with the P gel or placebo treated groups.

Tissue concentrations

The mean E_2 tissue concentrations were significantly higher in groups E_2 gel and $E_2 + P$ gel, than in the placebo or P gel group ($p < 0.01$). Due to large interindividual variations, P tissue concentrations did not vary significantly among the several groups ($p = 0.056$) *(Tables II and III)*.

Proliferation marker

The PCNA labeling index was 0.1% in the placebo group, significantly higher (11.5% ± 2.3) in the E_2 group. The P group showed also low levels (1.5% ± 0.6) of proliferation which were significantly higher than the placebo group. Finally, PCNA labeling index was reduced significantly in the $E_2 + P$ group (1.3% ± 1.1) in comparison with the E_2 group to reach levels identical to that of the P group *(Tables IV and V)*.

Table II. Hormone plasma and tissue levels.

Groups		Placebo	P	E_2	$E_2 + P$	Prob.	Concl.
Plasma progesterone (pg/ml)	n	8	13	10	7	< 0.001	S
	m	281.4	1265.6	300.2	952.1		
	sd	221.2	281.3	108.1	302.3		
	median	194.5	1432	287.5	830		
	min-max	126-863	830-1667	180-454	620-1400		
Plasma estradiol (pg/ml)	m	31.6	30.8	73.7	75.4	< 0.001	S
	sd	11	8.6	20.6	66.8		
	median	32.5	31	71.5	59		
	min-max	14-45	19-46	47-120	32-224		
Tissue progesterone (ng/g)	n	10	13	10	7	0.056	NS
	m	3.7	17.8	4.5	11.2		
	sd	2.4	20	1.8	8.2		
	median	3	12.2	4.2	9.1		
	min-max	1.6-9.8	5.4-82	2.4-7.3	4-29.1		
Tissue estradiol (pg/g)	n	10	10	9	7	0.010	S
	m	278.9	199.1	659	565.7		
	sd	104	67.8	462.67	355.4		
	median	283	207.5	470	588		
	min-max	76-435	100-320	208-1557	112-1096		

S: significant differences between the means among the 4 groups.
NS: non significant differences between the means.

Table III. Statistical comparison (« t » test).

Groups		Placebo	P	$E_2 + P$
Plasma progesterone (pg/ml)	E_2	NS (0.488)	< 0.001	< 0.001
	P	< 0.001		
	$E_2 + P$	< 0.001	NS (0.119)	
Plasma estradiol (pg/ml)	E_2	< 0.001	< 0.001	NS (0.745)
	P	NS (0.859)		
	$E_2 + P$	< 0.001	< 0.001	
Tissue estradiol (pg/ml)	E_2	0.019	0.002	NS (0.396)
	P	NS (0.335)		
	$E_2 + P$	NS (0.171)	S (0.031)	

Table IV. Proliferation marker.

Groups		Placebo	P	E_2	$E_2 + P$	Prob.	Concl.
	n	10	13	10	7		
PCNA	m	0.1	1.5	11.5	1.3	< 0.001	S
index	sd	0.1	0.6	2.3	1.1		
(%)	median	0.1	1.3	10.6	1		
	min-max	0-0.3	0.9-3	8.6-15.4	0-3.2		

S: significant differences between the means among the 4 groups.
NS: non significant differences between the means.

Table V. Statistical comparison (« t » test).

Groups		Placebo	P	$E_2 + P$
PCNA	E_2	< 0.001	< 0.001	< 0.001
index	P	< 0.001		
(%)	$E_2 + P$	0.003	NS (0.112)	

Discussion

This study was designed as a double blind randomized trial on 40 postmenopausal women undergoing breast surgery for plastic reasons or for benign breast mammary lesions. The daily percutaneous administration of P, E_2, P + E_2 or placebo for 14 days resulted in the expected changes in plasma and tissue concentrations of steroids.

E_2 considerably stimulated the proliferation of normal human breast epithelial cells in comparison with the placebo group (11.5% ± 2.3 *versus* 0.1% ± 0.1). This proliferation index was also considerably higher in comparison with the P group (1.5% ± 0.6) or P + E_2 group (1.3% ± 1.1). P administration thus dramatically reduced the E_2 induced proliferation of normal human breast epithelial cells.

The P group and P + E_2 group showed indeed low and identical levels of proliferation of galactophoric cells. This proliferation rate was significantly higher than in the placebo group (0.1% ± 0.1). This low level of PCNA positive cells could in fact reflect the capacity of P to engage breast epithelial cells in the G_1 phase of the cell cycle. Proliferating cell nuclear antigen immunostaining identifies all cycling cells from the G_1 to G_2 M phases. The interpretation of PCNA immunoreactivity is well documented [9, 10]. In contrast with the autoradiographic radiolabeling technique with ^{3}H-thymidine, it does not only measure those cells in the S phase but also detects cells in the G_1, G_2 and M phases.

The computerized detection of PCNA-labeled cells reduces subjectively, improves reproductibility and eases the workload. In addition, it allows the determination of objective tresholds of sensitivity. The intensity of PCNA labeling was significantly lower in the P or P + E_2 group than in the E_2 group. The PCNA positive cells in these two groups could therefore represent those cells in the G_1 phase of the cell cycle. Such cells are not necessarily committed to become mitotic and proliferative since cells in the G_1 phase may also undergo apoptosis.

Altogether, this study indicates that adding P to E_2 significantly reduces the proliferative effect of E_2 alone. Our data strongly support the previous observations by Barrat et al. [11] and Chang et al. [8] that P influences the control of the human breast epithelial cell cycle. It also suggests that P may have a therapeutic value to prevent breast epithelial hyperplasia when used for 14 days per month at substitutive doses.

References

1. Key DL, Pike M. The role of estrogens and progestogens in the epidemiology and prevention of breast cancer. *Eur J Cancer Clin Oncol* 1988; 24: 29-43.
2. Going J, Anderson T, Battersby S. Proliferative and secretory activity in human breast during natural and artificial menstrual cycle. *Am J Pathol* 1988; 130: 193-204.
3. Vorherr H. Fibrocystic breast disease: pathophysiology, pathomorphology, clinical picture, and management. *Am J Obstet Gynecol* 1986; 154: 161-79.
4. Colditz GA, Hankinson SE, Hunter DJ, Willett WC, Manson JE, Stampfer MJ, Hennekens Ch, Rosner B, Speizer FE. The use of estrogens and progestins and the risk of breast cancer in postmenopausal women. *N Engl J Med* 1995; 332: 1589-93.
5. Gambrell RD Jr. Use of progestogen therapy. *Am J Obstet Gynecol* 1987; 156: 1304-13.
6. Risch HA, Howe GR. Menopausal Hormone Usager and Breast Cancer. In: Saskatchewan: A record-Linkage-Cohort-Study.
7. Stanford J, Weiss WS, Voigt LF, Daling JR, Habel LA, Rossing MA. Combined estrogen and progestin hormone replacement therapy in relation to risk of breast cancer in middle-aged women. *JAMA*, 1995; 274: 137-42.
8. Chang KJ, Lee TTY, Linares-Cruz G, Fournier S, de Lignières B. Influences of percutaneous administration of estradiol and progesterone on human breast epithelial cell cycle in vivo. *Fertil Steril*, 1995; 663: 785-91.
9. Dietrich DR. Toxicological and pathological applications of proliferating cell nuclear antigen (PCNA), a novel endogenous marker for cell proliferation. *Crit Rev Toxicol* 1993; 23: 77-109.
10. Bravo R, Frank R, Bundell PA, MacDonald-Bravo H. Cyclin/PCNA is the auxillary protein of DNA polymerase-d. *Nature*, 1987; 326: 515-17.
11. Barrat J, de Lignières B, Marpeau L, Larue L, Fournier S, Nahoul K, Linares G, Giorgi H, Contesso G. Effet in vivo de l'administration locale de progestérone sur l'activité mitotique des galactophores humains. *J Gynecol Obstet Biol Reprod* 1990; 19: 269-74.

Clinical and biological prognostic factors in breast cancer diagnosed during postmenopausal hormone replacement therapy

P. Bonnier*, S.Romain**, P.L.Giacalone***, F.Laffargue***, P.M.Martin** and L.Piana*

* Service de Gynécologie et Obstétrique A, Hôpital de la Conception, Marseille, France;
** Laboratoire d'Oncologie et Biopathologie Tissulaire, Assistance publique à Marseille, France;
*** Service de Gynécologie et Obstétrique, Hôpital A. de Villeneuve, Montpellier, France

Abstract

Hormone replacement therapy is now widely used in postmenopausal women. Although this treatment does not increase the incidence of breast cancer, more and more cases are diagnosed concurrently. The purpose of this study was to ascertain the influence of hormone replacement therapy on clinical and biological prognostic factors in breast cancer.
Between 1976 and 1992 we treated 1,081 postmenopausal women for breast cancer at our institution. Of these 68 were undergoing postmenopausal hormone replacement therapy at the time of diagnosis. These patients were compared with a matched control group of 272 breast cancer patients who had not undergone prior hormone replacement therapy.
Patients who developed breast cancer during hormone replacement therapy had fewer locally advanced cancers (large tumors and extensive lymph node involvement) and more well-differentiated cancers (infiltrating lobular cancers and gradeI cancer). The number of patients with estradiol or progesterone receptors was lower in hormone-treated group. Metastasis-free survival curves showed a tendency ($p = 0.05$) for better prognosis in hormone-treated patients both overall and in stage T2.
We concluded that hormone replacement therapy per se does not affect the prognosis of breast cancer. Regular surveillance during hormone replacement therapy reduces the number of locally advanced cancers and thus improves survival. The higher number of well differentiated cancers and the distribution of hormone receptivity may reflect interaction between neoplastic tissue and exogenous hormones.

Hormone replacement therapy is now widely used in postmenopausal women. Numerous epidemiological surveys have studied the risk of breast cancer associated with use of estrogen replacement therapy [1-7]. Although this treatment has little or no effect on the incidence of breast cancer, more and more cases are diagnosed concurrently. Few data are available concerning the characteristics and outcome in this subgroup of hormone-treated breast cancer patients. Some evidence suggests that the characteristics of endometrial cancer in patients after hormone replacement therapy are different [6-8].

The purpose of this study was to determine if previous postmenopausal hormone replacement therapy changes prognosis and survival of patients. To answer this question we compared the clinical features, biological factors and survival rates of 68 patients that developed breast cancer during hormone replacement therapy with 272 matched breast cancer patients that did not undergo hormone replacement therapy. Mean follow-up was 49.5 months.

Materials and methods

During the period from 1976 to 1992, 1,081 postmenopausal women were treated for breast cancer at our institution by the same team using similar strategies. Patients presenting metastasis at the time of diagnosis, in situ lobular cancer, or inflammatory cancers, patients for whom the conditions of hormone therapy were not known and/or patients in whom hormone therapy had been discontinued in the months before diagnosis were not included. Based on these criteria, we obtained a cohort of 794 patients with a median age of 62.1 years (range: 34.7 to 90.2).

Hormone replacement therapy is usually initiated after only a few months of amenorrhea especially in patients complaining of « hot flashes ». For this reason we considered patients as menopausal after a 6-month period of amenorrhea. This contrasts with the classic definition of menopause which requires a 1- to 2-year period of amenorrhea unless ovaries had been surgically removed.

The cohort of 794 patients was divided into three groups of patients as follows:

Group 1: 68 patients who developed breast cancer during postmenopausal hormone replacement therapy. Mean age in this group was 55.6 years and median age was 55.3 years (range: 39.6-71.6 years). The mean duration of hormone replacement therapy was 61.3 months (6-153 months). An estrogen-progestogen combination was used in 84% of cases and estrogen alone in 12%. The estrogens used were 17β estradiol (66%), estradiol valerate (12%), synthetic estrogens (10%), and conjugated estrogen and natural estrogen (2%). Progesterone and derivatives of 17hydroxyprogesterone were used in 36% of patients, derivatives of 19nortestosterone in 36% and derivatives of 19 norprogesterone in 28%.

Group 2: 272 patients who developed cancer with no previous hormone replacement therapy and in whom age and date of onset of cancer treatment was comparable to that observed in Group1. Matching based on age and on date of onset of cancer treatment takes into account both age related variations in prognostic factors and the recent use of routine mammography screening as well as progress in adjuvant therapy. Thus the age distribution and date of onset of cancer treatment in Group2 was the same as in Group 1. Mean age in this group was 56 years and median age was 55.5 years (range: 39.4-72.2 years).

Group 3: 726 who developed cancer with no previous hormone replacement therapy. Mean age in this group was 63.6 years and median age was 62.9 years (range: 39.4 to 90.2 years). Group 2 was drawn from this group.

Treatment methods evolved over the years but the basic principles were similar in all groups. Conservative surgery was performed in most cases (73.2%). Radical modified mastectomy was used for large tumors and in cases in which the margins were pathologic. Lymph node dissection was performed in 91.5%. The breast or chest wall was irradiated in 91.7% (mean dose: 49.7 grays). A boost on the tumor bed in 47.7% of patients (mean dose: 10.6 grays). Internal mammary lymph nodes were irradiated in patients with tumors involving the central and internal quadrants. The supraclavicular and internal mammary lymph nodes were irradiated in patients with axillary lymph node involvement (mean dose: 45 grays). Adjuvant therapy was administered when any of the following poor prognostic factors were present: large tumor, lymph node involvement, histoprognostic grade III, or negative steroid receptor. Chemotherapy was used in patients with negative hormone receptors or involvement of more than 4 lymph nodes. The most common protocols were a combination of either cyclophosphamide, methotrexate, and 5-FU or of adriblastine, cyclophosphamide and 5-FU. Chemotherapy was performed in 19.7% of patients. Hormone therapy with tamoxifen was administered for 1 to 5 years to patients with positive hormone receptors. Hormone therapy was used in 23.9% of patients. There was no difference between the groups 1 and 2 with regard to adjuvant treatment.

The mean duration of surveillance in the 3 groups was 45.1, 47.8, and 50.8 months respectively and median follow-up was 32.3, 34.3 and 41.2 months respectively. In most patients surveillance consisted in clinical examination 3 times a year and annual mammography, liver ultrasonography, and bone scintiscan. Tumor marker assays, CT-scan, and MRI were performed only in symptomatic patients.

One or more metastases were observed in 127 patients, local recurrences in 51 and contralateral cancer in 22. Of the 90 deaths that occurred, the cause was breast cancer in 74 cases, concomitant cancer in 4, therapeutic complications in 1 and other causes in 11.

The following clinical data were noted: diagnostic modality (clinical examination or X-ray), delay between the first sign and histological confirmation of cancer, clinical tumor size, disease stage, and surgical methods. The histological data were anatomical size, histological type, degree of infiltration, histoprognostic grade (Scarff, Bloom and Richardson) and lymph node involvement.

Estradiol receptor and progesterone receptor levels were determined either by radioligand binding assay or by enzyme immunoassay. All assays were carried out in the same laboratory [9]. Both techniques measure bound and unbound receptors; in case of radioligand binding assay this was achieved by an exchange technique. The cut-off point was 10 fmol/mg protein for radioligand binding assay and 15 fmol/mg protein for enzyme immunoassay. Radioligand binding assay was performed using the dextran-coated charcoal procedure with a single saturating dose assay. Enzyme immunoassay was performed using Abbott kits (Abbott Laboratories, Chicago, IL, USA). Quality control was ensured by frequent testing within the framework of the European Organization for Research and Treatment of Cancer (EORTC) and by internal laboratory standards according to the recommendations of the Receptors and Biomarkers EORTC Group [10-16].

Only data from groups 1 and 2 were compared. Findings from group 3 are given for reference. Group 2 was extracted from group 3 (patients without prior hormone replacement therapy) using a hazard table to identify patients whose age distribution and date of onset of cancer treatment matched those in group 1. The highest usable matching factor was 4. Variable frequency was compared using the Chi-square test and medians using the Wilcoxon test. Survival curves were calculated according to the Kaplan and Meyer method [17] and compared using the Log-Rank test [18]. As recommended by Arriagada et al. [19] survival curves were calculated excluding patients who presented a contralateral breast tumor or another primary malignancy. This was done in order to avoid overestimating the rate of local recurrence, metastasis and death attribuable to the primary breast cancer. The duration of recurrence-free survival, metastasis-free survival and overall survival were calculated from the date of onset of cancer treatment. Recurrence was defined as local recurrence in the homolateral breast or chest wall. Only deaths related to breast cancer were taken into account in the calculation of overall survival.

Results

There was no significant difference between groups 1 and 2 with regard to the diagnostic modality but it should be noted that X-ray detection was more common in group 2 *(Table I)*. Hormone replacement therapy did not change the radiologic features of cancer. Glandular opacities were observed in 66.6% of patients in group 1 and 58.7% in group 2 and microcalcifications in 20.4% and 21.6% respectively. Opacity associated with microcalcifications were observed in 13% and 19.7% respectively.

The delay between the first symptom and histological confirmation of cancer was not significantly different in groups 1 and 2 *(Table I)*. Similarly overall distribution of clinical stage (TNM classification) and clinical tumor size were not statistically different but it should be noted that the number of stage T3 and T4 as well as tumors larger than 40 mm was lower in group 1 ($p = 0.01$) *(Table II)*. Conservative surgery was more common in group 1 ($p = 0.03$) *(Table III)*.

There was no significant difference between groups 1 and 2 as to the macroscopic tumor size or the proportion of infiltrating and in situ cancer *(Table IV)*. Similarly no significant difference was found as to histological type or histoprognostic grade although it should be noted that group 1 contained a higher proportion of infiltrating lobular cancer (21.5% *versus* 16.2%) and grade 1 cancer (30.9% *versus* 19.4%). There was no significant difference between groups 1 and 2 with regard to lymph node involvement. The number of patients with no lymph node involvement was the same in both groups but the number of cases with extensive involvement (4 or more nodes) was lower in group 1 (9.1% *versus* 18.0%) *(Table IV)*.

Assessment of hormone receptivity revealed a positive and negative population. There was no significant difference in receptor status regardless of whether estradiol receptor and progesterone receptor were studied separately or together. However the number of negative patients was higher in group 1 *(Table V)*.

There was no significant difference in the distribution of ER and PR levels. However it should be noted that ER levels were higher in group 2 (median levels: 89.5 versus 31.5). Median PR values were 20 fmol/mg in group 1 and 26 fmol/mg in group 2 *(Table VI)*.

Metastasis-free survival curves showed that prognosis tended to be better ($p = 0.05$) in hormone-treated patients both overall and in stage T2 *(Figures 1 and 2)*. There was no significant difference between groups 1 and 2 with regard to the probability of recurrence-free survival and overall survival. This lack of significance could be due to the small number of patients. Three-year local recurrence free survival was 0.95 in groups 1 and 2. Three-year metastasis-free survival was 0.93 in group 1 and 0.86 in group 2. Three-year overall survival was 0.98 in group 1 and 0.93 in group 2.

Discussion

Hormone replacement therapy is now widely used in postmenopausal women. Although this treatment does not increase the incidence of breast cancer, more and more cases are diagnosed concurrently. Some evidence suggests that hormone therapy may modify features and outcome

Table I. Method of detection of cancer and delay between the first sign and histological confirmation.

	Group 1 (n = 68 cases)	Group 2 (n = 272 cases)	p value	Group 3 (n = 726 cases)
Method of detection				
clinical	74.6%	67.4%	NS	76.0%
x-ray	25.4%	32.6%		24.0%
Delay for diagnosis (months)				
median	1.6	2.2	NS	2.2
mean	5.7	7.8		7.2

Group 1: breast cancer detected in patients undergoing hormone replacement therapy for menopause.
Group 2: breast cancers detected in patients with no previous hormone replacement therapy and matched to group 1.
Group 3: breast cancers detected in patients with no previous hormone replacement therapy.
NS: not significant.

Table II. Clinical stage (TNM), tumor size distribution, and mean clinical tumor size.

	Group 1 (n = 68 cases)	Group 2 (n = 272 cases)	p value	Group 3 (n = 726 cases)
Stage				
T0	17.9%	21.7%		16.6%
T1	20.9%	21.7%		18.7%
T2	52.2%	40.8%	N.S.	49.1%
T3	6.0%	8.6%		8.0%
T4	3.0%	7.1%		7.6%
Clinical size distribution				
<10	16.4%	25.3%		19.9%
10-19	16.4%	17.7%		15.1%
20-39	55.7%	37.1%	NS	43.5%
40-59	4.9%	11.8%		13.6%
>60	6.6%	8.1%		7.9%
There new significantly more tumors greater than 40 mm in group 2 (p = 0.01).				
Mean tumor size (mm)	24.2	23.9	NS	26.5

NS: not significant.

Table III. Surgical methods.

Treatment	Group 1 (n = 68 cases)	Group 2 (n = 272 cases)	p value	Group 3 (n = 726 cases)
Lumpectomy	83.8%	70.6%	p = 0.03	65.6%
Mastectomy	16.2%	29.4%		34.6%

Table IV. Histological type, degree of infiltration, histoprognostic grade (Scarff-Bloom and Richardson) and lymph node involvement.

	Group 1 (n = 68 cases)	Group 2 (n = 272 cases)	p value	Group 3 (n = 726 cases)
Mean histological size (mm)	20.8	21.2	NS	21.6
Degree of infiltration				
Infiltrating	93.8%	90.6%	NS	90.4%
In situ and microinfiltrating	6.2%	9.4%		9.6%
Histological type				
Ductal	73.8%	79.3%	NS	77.8%
Lobular	21.5%	16.2%		17.6%
Other	4.7%	4.5%		4.6%
Histoprognostic grade				
I	30.9%	19.4%	NS	20.9%
II	43.6%	50.7%		51.0%
III	25.5%	29.9%		28.1%
Number of involved lymph nodes*				
0	60.6%	59.6%	NS	56.9%
1-3	27.3%	22.4%		23.6%
4-7	4.5%	7.8%		7.7%
> 7	4.6%	10.2%		11.8%

NS: not significant.
* the mean number of lymph nodes studied per patient was 15.1.

Table V. Estradiol receptor (ER) and progesterone receptor (PR) levels.

	Group 1 (n = 68 cases)	Group 2 (n = 272 cases)	p value	Group 3 (n = 726 cases)
ER-	33.3%	21.9%	NS	22.3%
ER+	66.7%	78.1%		77.7%
PR-	42.9%	40.4%	NS	37.8%
PR+	57.1%	59.6%		62.2%
ER-,PR-	28.6%	20.5%	NS	18.8%
ER+,PR+	51.4%	58.4%		58.7%
ER-,PR+	5.7%	1.2%		3.0%
ER+,PR-	14.3%	19.9%		19.6%

NS: not significant.

Table VI. Distribution of estrogen and progesterone receptor levels (fmol/mg protein).

	Group 1 (n = 68 cases)	Group 2 (n = 272 cases)	p value	Group 3 (n = 726 cases)
Estradiol receptors				
25th percentile	7.0	16.0	NS	19.7
median	31.5	89.5		104.0
75th percentile	207.5	266.0		286.2
mean	127.25	179.45		186.0
SD	29.8	20.7		9.2
Max. value	649	2 425		2 425
ER>100	33.3%	46.4%	NS	50.5%
Progesterone receptors				
25th percentile	6.25	2.75		3.0
median	20.0	26.0	NS	27.0
75th percentile	66.5	119.5		129.7
mean	48.43	97.47		121.4
SD	13.7	13.6		8.8
Max. value	444	1 120		1 429
PR>100	14.3%	27.9%	NS	29.5%

NS: not significant.
ER and PR cut-off: RLBA = 10 fmol/mg protein; EIA = 15 fmol/mg protein.

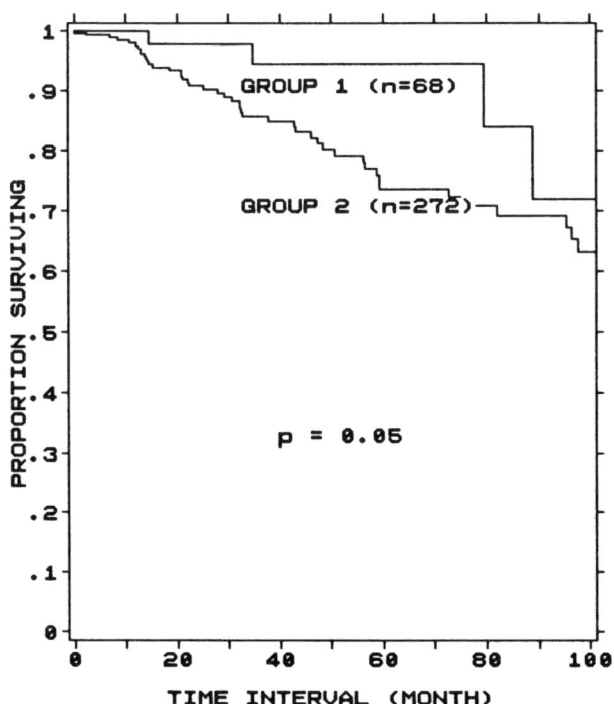

Figure 1. Kaplan-Meyer estimates of the probability of metastasis-free survival in patients who developed breast cancer during hormone replacement therapy (group 1) and controls (group 2).

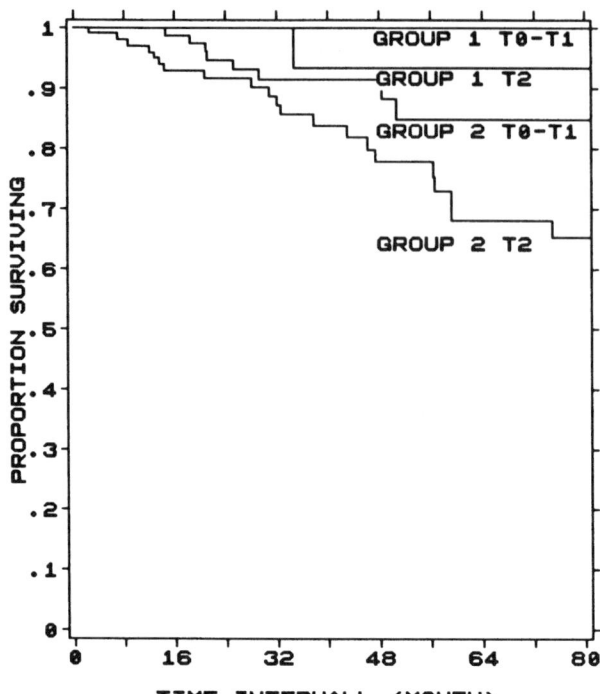

Figure 2. Kaplan-Meyer estimates of the probability of metastasis-free survival according to stage in patients who developed breast cancer during hormone replacement therapy (group1) and controls (group 2).
Group 1 T0-T1: 28 cases. Group 1 T2: 34 cases. Group 2 T0-T1: 116 cases. Group 2 T2: 109 cases. p = 0,05 between stage T2 patients in groups 1 and 2; no significant difference between stage T0-T1 patients in groups 1 and 2.

of disease. Estrogens are known to enhance the growth rate of breast cancer [20-24]. Hormone therapy has been used as an adjuvant or palliative treatment [25]. The relationship between steroïd receptor status, the degree of differentiation and the activity of carcinomas [26, 27] as well as the correlation between receptor levels and outcome of disease [28-31] have been described previously.

In this study we compared two groups of postmenopausal breast cancer patients. One group had undergone hormone replacement therapy for menopause and the other group had not undergone such treatment. The two groups were matched with regard to age and date of onset of cancer therapy. The purpose of this study was to detect any differences in clinical or biological prognostic factors.

Few studies [32, 33] have reported clinical, histological and biological factors in patients who develop breast cancer during hormone replacement therapy. Skimpy data comes from cohort studies and case-control studies [1-5, 34-38] designed to evaluate the risk of breast cancer associated with hormone replacement therapy. These studies do not give clinical and histological prognostic factors concerning breast cancer occurring during hormone replacement therapy. In addition they do not allow analysis in function of stage and age.

Current evidence seems to indicate a better prognosis in patients who develop breast cancer during hormone replacement therapy. Two possible explanations can be proposed. The first is that since these patients are kept under regular surveillance, diagnosis is achieved earlier [3, 32, 33, 37, 39]. In our study X-ray detection was not more frequent in patients undergoing hormone replacement therapy. The delay between the first symptom and histological confirmation of cancer was slightly but not significantly shorter in group 1. Analysis of the distribution of clinical tumor size and TNM stage showed that there were fewer large tumors (greater than 40 mm) and stage T3 and T4 tumors in group1. Unexpectedly the number of unpalpable and small tumors (T0-T1) was higher in group 2. Although it was not significant, this difference could be related to a well-organized program of mass screening with mammography in our region [40]. Thus regular clinical surveillance may reduce the number of large tumors, as well as the incidence of extensive lymph node involvement (3 or more nodes). Similar results regarding tumor distribution and lymph node involvement have been reported by Strickland *et al.* [33].

The second possible explanation for the better prognosis in hormone treated patients is a higher incidence of differentiated cancers. Lobular cancers and histoprognostic grade 1 cancers were more frequent in patients undergoing hormone replacement therapy than in their counterparts that had not been undergone hormone therapy (21.5% *versus* 16.2% and 30.9% *versus* 19.4% respectively).

To evaluate the relationship between hormone replacement therapy and differentiated tumors, we studied estrogen and progesterone receptor levels. Unexpectedly tumors with no receptors were more frequent in patients that underwent hormone therapy. This finding which contrasts with the greater degree of differentiation could be related to the fact that the estrogen and progesterone receptor levels in treated patients are closer to those observed in premenopausal women [26, 27]. Differences in receptor distribution according to menopause status was confirmed in a recent EORTC study including 48,000 tumors (R. Leake, 1993, personal communication). The lower steroid receptor status could not have been due to a technical biais since both the measurement techniques used in our study (enzyme immunoassay and radioligand exchange assay) detect both free and bound receptors. The most likely explanation would be that natural processes triggered by receptor binding reduces intracellular receptor levels. In this regard, hormone receptivity in premenopausal women is known to be correlated with circulating steroid hormone levels [41]. In agreement with this explanation, hormone receptor status in tumors detected in patients undergoing hormone replacement therapy documents responsivenes to exogenous hormones. This interaction which is more frequent with lobular and grade1 cancer is directly proportional to the degree of tissue differentiation. A similar interaction has already been described with regard to the greater differentiation and better prognosis of endometrial cancer occurring during hormone therapy [6-8]. It remains unclear as to whether this is due to promotion or selection of hormone sensitive tumoral clones. It should be noted that Strickland *et al.* [33] reported that, while there was no difference with regard to estrogen receptor levels, the number of patients with progesterone receptors was significantly higher after hormone replacement therapy.

In our study the probability of metastasis-free survival tended to be better in hormone-treated patients. Strickland *et al.* [33] reported a significantly higher survival rate in patients that developed breast cancer during hormone replacement therapy, but this difference disappeared for tumors of the same stage. It has been suggested that the differences observed are correlated with differences in clinical stage and tumor size. Bergvist *et al* [32] reported relatively longer survival in patients undergoing hormone replacement therapy but his control group was not matched with the treated group and menopausal status was not taken into account for stratification. Without clinical and laboratory data, stage cannot be taken into account for stratification. Nevertheless Bergwist [32] suggested that female sex hormone has a favorable effect on the natural course of breast tumors by prolonging the premetastatic phase. Further study will be necessary to understand the interaction between malignant tissue and exogenous steroids.

The most clinically important finding of this study is that hormone replacement therapy is not an unfavorable factor for breast cancer. This finding supports the safety of widespread use of hormone replacement therapy.

Acknowledgements

We are grateful to Professor C. Charpin, Dr. C. Lejeune, and Dr. N. Tubiana for their expert advice and to Andy Corsini for his linguistic assistance.

References

1. Brinton LA, Hoover RN, Fraumeni JF. Menopausal estrogens and breast cancer risk: an expand case-control study. *Br J Cancer* 1986; 54: 825-32.
2. Buring JE, Hennekens CH, Lipnick RJ *et al*. A prospective cohort study of postmenopausal hormone use and risk of breast cancer in US women. *Am J epidem* 1987; 125: 939-47.
3. Bergwist L, Adami HO, Personn I, Hoover R, Schairer C. The risk of breast cancer after estrogen and estrogen-progestin replacement. *N Eng J Med* 1989; 321: 293-7.
4. Dupont W, Page D. Menopausal estrogen replacement therapy and breast cancer. *Arch Intern Med* 1991; 151: 67-72.
5. Steinberk KK, Thacker SB, Smith SJ, *et al*. A meta-analysis of the effect of estrogen replacement therapy on the risk of breast cancer. *JAMA* 1991; 265: 1985-90.
6. Henderson BE. The cancer question: an overview of recent epidemiologic and retrospective data. *Am J Obstet Gynecol* 1989; 161: 1859-64.
7. Persson I. The risk of endometrial and breast cancer after estrogen treatment. A review of epidemiological studies. *Acta Obstet Gynecol Scand* (Suppl) 1985; 66: 59-66.
8. Persson I, Adami HO, Bergwist L, Lindgren A, Pettersson B, Hoover R, Schairer C. Risk of endometrial cancer after treatment with progestogens: results of a prospective study. *Br Med J* 1989; 298: 147-51.
9. Spyratos F, Martin PM, Hacene K, Romain S, *et al*. Multiparametric prognostic evaluation of biological factors in primary breast cancer. *J Natl Cancer Inst* 1992; 84: 1266-72.
10. Breast Cancer Cooperative group. Standards for the assessment of hormone receptors in human breast cancer. *Europ J Cancer* 1973; 9: 379-81.
11. Breast Cancer Cooperative group. Revision of the standards for the assessment of hormone receptors in human breast cancer. *Eur J Cancer* 1980; 16: 1513-5.
12. Koenders A, Thorpe SM on behalf of the EORTC Receptor group. Standardisation of steroid receptor assays in human breast cancer. I Reproducibility of oestradiol and progesterone receptor assays. *Eur J Cancer Clin Oncol* 1983; 19: 1221-9.
13. Thorpe SM on behalf of the EORTC Receptor group. Standardisation of steroid receptor assays in human breast cancer. II Samples with low recptor content. *Eur J Cancer Clin Oncol* 1983; 19: 1467-72.
14. Koenders A, Thorpe SM on behalf of the EORTC Receptor group. Standardisation of steroid receptor assays in human breast cancer. III Selection of reference material for intra and inter laboratory quality control. *Eur J Cancer Clin Oncol* 1986; 22: 939-44.
15. Koenders A, Thorpe SM on behalf of the EORTC Receptor group. Standardisation of steroid receptor assays in human breast cancer. IV Long term within- and between- laboratory vatiation of oestrogen and progesterone receptor assays. *Eur J Cancer Clin Oncol* 1986; 22: 945-52.
16. Blankenstein MA, Benraad TJ. Multilaboratory assessment of tissue prognostic factors in breast cancer: the EORTC Receptor Study Group experience. *Canadian J Oncol* (Suppl) 1992; 3: 58-64.
17. Kaplan EL, Meier P. Non-parametric estimation from incomplete observation. *J Am Stat Assoc* 1971; 53: 457-81.
18. Peto R, Peto J. Asymptomatically efficient rank invariant test procedures. *J R Stat Soc A* 1972; 135: 185-98.
19. Arriagada R, Rutquist LE, Kramar A, Johanson H. Competing risks determining event-free survival in early breast cancer. *Br J Cancer* 1992; 66: 951-7.
20. Harris JR, Lippman ME, Veronesi U, Willet W. Breast cancer. *N Eng J Med* 1992; 5: 319-28 Part I; 6: 390-8 Part II; 7: 473-82 Part III.
21. Moolgavkar SH. Hormones and multistage carcinogenesis. *Cancer Surveys* 1986; 5, 3: 635-48.

22. Macmahon B, Cole P, Brown J. Etiology of human breast cancer: a review. *J Natl Cancer Inst* 1973; 50: 21-42.
23. Waard F. Premenopausal and postmenopausal breast cancer: one disease or two? *J Natl Cancer Inst* 1979; 63: 549-52.
24. Key TJA, Pike MC. The role of oestrogens and progestagens in the epidemiology and prevention of breast cancer. *Eur J Clin Oncol* 1988; 24: 29-43.
25. Senn HJ, Goldhirsh A, Gelber RD, Osterwalder B. Adjuvant therapy of primary breast cancer. Berlin Heidelberg: Springer-Verlag, 1989.
26. Martin PM, Rolland P, Jacquemier J, Rolland AM, Toga M. Multiple steroid receptors in human breast cancer. Estrogen and progesterone receptors in 672 primary tumors. *Cancer Chemother Pharmacol* 1979; 2: 107-13.
27. Martin PM, Rolland P, Jacquemier J, Rolland AM, Toga M. Multiple steroid receptors in human breast cancer. Relationships between steroïd receptors and the state of differentiation and the activity of carcinomas throughout the pathologic features. *Cancer Chemother Pharmacol* 1979; 2: 115-20.
28. Thorpe SM. Estrogen and progesterone receptor determinations in breast cancer. Technology, biology and clinical signifiance. *Acta Oncologica* 1988; 27: 1-19.
29. Rose C, Thorpe SM, Andersen KW *et al*. On behalf of the Danish Breast Cancer Cooperative Group. Beneficial effect of adjuvant tamoxifen therapy in primary breast cancer patients with high oestrogen receptor values. *Lancet* 1985; 1: 16-20.
30. Black R, Prescott R, Bers K, Hawkins A, Stewart H, Forrest P. Tumour cellularity, oestrogen receptors and prognosis in breast cancer. *Clin Oncol* 1983; 9: 971-7.
31. Thorpe SM, Christensen IJ, Rasmussen BB, Rose C. Short recurrence-free survival associated with high oestrogen receptor levels in the natural history of postmenopausal, primary breast cancer. *Eur J Cancer* 1993, 29: 971-7.
32. Bergvist L, Adami HO, Persson I, Bergstrom R, Krusemo UB. Prognosis after breast cancer diagnosis in women exposed to estrogen and estrogen-progestogen replacement therapy. *Am J Epidemiol* 1989; 130: 221-8.
33. Strickland DM, Con Gambrell R, Butzin CA, Stickland K. The relationship between breast cancer survival and prior postmenopausal estrogen use. *Obstet Gynecol* 1992; 80: 400-4.
34. Brinton LA. The relationship of exogenous estrogens to cancer risk. *Cancer Det Prev* 1984; 7: 159.
35. Henderson BE, Paganini-Hill A, Rass RK. Decreased mortality in users of estrogen replacement therapy. *Arch Intern Med* 1991; 151: 75-8.
36. Hunt K, Vessey M, McPherson K. Mortality in a cohort of long term users of hormone replacement therapy, an update analysis. *Br J Obstet Gynecol* 1990; 97: 1080-6.
37. Gambrell JR. Role of hormones in the etiology and prevention of endometrial and breast cancer. *Acta Obstet Gynecol Scand* Suppl 1982; 106: 37-46.
38. Burch JC, Byrd BF, Vaugh WK. The effect of long term estrogen to hysterectomised women. *Am J Obstet Gynecol* 1974; 118: 778-82.
39. Tabar L, Fagerber CJG, Gad A, *et al*. Reduction in mortality from breast cancer after mass screening with mammography. *Lancet* 1985; 1: 829-32.
40. Enel P, Seradour B, Dubuc M, Manuel C *et al*. Evaluation de la mammographie de dépistage du cancer du sein dans la campagne des Bouches-du-Rhône. *Santé Publique* 1993; 2: 54-61.
41. Saez S, Martin PM, Chouvet C. Estradiol and progesterone receptor levels in human breast adenocarcinoma in relation to plasma estrogen and progesterone levels. *Cancer Res* 1978, 30: 3468-73.

Estrogen replacement therapy in breast cancer survivors

Philip J. DiSaia

University of California, Irvine, Clinical Cancer Center, 101 The City Drive, Orange, CA 92668

The author is currently following a group of 110 breast cancer survivors who have elected HRT for themselves. All of these patients were thoroughly counseled regarding the theoretical hazards and the well-substantiated benefits. Patients were not excluded because of positive node status or positive estrogen receptor status. Every patient understood that HRT would not prevent a recurrence of their malignant disease. The patients also understood that this author is convinced that currently, there is no solid clinical evidence that such therapy will adversely affect the outcome of their malignant disease. To date, there have been seven recurrences of breast cancer (6%) among this group of 110 patients. A preliminary analysis of the first 77 patients was reported in a letter to the editor in Lancet, 1993 [1]. What follows is a more detailed analysis of that group of 77 patients who have had the longest follow-up.

The median age at diagnosis in the group was 50 years (range 26-88). A large majority of the patients were between 40 and 60 *(Table I)* years of age. Interestingly, seven of the patients previously had a second primary gynecological cancer, (4 endometrial, 2 ovary, and 1 cervix). Fifty-six percent of the patients were Stage I, and 22 percent of the patients were Stage II *(Table II)*. Eighteen percent of the patients had positive lymph nodes at the time of initial therapy, and 62 percent had a histological diagnosis of ductal carcinoma.

Table I. Demographics for estrogen users and their controls [2].

Variable	Estrogen users n = 90	Controls n = 180
Age at diagnosis (yr)	47(24 - 71)	48(27 - 96)
Max. tumor diameter (cm)	1.8(0.40 - 7.0)	1.5(0.20 - 10.0)
Nodes involved	0(0-18)	0(0-18)
Tamoxifen usage	12(13%)	39(22%)
ER measured	22(24%)	42(23%)
Total follow-up (yr)	7(0.3-30)	6(0.3-29)
Deaths	0	11(6%)

Table II. Characteristics of 77 patients who received HRT after breast cancer therapy [1].

	Total patients	Recurrence (%)	Alive NED
Stage			
0	6		6
I	43	4 (9)	41
II	17	3 (18)	14
III	5		4
Unknown	6		6
Receptor status			
ER+/PR+	20	2 (10)	18
ER+/PR-	8	2 (25)	7
ER-/PR+	3	1 (33)	2
ER-/PR-	9		9
Unknown	37	2 (5.4)	35
Histology			
Ductal	48	9 (19)	42
Non-ductal	29	1 (3)	29
Lymph node status			
Negative	58	5 (9)	55
Positive	13	2 (15)	10
Unknown	6		6

* NED = no evidence of disease; ER = estrogen receptor; PR = progesterone receptor; + = positive; - = negative.

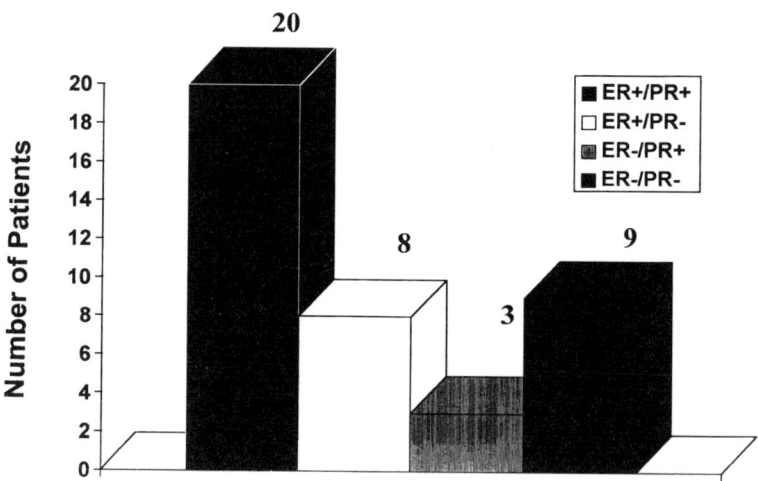

Figure 1. Oestrogen receptor status.

Receptor status was known on only 40 of the patients *(Figure 1)*. Receptor status was not a consideration in prescribing HRT. In fact, out of the 40 patients whose receptor status was known, 28 patients (70%) were estrogen receptive positive. Nearly 50 percent of the patients were individuals who became menopausal during or shortly following adjuvant chemotherapy. An additional 28 patients (36%) had been on postmenopausal HRT at the time of the diagnosis of breast cancer. Interestingly, 25 of the 28 patients, who were users of HRT at the time of diagnosis, had negative nodes. This may represent a clinical bias since patients on HRT may be monitored more carefully *(Figure 2)*.

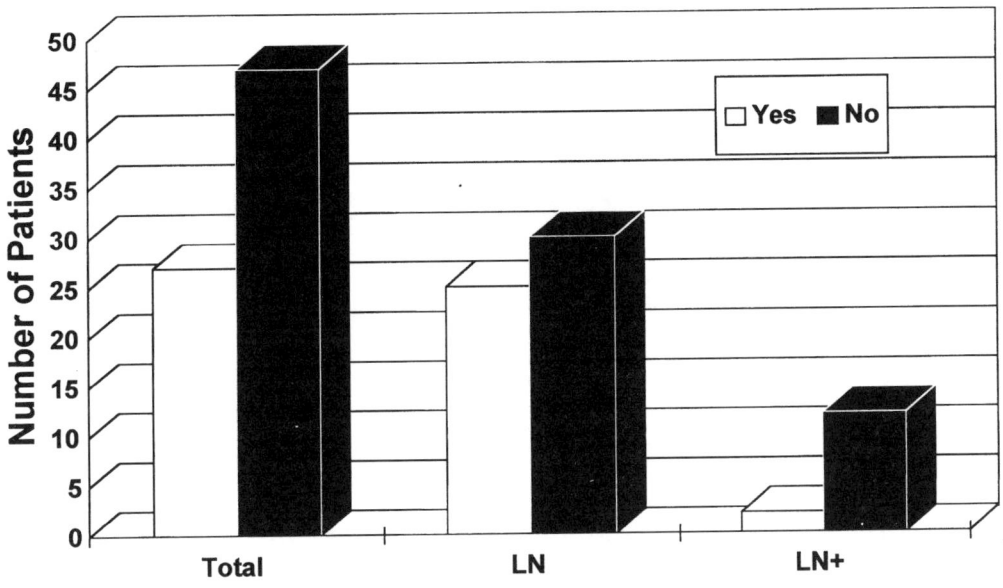

Figure 2. Lymph node status.

The median interval between diagnosis and the start of HRT was 24 months, with 37 (48%) of the patients starting within 24 months *(Figure 3)*. All but 13 of the patients received a combination of estrogen plus progestin. Most of the patients received HRT as conjugated estrogen with three of the patients using estradiol patches. Some 30 patients (39%) were on concomitant tamoxifen therapy during some interval of HRT. Tamoxifen was considered a chemotherapeutic agent and was continued as long as desired by the patient and her oncologist. Those patients on HRT and tamoxifen did not differ clinically from patients on HRT alone; hot flushes and vaginal dryness disappeared and the patients appeared optimally estrogenized. The median follow-up from diagnosis was 59 months, and the median disease-free survival was 53 months.

Seven women had a breast cancer recurrence after starting HRT (average interval from diagnosis to relapse was 45.3 months). Of these seven patients, five were still taking HRT at the time of recurrence, whereas two had stopped HRT before recurrence was diagnosed. Four of the five patients, who were still on HRT at the time of recurrence, stopped HRT at the time of the diagnosis of recurrence; one is alive with no evidence of disease; two are alive with disease, and one died of disease. The fifth patient continued treatment with HRT despite having relapsed; she is alive with no evidence of disease. Eighteen months have elapsed since the initial report, and there have been no further recurrences, nor have there been any recurrences in the 33 additional patients accrued to this study since the initial report.

Of the initial 77 patients started on HRT, 72 (92%) have no evidence of disease. Two patients (3%) are alive with disease; three have died, one of complications from chemotherapy (at autopsy she was free of demonstrable disease), and two of progressive disease. Among the

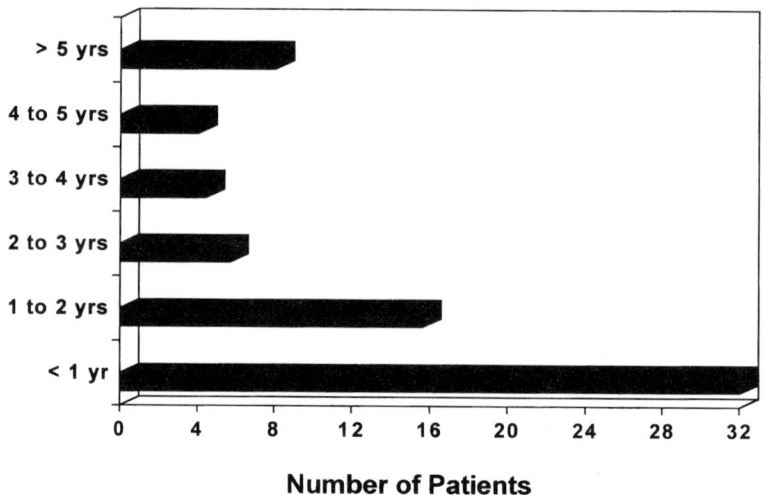

Figure 3. Interval from diagnosis to onset of HRT.

70 patients with no evidence of recurrence, only three have stopped taking HRT. The interval between the onset of HRT and recurrence was carefully examined. Two patients recurred 8 and 10 months after initiation of HRT; the other 5 patients recurred at 27, 36, 36, 60 and 80 months.

Eden [2] reported a case control study of combined continuous HRT among women with a personal history of breast cancer. His objective was to examine the effect on general mortality and tumor recurrence rate of combined continuous HRT given to symptomatic menopausal women with a personal history of breast cancer. He performed a case-controlled study in a cohort of women with a personal history of breast cancer. The entire database comprised 901 women with surgically confirmed breast cancer attending one of three teaching hospitals in south-eastern Sidney, Australia. Ninety had taken estrogen for relief of severe menopausal symptoms after their diagnosis and treatment of breast cancer. Most were using combined continuous HRT, usually an oral estrogen with a moderate dosage progestin. Controls were matched subjects from the same database who had not taken sex hormones after their diagnosis of cancer. The main outcome measures were all-cause mortality and recurrence of breast cancer (or new contralateral breast cancer). Relative risks were then calculated comparing sex-hormone users with matched controls. Among the 90 estrogen users, there were no deaths and only seven percent developed a recurrence, compared to 17% of the nonusers (using two matched controls; RR = 0.40). These results suggest that short-term usage of combined continuous HRT by women with a personal history of breast cancer may be safe and might even reduce the risk of recurrence. They also concluded that a formal prospective double-blind study is needed to confirm their results.

References

1. DiSaia PJ, Odicino F, Grosen EA, Cowan B, Pecorelli S, Wile A, Creasman WD. Hormone replacement therapy in breast cancer [Letter]. *Lancet* 1993; 342: 1232.
2. Eden JA, Bush T, Nand S, Wren EG. A case-control study of combined continuous estrogen-progestin replacement therapy among women with a personal history of breast cancer. *Menopause* 1995; 2: 67-72.

Breast cancer in young women: the University of Pennsylvania experience

Lawrence J. Solin[1], Jonathan Haas[1] and Delray J. Schultz[2]

[1]Department of radiation oncology, University of Pennsylvania, School of Medicine, Philadelphia, PA, USA;
[2]Department of Mathematics, Millersville University, Millersville, PA, and the University of Pennsylvania Cancer Center, Philadelphia, PA, USA

The outcome after treatment of breast cancer in younger women has been reported in a number of studies. In general, most studies have reported that younger age is associated with an increased risk of local recurrence after breast-conserving surgery plus definitive breast irradiation in comparison to older patients. However, the magnitude of increased risk of local recurrence after breast-conservation treatment has been somewhat variable. This lack of consistency may be related to differences in definitions of young age, which have ranged from ≤ 30 years to ≤ 40 years. A prior report from the University of Pennsylvania has demonstrated a higher rate of local recurrence after breast-conserving surgery plus definitive breast irradiation; the local recurrence at 8 years was 24% for women age ≤ 35, compared to 14% for age 36-50 and 12% for age ≥ 51 ($p = .001$) [2].

The impact of younger age on survival after breast-conservation treatment is less well established. While some series have shown a decreased survival for younger women, other studies have not shown any adverse effect on age relative to outcome. A prior report from the University of Pennsylvania has demonstrated a decreased 8 year survival for younger women age ≤ 35 compared to older women [2].

These results suggest that there are major differences in the patterns of local and systemic recurrence based on age of the patient at presentation. The present study reports updated results based on patient age from the University of Pennsylvania.

Methods and materials

From 1977 to 1992, 1,021 women of all ages underwent breast-conservation treatment for early-stage breast cancer at the hospital of the University of Pennsylvania. All women presented with American Joint Committee on Cancer (AJCC) clinical stages I-II breast cancer [1].
Surgical treatment consisted of a complete gross excision of the primary tumor plus an axillary lymph node dissection. Re-excisional biopsy was performed in 53% of the patients. Radio-

therapy was delivered to breast tangential fields to a dose of 45-50 Gy, using 1.8-2.0 Gy fractions, followed by an iridium implant or electron boost to a total dose of $\leq$ 60 Gy. Whole breast irradiation was delivered using 6 MV photons for most patients, although patients with larger separations were treated with 10 or 15 MV photons. Supraclavicular irradiation was delivered to 27% of the patients, generally for positive axillary lymph nodes. Chemotherapy was delivered to 30% of the patients. The chemotherapy was usually CMF (cyclophosphamide, methotrexate, and 5-fluorouracil), although adriamycin-based chemotherapy was used later in the study. Tamoxifen was given to 25% of the patients, mainly for hormone receptor positive tumors.

Patients were divided for analysis by age into three groups: (1) age $\leq$ 40 years; (2) age 41-50 years; and (3) age $\geq$ 51 years. The number of patients in each of these three age groups was 171, 286, and 564, respectively. Actuarial curves were determined using the Kaplan-Meier method [3], and comparisons between curves were performed using the Mantel-Cox test [4]. Median follow up after treatment was 6.1 years (mean = 6.5 years; range = 0-16.1 years).

Results

Patient and tumor characteristics are shown in *Table I*. There was no difference among the three age groups for pathologic nodal status. However, women age $\leq$ 40 years had an increased number of T2 lesions. Tumors in younger women were more commonly estrogen receptor negative, but there was no difference for progesterone receptor status.

Actuarial 10-year outcome is shown in *Table II* for the three age groups. There was a higher 10-year rate of deaths from breast cancer for women age $\leq$ 40 years in comparison to the older age groups (p = .007). As expected, deaths from intercurrent disease were lower in the younger age group in comparison to the older women (p = .08). The 10-year local failure was higher for women age $\leq$ 40 years (22%) compared to women age 41-50 (18%), and age $\geq$ 51 years (12%), although this difference was of borderline statistical significance (p = .10). The impact of family history of breast cancer relative to outcome for younger women was analyzed to assess the potential interaction of family history of breast cancer and young age *(Table III)*. These results show that family history was not significantly related to outcome for younger women (all p $\geq$ .16).

Discussion

The present study has confirmed the results of breast-conservation treatment in younger breast cancer patients, and extended these results to assess the impact of family history on outcome. Consistent with previous studies, the 10-year rate of local failure rate was higher in younger women age $\leq$ 40 years (22% at 10 years) in comparison to older age groups. The present study has shown a significantly increased risk of deaths from breast cancer in younger women age $\leq$ 40, although there was a lower rate of deaths from intercurrent disease. Thus, the overall survival rate in breast cancer as a function of age is an interaction of the two competing risks of deaths from cancer and non-cancer causes. The direction of these competing risks of death for younger patients are in opposite directions (*i.e.*, higher for deaths from breast cancer,

Table I. Patient and tumor characteristics.

	Age			
	≤ 40	41-50	≥ 51	
	No. (%)	No. (%)	No. (%)	p value
Clinical T stage				.01
T1	98 (57)	203 (71)	373 (66)	
T2	73 (43)	83 (29)	191 (34)	
Pathologic lymph node status				.22
N0	115 (67)	203 (71)	410 (73)	
N1				
1-3 positive	47 (27)	61 (21)	110 (20)	
≥ 4 positive	9 (5)	22 (8)	44 (8)	
Final pathology margin of the primary tumor excision				.30
Negative	83 (49)	147 (51)	288 (51)	
Positive	17 (10)	32 (11)	75 (13)	
Close	12 (7)	26 (10)	58 (10)	
Unknown	59 (35)	81 (28)	143 (25)	
Estrogen receptor status				< 0001
Negative	55 (32)	60 (21)	80 (14)	
Positive	72 (42)	144 (50)	334 (59)	
Not done/unknown	44 (26)	82 (29)	150 (27)	
Progesterone receptor status				.45
Negative	48 (28)	60 (21)	129 (23)	
Positive	60 (35)	120 (42)	227 (40)	
Not done/unknown	63 (37)	106 (37)	208 (37)	

Table 2. 10-year actuarial outcome.

	Age			
	≤ 40	41-50	≥ 51	p value
Survival				
Overall	74%	82%	82%	.12
NED	69%	75%	77%	.19
Relapse-free	53%	70%	70%	.007
Deaths				
From breast cancer	25%	16%	14%	.007
From intercurrent disease	1%	2%	4%	.08
Local failure	22%	18%	12%	.10

NED = No evidence of disease.

Table III. 8-year actuarial outcome for women age ≤ 40 years relative to family history of breast cancer.

	Family History		p value
	Positive	Negative	
Survival			
Overall	79%	77%	.68
NED	81%	71%	.36
Relapse-free	67%	61%	.27
Deaths			
From breast cancer	21%	22%	.79
From intercurrent disease	0%	2%	.45
Local failure	13%	19%	.16

but lower for deaths from intercurrent disease), which may account for the lack of survival difference for younger patients in some series.

The results of the present study have been further analyzed to assess the impact of family history of breast cancer in younger women. There is no impact of family history on outcome. These results suggest that positive family history in younger women does not represent a contraindication to breast-conservation treatment.

In summary, younger women with early stage breast cancer can be adequately treated with breast-conservation treatment, although with a higher risk of local and systemic recurrence. Neither young age alone nor young age plus a positive family history should preclude the use of breast-conservation treatment for appropriately selected patients.

References

1. American Joint Committee on Cancer. Manual for staging of cancer. Fourth edition. Philadelphia, PA. JB Lippincott Co 1992; 149-54.
2. Fowble BL, Schultz DJ, Overmoyer B, *et al.* The influence of young age on outcome in early stage breast cancer. *Int J Radiat Oncol Biol Phys* 1994; 30: 23-33.
3. Kaplan EL, Meier P. Nonparametric estimation from incomplete observations. *J Am Stat Assoc* 1958; 53: 457-81.
4. Mantel N. Evaluation of survival data and two new rank order statistics arising in its consideration. *Cancer Chem Rep* 1966; 50: 163-70.

Author index

Acres B., 303, 315
Allemand H., 77
Ancelle-Park R.A., 77
Anderson E., 225
Apostolopoulos V., 315
Awada A., 257
Azzli N., 273

Baert J.L., 115
Balloul J.M., 303
Barnabas N., 33
Basset P., 111
Baum M., 235
Bellocq J.P., 111
Bender H.G., 289
Bishop W.R., 159
Bissery M.C., 265
Bizouarne N., 303
Boer M., 281
Bole-Feysot C., 131
Bonnier P., 335
Borg-Olivier O., 273
Bougnoux Ph., 59
Box G., 147
Boyd N.F., 45
Brouillet J.P., 183
Brünner N., 201
Burchell J., 309
Byrne J., 111

Carr D.M., 159
Carter P., 139
Catino J.J., 159
Chajes V., 59
Charlier C., 97
Chenard M.P., 111
Chotteau A., 115
Clark G.M., 217
Cognault S., 59
Colin C., 329
Coombes R.C., 289
Cottu P., 245
Coutte L., 245
Cuvier C., 245

de Valeriola D., 257
Dean C., 147

Defossez P.A., 115
Delecroix V., 273
Denoo X., 329
Derocq D., 183
Desreux J., 329
Di Leo A., 257
DiSaia P.J., 347
Dive V., 111
Doll R.J., 159

Eccles S., 147
Espie M., 245
Extra J.M., 245

Ferrag F., 131
Fety R., 273
Foekens J.A.F., 201, 209
Foidart J.M., 329
Fournier S., 329
Frouge C., 93
Fumoleau P., 273

Gampietro Gasparini M.D., 167
Garcia M., 183
Garusi C., 105
Gazet J.C., 289
Germain E., 59
Giacalone P.L., 335
Goffin V., 131
Gomm J., 289
Gore M., 147
Graeff H., 191
Graham R., 309
Greenberg C., 45
Grey K., 159

Haas J., 351
Heukamp L., 309
Higgy N., 33
Hikish T., 147
Hilkens J., 281
Höfler H., 191
Holmberg L., 23
Holst-Hansen C., 201
Hortobagyi G.N., 251
Howell A., 225

Hoyer-Hansen G., 201
Hwang L., 315

Ip C., 53

Jackson E., 147
James L.J., 159
Jänicke F., 191

Kannan R., 111
Karanikas V., 315
Kelly P.A., 131
Kiaris H., 27
Kieny M.P., 303
Kirschmeier P.T., 159
Klijn J.G.M., 209
Koffa M., 27
Kruger K.H., 289

Laffargue F., 335
Laget M.P., 115
Launoit Y. de, 115
Laurent V., 183
Lavelle F., 265
Leenders F., 115
Lees A.W., 81
Lees C., 315
Lerman C., 11
Lhuillery C., 59
Liaudet E., 183
Lignières B. de, 329
Lockwood G., 45
Look M.P., 209
Louboutin J.P., 273
Luqmani Y., 289
Lynch H., 11
Lynge E., 67

Maas M.C.E., 281
Maaskant R., 131
Magdolen V., 191
Malavaud B., 175
Martin L., 45
Martin P.M., 335
Marty M., 245
Maugard C., 273
McKenzie I.F.C., 315
Meijer-van Gelder M.E., 209

Miles D., 309
Miller W.R., 123
Modjtahedi H., 147
Monte D., 115
Moon R.C., 19
Mullen P., 123

Njoroje F.G., 159
Noël A., 111

Okada A., 111
Ong C.S., 315
Ortega N., 175
Osinski C., 315

Patnick J., 73
Pedersen A.N., 201
Pelczar H., 115
Perkins L.M., 159
Perrocheau G., 273
Peterse J., 281
Petit J.Y., 105
Piana L., 335
Piccart M.J., 257
Pietersz G.A., 315
Platet N., 183
Plouet J., 175
Popovski V., 313
Potier P., 279
Pujol H., 97
Pyke C., 201

Reuning U., 191
Rietjens M., 105
Rio M.C., 111
Riva A., 273
Rochefort H., 183
Romain S., 335
Rouanet P., 97
Rougeot C., 183
Russo I.H., 33
Russo J., 33

Sacks N., 289
Salicioni A.M., 33
Schaffer P., 77
Schatz C., 303
Schipper H., 235
Schmitt M., 191
Schoenfeld A., 289
Schultz D.J., 351
Seradour B., 77
Shattuck-Eidens D., 3
Shearer M., 309
Sinnet H.D., 289
Skolnick R.M., 3
Smith I., 147
Smith M., 309
Solin L.J., 351
Sordello S., 175
Sourvinos G., 27
Spandidos D.A., 27

Stanford J.L., 321
Stephens R.W., 201
Stoll I., 111
Storm J., 281

Taylor-Papadimitriou J., 309
Thomssen C., 191
Thynne G., 315
Tritchler D.L., 45
Turley E.A., 235

Ulm K., 191

Van der Valk S.W., 281
Van Putten W.L.J., 209
Vaughan H.A., 313
Veronesi P., 105
Vincent V., 131
Voigt L.F., 321
Vos H.L., 281
Vrignaud P., 265

Wait S., 87
Weimann E., 131
Weiss N.S., 321
Wesseling J., 281
Whyte D., 159
Wilhelm O., 191
Wu Y.L., 33

Xing P.X., 315

Zhang F., 159

Subject index

The numbers indicate the first page of the chapter concerned

α linolenic acid, 59
Adhesion, 281
Adipose tissue, 59, 123
Adjuvant chemotherapy, 217
Adjuvant endocrine therapy, 217
Adjuvant treatment, 257
Advanced breast cancer, 257, 273
Advanced breast cancer treatment, 251
Angiogenesis, 167, 175
Angiostatin, 167
Anti-p185^{HER2}, 139
Antiangiogenic treatment, 175
Antioestrogens, 225
Aromatase, 123
Autologous reconstruction, 105

bcl 2, 217
Biological prognostic factors, 209, 217
Bispecific antibodies, 139
BRCA1, 3
BRCA2, 3
Breast cancer survivors, 321, 347
Breast cancer susceptibility, 11
Breast cancer susceptibility gene, 3
Breast reconstruction, 105

c-myc, 27
Cancer prevention, 53
Cathepsin D, 183
Cathepsins, 191
Cellular immunity, 303
Cellular transformation, 115
Chemotherapy, 97, 235, 245
Circulating cells, 289
Circumvention of antioestrogen resistance, 225
CNAMTS, 77
Combination chemotherapy, 245
Combination therapy, 251, 257, 265, 273
Conjugated linoleic, 53
Conservative treatment, 351
Cost, 87
Cyclophosphamide, 245
Cytokines, 123, 131
Cytotoxicity, 281

Dendritic cells, 309
Diagnosis, 73, 81
Diet, 45, 53
Dietary intake, 59
Differentiation, 235
DMBA, 19
Docetaxel, 257, 265, 273, 279
Dose densification, 245
Dose intensification, 245
Dose intensity, 235, 251, 257
Drug targeting, 159
Ductal carcinoma, 97

Early detection, 93
EGF receptors, 147
Endocrine therapy, 225
Endogenous hormones, 45
Epidemiology, 67
Epirubicin, 245
Estrogen receptor, 335
Estrogen replacement therapy, 321
Ets, 115
Exogenous hormones, 335
Experimental carcinogenesis, 19
Experimental chemoprevention, 19
Experimental models, 19
Experimental paradigms, 19, 23
Experimental therapy, 265
Extracellular growth factors, 183

Factor integration, 217
Familial breast cancer, 11
Familial screening, 3
Farnesyl transferase inhibitors, 159
Fat, 53
FGF, 175
Fibrous reaction, 93

Gelatinase A, 111
Genetic alterations, 27, 33
Genetic testing, 11
Geographical distribution, 81
Growth factors, 123, 167

H-ras, 27, 33, 159
HER2/neu, 139
Histopathology, 335
Hormone replacement therapy, 235, 335, 347
Hospital, 81
Host response, 235
Human experiments, 23

ICI164384, 225
Immortalization, 33
Immunogens, 309
Immunohistochemistry, 289
Immunotherapy, 139, 147, 303, 315
Implant, 105
In vitro model, 33
Interleukin 2, 303
Invasion, 115, 167, 191

K19, 289

LAK, 281
Lipoperoxides, 59
Lobular carcinoma, 77
Local recurrence, 351

357

Macrophages, 201
Magnetic resonance imaging, 93
Mammary tumors, 53
Mammography, 67, 93
Management of risk factors, 11
Mannan, 315
Mechanism of action, 131
Menopause, 45
Meta-analysis, 321
Metalloprotease inhibitors, 111
Metalloproteases, 111, 191
Metastasis, 167, 191, 281, 351
Microcalcification, 93
Microinvasive carcinoma, 97
Micrometastases, 289
Microsatellite instability, 27, 33
Microvessel, 167
Minimal breast cancer (MBC), 93, 97, 105
MNU, 19
Mouse models, 309
Mouse tumours, 315
MT-MM P 1, 111
MUC 1, 281, 303, 309, 315
Mucines, 303
Multiparameter analysis, 209
Mutations, 3
Myelosuppression, 245

n-3 polyunsaturated fatty acid, 59
Natural compounds, 279
Navelbine, 273, 279
Non-small cell lung cancer, 251

Oestradiol, 329
Oestrogen, 123
Oncogene activation, 27

Ovarian cancer susceptibility gene, 3
p53, 33
PA2-1, 191
Paracriny, 123
Participation rate, 77
PCNA, 329
PEA3, 115
Percutaneous administration, 329
Phagocytosis, 183
Phase II study, 273
Phase II trials, 257
Plasma uPA receptor, 201
Plastic surgery, 105
Policy, 87
Population screening, 81
Postmenopausal breast cancer, 321, 335
Predictive factors, 217
Prevention, 77
Prodrug, 139
Progesterone, 329
Progesterone and estrogen replacement therapy (PERT), 321
Progesterone receptors, 335
Prognostic markers, 183
Progression, 123, 167
Prolactin receptors, 131
Proliferation, 329
Prospective study, 59
Psychological aspects, 11

Quality of life, 11

Ras dependent cascade, 115
Receptor isoforms, 131
Relapse, 321
Relative hazard rate, 209
Resistance, 225
Review, 321
Risk factor, 3, 19, 23, 45, 67
Risk reduction, 67
RT-PCR, 289

Sanitary organisation, 81
Screening, 67, 87, 97
Sequential chemotherapy, 245
Signal transduction, 159
Silicon prothesis, 105
Sonography, 93
Statistical models, 209
Steroid metabolism, 123
Stromal cells, 111
Stromal-epithelial interactions, 281
Stromelysin-3, 111
Surgery, 97
Survival, 321

T cell, 281
Tamoxifen, 225
Targeting, 139, 147
Taxanes, 257, 273
Taxol, 279
Taxotere, 273
Transcription activation, 131
Transcription factors, 115
Transformation, 33
Tubulin, 265
Tumor cell kill, 235
Tumor evolution, 27
Tumor growth and metastasis, 183
Tumor progression, 115
Tumor rejection, 303
Tumor suppression genes, 27
Tyrosine kinase inhibitors, 147
Tyrosine kinases, 131
Tyrosine phosphatases, 131

United Kingdom, 81
uPA, 191, 201
Urokinase, 191

Vaccinia, 303
VEGF, 175
Vinca alcaloides, 251, 279
Vinorelbine, 251, 265, 273

Contents

Foreword IX

1. Predisposition to breast cancer, Carcinogenesis Early breast cancer screening and management 1

Breast and ovarian cancer susceptibility: implications for presymptomatic testing and screening
M. Skolnick and D. Shattuck-Eidens 3

Psychological aspects of familial breast cancer
H. Lynch and C. Lerman 11

Experimental breast cancer studies: paradigms for human breast cancer
R.C. Moon 19

Human breast cancer risk factors: development of experimental paradigms
L. Holmberg 23

Oncogenes and onco-suppressor genes in the prevention and therapy of breast cancer
D.A. Spandidos, M. Koffa, G. Sourvinos and H. Kiaris 27

Molecular basis of human breast epithelial cell transformation
J. Russo, N. Barnabas, N. Higgy, A.M. Salicioni, Y.L. Wu and I.H. Russo 33

Diet and endogenous hormones as risk factors for cancer of the breast: intervention studies
N.F. Boyd, L. Martin, G. Lockwood, C. Greenberg, D.L. Tritchler 45

Multiple mechanisms of conjugated linoleic acid in mammary cancer prevention
C. Ip 53

n-3 polyunsaturated fatty acids and breast cancer
C. Lhuillery, S. Cognault, E. Germain, V. Chajes and Ph. Bougnoux ... 59

Breast cancer screening. The scientific basis and the Danish programme
E. Lynge 67

Breast cancer screening. The relations with the hospitals and sanitary organisations in the United Kingdom
J. Patnick 73

The French national breast cancer screening programme
R.A. Ancelle-Park, B. Seradour, P. Schaffer and H. Allemand 77

Breast cancer screening in Canada
A.W. Lees 81

The cost-effectiveness of breast cancer screening in France: from research to policy
S. Wait 87

Minimal breast cancer: diagnosis, strategy and decisional trees
C. Frouge 93

Is there now a consensus on the treatment of minimal breast cancer?
P. Rouanet, C. Charlier and H. Pujol 97

Minimal breast cancer: place of the plastic surgery
J.Y. Petit, M. Rietjens, C. Garusi and P. Veronesi 105

2. Tumor biology. Prognostic factors 109

Molecular and clinical aspects of metalloproteases in breast cancer
P. Basset, A. Okada, R. Kannan, J. Byrne, I. Stoll, A. Noël, V. Dive, M.P. Chenard,
J.P. Bellocq and M.C. Rio 111

Characterization of the PEA3 group of ets-related transcription factors: role in breast cancer
Y. de Launoit, J.L. Baert, A. Chotteau, D. Monte, P.A. Defossez, L. Coutte, H. Pelczar,
M.P. Laget and F.Leenders 115

Steroid metabolism in normal and malignant breast tissue compartments
W.R. Miller and P. Mullen 123

Signal transduction of prolactin and cytokine receptors
V. Goffin, C. Bole-Feysot, F. Ferrag, R. Maaskant, V. Vincent, E. Weimann
and P.A. Kelly 131

Targeting the product of the HER2/*neu* protooncogene for therapy
P. Carter... 139

Targeting of EGF receptors: approaches and clinical results
C. Dean, H. Modjtahedi, S. Eccles, E. Jackson, G. Box, T. Hikish, I. Smith
and M. Gore 147

Pharmacological targeting of signal transduction processes
P.T. Kirschmeier, J.J. Catino, R.J. Doll, F.G. Njoroje, D.M. Carr, L.J.James, K. Grey,
L.M. Perkins, D. Whyte, F. Zhang and W.R. Bishop 159

The role of angiogenesis in tumour progression of breast cancer
M.D. Giampietro Gasparini.. 167

VEGF and breast cancer
J. Plouet, S. Sordello, B. Malavaud and N. Ortega 175

Why is cathepsin D involved in breast cancer? A 1996 overview
H. Rochefort, V. Laurent, E. Liaudet, N. Platet, D. Derocq, C. Rougeot, J.P. Brouillet
and M. Garcia 183

Clinical significance of the serine protease uPA (urokinase) and its inhibitor PAI-1 as well as the cysteine proteases cathepsin B and L in breast cancer
M. Schmitt, C. Thomssen, F. Jänicke, H. Höfler, K. Ulm, V. Magdolen, U. Reuning,
O. Wilhelm and H. Graeff 191

Urokinase plasminogen activator receptor in breast cancer
N. Brünner, C. Holst-Hansen, A.N. Pedersen, C. Pyke, G. Hoyer-Hansen, J. Foekens
and R.W. Stephens 201

Mutiparameter analysis of prognostic factors in breast cancer
W.L.J. van Putten, J.G.M. Klijn, M.E. Meijer-van Gelder, M.P. Look and J.A. Foekens 209

Interpretation of data in prognostic studies
G.M. Clark 217

3. Therapy 223

Clinical circumvention of antioestrogen resistance
A. Howell and E. Anderson 225

Breast cancer: should we control rather than kill tumor cells?
H. Schipper, M. Baum and E.A. Turley 235

High dose sequential chemotherapy in poor prognosis breast cancer patients
J.M. Extra, C. Cuvier, M. Espie, P. Cottu and M. Marty 245

Summary of clinical results of vinorelbine (Navelbine®) in the treatment of breast cancer
G.N. Hortobagyi 251

Docetaxel in the treatment of breast cancer: current status, ongoing trials and future directions
M.J. Piccart, A. Di Leo, A. Awada and D. de Valeriola 257

In vivo evaluation of docetaxel (Taxotere®) and vinorelbine (Navelbine®) as single agents and in combination in mammary tumor models
M.C. Bissery, P. Vrignaud and F. Lavelle 265

Clinical data of Navelbine-Taxotere association in breast cancer patients
P. Fumoleau, V. Delecroix, G. Perrocheau, O. Borg-Olivier, C. Maugard, R. Fety, N. Azzli, J.P. Louboutin and A. Riva 273

A short history of drug discovery
P. Potier 279

The expression levels of episialin in human carcinomas are sufficiently high to potentially interfere with adhesion and promote metastasis
J. Hilkens, H.L. Vos, J. Wesseling, J. Peterse, J. Storm, M. Boer, S.W. van der Valk and M.C.E. Maas 281

The detection of micrometastases in the lymph nodes, peripheral blood and bone marrow of patients with breast cancer using immunohistochemistry and the polymerase chain reaction
A. Schoenfeld, K.H. Kruger, J. Gomm, H.D. Sinnett, J.C. Gazet, N. Sacks, H.G. Bender, Y. Luqmani and R.C. Coombes 289

Immunotherapy of breast cancer using a recombinant Vaccinia virus expressing the human *MUC1* and *IL2* genes
N. Bizouarne, J.M. Balloul, C. Schatz, B. Acres and M.P. Kieny 303

The *MUC1* gene as an immunogen: use of naked DNA and role of dendritic cells
J. Burchell, R. Graham, M. Shearer, M. Smith, L. Heukamp, D. Miles and J. Taylor-Papadimitriou 309

Tumour immunotherapy against MUC1 expressing tumours using mannan MUC1
V. Apostolopoulos, G.A. Pietersz, B. Acres, C. Osinski, G. Thynne, P.X. Xing,
V. Karanikas, H.A. Vaughan, L. Hwang, V. Popovski, C. Lees, C.S. Ong
and I.F.C. McKenzie 315

Review of the epidemiologic data on hormone replacement therapy in relation to the risk of breast cancer
L.F. Voigt, N.S. Weiss and J.L. Stanford 321

Influence of percutaneous administration of estradiol and progesterone on the proliferation of human breast epithelial cells
J.M. Foidart, C. Colin, X. Denoo, J. Desreux, S. Fournier and B. de Lignières 329

Clinical and biological prognostic factors in breast cancer diagnosed during postmenopausal hormone replacement therapy
P. Bonnier, S. Romain, P.L. Giacalone, F. Laffargue, P.M. Martin and L. Piana 335

Estrogen replacement therapy in breast cancer survivors
P.J. DiSaia 347

Breast cancer in young women: the University of Pennsylvania experience
L.J. Solin, J. Haas, D.J. Schultz 351

Author index 355

Subject index 357